Obesity
A Clinical Review

"The difference between the right word and the almost right word is the difference between lightning and a lightning bug". Mark Twain

Mark W DelBello MD FACP CDE

Published by Mark W DelBello, M.D.

ISBN: 9781545586181

Printed in the United States of America.

Table of Contents

Preface

My initial preface was boring and talked about studying to pass the obesity boards. A good preface grabs the reader's attention and makes him turn to the next page. As a doctor, we are taught to show respect, provide accurate information and "do no harm". "Mrs. And Mr. American waste valuable dollars and invaluable time in the pursuit of slimness through get-thin-quick drugs and dreams. The physician has to doff the robes of medicine and don the flannels of Madison Avenue. He has to be a counter-salesman, battling all the sources of misleading misinformation with convincing, correct, information. He has to prove to his patient that "reducing" foods do not reduce, that there are no "fattening" foods or "slimming" foods, just too much food." (Alexander & Stare, 1967)

My book talks about the dangers and treatment of having extra weight that can lead to medical issues and shorten one's lifespan. **More than 60 diseases and 12 cancers are associated with obesity.**

Dr Edward Mason "the Father of Gastric Bypass Surgery" said in 1977 **"Obesity is a disease that can be fatal. Why the insurance companies will charge extra or not even give insurance to people that are grossly obese and then turn around and refuse to pay for an operation that treats that condition is beyond me. This is not cosmetic surgery. This is a disease. It is potentially lethal.**

Obesity is complicated with many different concepts and treatments. Weight loss is hard. Mark Twain wrote **"A little starvation can really do more for the average sick man than can the best medicines and the best doctors. I do not mean a restricted diet; I mean total abstention from food for one or two days".** Mark Twain also said **"Be careful about reading health books. You may die of a misprint"**

1

Something that is not hard to understand are vaccines. Unlike obesity or diabetes, they are not complicated and don't require 400 pages of research. They are not controversial. They save lives. Vaccines are one of the great success stories in medicine. This simple one paragraph hopefully will save lives. If you do not believe in vaccines, please do not buy this book. Anti-vaccine propaganda is a cancer that needs to be permanently terminated. I am glad I changed my preface.

Introduction

Sometimes the highlight of my day is eating a chocolate muffin and 2 skim milks for breakfast. I love to eat like many others. As I age, I am not going to have the luxury of eating whatever I want and maintain a healthy weight. A healthy weight varies among people and is best defined as a weight which does not promote diseases. **Excess adipose tissue (obesity) has been shown to be deleterious for multiple body organ systems through thrombogenic, atherogenic, oncogenic, hemodynamic and neurohumoral mechanisms and has been linked to multiple medical conditions, such as diabetes, heart disease and several types of cancer. In fact, obesity has been recently labeled as the number one killer worldwide replacing smoking in this matter** (Romero-Corral, et al., 2008). That is a serious paragraph and I have used some fancy intimidating words already within the first 200 words of the book. The rest of the book is like talking to an old friend or listening to Morgan Freeman narrate a documentary; so let's start.

Weight is determined by many factors. Genetic factors play a large role. For example, a child has a 50% chance of being obese if one parent is obese and an 80% chance if both parents are obese (Blackburn Course in Obesity Medicine, 2014). Studies show a similar risk of obesity in identical twins raised in separate environments compared with those raised in the same household. Adoptees have been shown to mirror the BMIs of their biological parents rather than their adoptive parents (Wardle, Carnell, Haworth, & Plomin, 2008). Although multiple genetic markers have been identified, the 32 most common genetic variants associated with obesity are responsible for less than 1.5% of the overall interindividual variation in BMI (Speliotes, et al., 2010). People are judged by their weight every day; the "skinny nervous kid", the "fat truckdriver". No one blames one for being short or tall, but people feel and act differently when it comes to a person's weight. Height is mostly genetic, but weight is due to genetics and environment. Lifestyle modification is the term used to treat obesity. Unfortunately, this approach has failed for several decades despite different dietary and multidisciplinary ideas. (Dansinger, Tatsioni, Wong, Chung, & Balk, 2007) (Leblanc, O'Connor, Whitlock, Patnode, & Kapka, 2011). Several medicines have been tried to help lose weight. Many weight loss medicines have been removed from the market due to complications resulting in a field of study with "medical baggage." Convincing anyone to look past prior misconceptions and half-truths is a dauting task, whether in medicine or any field. Sir Winston Churchill stated, "kites rise highest against the wind, not with it." Questioning ideas and principles promotes innovation and discoveries. Doing the same thing and expecting different results is what Albert Einstein described as "insanity". It's easy to convince people that sugar causes tooth decay, but much harder to convince them that it also causes decay in multiple organs due to diabetes and obesity. The use of anti-obesity medications helps the overall response in losing weight. Unfortunately, obesity medicines are under-utilized. (Bray, Frühbeck, Ryan, & Wilding, 2016) (Apovian, et al., 2015) (Halpern & Halpern, 2015). The public, many medical professionals and many countries believe obesity is a life choice. Most weight loss medicines approved in the United States are not approved in Europe. The FDA does an outstanding job in making sure drugs are safe to the public. Only a very small percentage of drugs are approved each year. For instance, from 2007 to 2017, the number of drugs approved ranged from 18 to 46 drugs per year. In 2018, 59 drugs were approved with 34 labeled as orphan drugs (drugs for very rare diseases). Getting a drug approved from idea to pharmacy can take approximately 12 to 18 years and often costs well over $1 billion.

Weight loss is very complicated, very hard, and potentially can help not just millions of people but billions of people. In 2014, more than 1.9 billion adults were overweight with over 600 million considered obese. More than 41 million children under 5 years old are overweight or obese (WHO, 2016). Since the numbers involved are massive, safety is of paramount importance, but the potential upside is even more promising. A survey of obesity specialists (published before the availability of fixed dose combination weight loss medicines) found that 85% prescribed combination treatments despite limited evidence of efficacy and safety (Hendricks, Rothman, & Greenway, How physician obesity specialists use, 2009). In obesity, "one size fits all" approach simply does not work (Field, Camargo, & Ogino, 2013).

A recent article published in the New England Journal of Medicine in March 2017 looked at more than 27,500 people regarding cardiovascular events using a new cholesterol lowering agent costing more than $14,000 a year. It decreased the risk of a major cardiovascular event by 15-20%. For every 200 patients treated for 2 years with the new drug, three fewer people would suffer from a major cardiovascular event. Even though long-term sustained weight loss is difficult with the majority being unsuccessful, the statistics are still better than this example. Compared with normal-weight people, obese individuals are responsible for 46% higher inpatient costs, 27% more outpatient visits, and 80% higher spending on prescription medications (Finkelstein, Trogdon, Cohen, & Dietz, 2009).

Weight loss has so-much upside regarding decreasing insulin resistance, lipids, unfavorable mechanical stress and the toxicity of adiposity/inflammation yet it is often treated in a nihilistic or unconquerable attitude. Weight loss should be an easy sell to patients since they can see the results in the mirror themselves.

A surgical policy that is present now and will be implemented more aggressively in the future are shorter hospital stays for common surgical procedures. Surgeries that would require 1-3 days hospitalizations in the past are now completely outpatient or patients are only kept overnight. Obese patients may fail this policy since they are at risk for more complications and longer length of stays. This will probably translate to more obese patients transferring from the hospital to skilled nursing facilities. A study by Regenbogen et al., accepted in JAMA March 22, 2017, **Costs and Consequences of Early Hospital Discharge After Major Inpatient Surgery in Older Adults,** looks at early postoperative discharge practices. Analysis looked at Medicare beneficiaries undergoing colectomy (189,229 patients at 1,876 hospitals), Coronary Artery Bypass Grafts (CABG) (218,940 patients at 1,056 hospitals), or total hip replacement (231,774 patients at 1,831 hospitals) between Jan 1, 2009 and June 30, 2012. A shorter length of stay protocol did not result in higher post-discharge costs, or readmission rates. Payments were statistically lower for all three surgeries ($26,482 vs $29,250 for colectomy, $44,777 vs $47,675 for CABG, and $24,553 vs $27,927 for total hip replacement. The study looked at older patients and postoperative care protocols. Obese patients are at higher risk to become outliers in many standardized protocols for early hospital discharges. (Regenbogen, et al., 2017).

A basic principle in weight loss and overall good health is lifestyle modification. This means healthier eating and routine exercise/physical activity. It promotes longevity and a better quality of life. **If someone struggles with diet and exercise over and over again, there is a 95% chance that he will continue to fail** (Blackburn Course in Obesity Medicine, 2014). About 80% will initially lose at least 10% body weight, but more than 95% will regain all of the lost weight or more within the next 2-5 years (Blackburn Course in Obesity Medicine, 2014). Only 17% of patients maintain 10% weight loss after one year and only 10-20% maintain 5% weight loss after several years (Blackburn Course in Obesity Medicine, 2014). Intensive lifestyle interventions generally result in a weight-loss of only 5-10%. **63% of obese Americans attempt weight loss each year**. These are not encouraging statistics.

Because weight loss is very difficult, adjunctive medications can be added to lifestyle modification. Obesity drugs approved for long-term use result in additional weight loss relative to placebo ranging from approximately 3-9% at 1 year. Mean total weight loss can be 1-5% greater with medicines and **some of the medications have been able to achieve weight loss of 5-20%**. An approach to weight loss medication has evolved similar to the approach with chronic illnesses. Because chronic illnesses are complicated and involve interaction with many mechanisms and organ systems, the same philosophy is developing with weight loss medications. Combination pharmacotherapy for obesity deploys medications with differing mechanisms of action offering the prospect of overcoming the counter-regulatory mechanisms which manifest in the weight-losing state. We use this strategy daily in combating diabetes, heart disease and cancers. By using several drugs, we can theoretically decrease the dose and possible side effects. With the majority of people with type 2 diabetes not achieving the desired glucose control, lipid control and blood pressure control over the last several decades, one wonders if thinking outside the polypharmacy box needs to be considered. Weight loss is without question or controversy the best treatment in most people with type 2 diabetes. **The selling point for adding medications is the higher success rate and greater potential for larger weight loss.** It is simply a tool to increase success like higher education. Going to college does not get you a job but improves your chances. It is a bridge to help short-term and long-term goals. Many people exhibit initial weight loss only to return to the same weight or even higher months later. A weight chart would look like a U-shaped curve, initial weight loss followed by rebound increase. For weight-loss success, the acquisition of a habit takes 4 weeks to install and 1-2 years to make permanent. I define weight loss success, not at 6 months, but after 2 years.

Chapter 1: Highlight Reel

"It's like déjà vu all over again" Yogi Berra

The most important ideas and concepts of the book have been highlighted below. This promotes better learning and retention.

- Excess adipose tissue (obesity) has been shown to be deleterious for multiple body organ systems through thrombogenic, atherogenic, oncogenic, hemodynamic and neurohumoral mechanisms and has been linked to multiple medical conditions, such as diabetes, heart disease and several types of cancer. In fact, obesity has been recently labeled as the number one killer worldwide replacing smoking in this matter (Romero-Corral, et al., 2008).
- A child has a 50% chance of being obese if one parent is obese and an 80% chance if both parents are obese (Blackburn Course in Obesity Medicine, 2014). Studies show a similar risk of obesity in identical twins raised in separate environments compared with those raised in the same household. Adoptees have been shown to mirror the BMIs of their biological parents.
- As Joslin (pioneer physician in diabetes) described almost a century ago, genetics probably loads the gun, while lifestyle in our obesogenic environment pulls the trigger for the spreading of the obesity epidemic.
- By 2006, only 20% of American jobs required high levels of physical activity, thus representing a huge drop from the 1960s when more than 50% of jobs required levels of physical activity that met the current daily physical activity goals

- If someone struggles with diet and exercise over and over again, there is a 95% chance that he will continue to fail (Blackburn Course in Obesity Medicine, 2014).

- A simple anecdotal observation will help understand that obesity is complicated and requires openness and objectivity in treating this newly designated disease. Most people, both doctors and non-professionals, would agree that people with grey hair have more heart disease and cancer then people without grey hair. Therefore, grey hair must cause heart disease and cancer and the best treatment for these ailments would be simply cutting grey hair. We know this is not true but sometimes we think this way towards obesity. We look for simple solutions to complicated questions. It is not just overeating and being lazy.

- Between 1975 and 2014 the global prevalence of obesity increased from 3.2% to 10.8% for men and from 6.4% to 14.9% for women. The United States and United Kingdom have among the highest rates of obesity in the world: 69% of US adults are overweight or obese and 36% are obese, and 61% of UK adults are overweight or obese. Once obesity is established, it is difficult to achieve substantial and sustained weight loss.

- 63% of obese Americans attempt weight loss each year.

- Health care costs for obese patients were on average $1,429 higher than for patients of normal weight.

- With many people with type 2 diabetes not achieving the desired glucose control, lipid control and blood pressure control recommended by multiple medical organizations, one wonders if thinking outside the polypharmacy box needs to be considered.

- The selling point for adding medications is the higher success rate and greater potential for larger weight loss. Some of the medications for chronic weight management have been able to achieve weight loss of 5-20%.

- On June 21, 2013, the American Medical Association declared obesity a disease. Despite this declaration, most states do not provide coverage for newer obesity medicines as of 2019. Among 136 marketplace health insurance plans, 11% had some coverage for the specified drugs in only nine states. Medicare policy strictly excludes drug therapy for obesity. Only seven states have Medicaid programs to provide drug coverage for obesity.

- Weight loss of 5-10% is clinically significant to reduce disease risk.

- Bariatric surgeries involving vertical sleeve gastrectomy reduce plasma ghrelin levels close to 60% over time. Ghrelin plasma concentration increases as people age, which may contribute to the tendency for people to gain weight as they get older (Cummings, et al., 2001).

- When one diets, our body thinks we are still in the stone-age and that dieting is not a voluntary act, but a threat to our survival. Our body releases counter measures to decrease our success.

- Our body does not like change and will do everything to prevent this. The physiological control of appetite regulation involves circulating hormones with orexigenic (appetite-stimulating) and anorexigenic (appetite-inhibiting) properties that induce alterations in energy intake via perceptions of hunger and satiety. Orexigenic and anorexigenic neuropeptides are constantly orchestrating are responses to food and attempts at dieting (Hazell, Islam, Townsend, Schmale, & Copeland, 2016).

- Twin studies point towards an obesity inheritance pattern of 60-70 %. Twin studies suggest that genetics at birth can predict 25% of lifespan thus showing how important our reaction to the environment is. If obesity was totally genetic, you would not have seen the epidemic in obesity develop in the last 20-30 years since genetics do not evolve that rapidly

- Many weight loss medicines work on the dopamine/norepinephrine/epinephrine neurotransmitter systems. Many psychiatric medicines work on this system also but in a different manner which helps explain why many psychiatric medicines have weight gain as a major side-effect. Body weight is regulated in the hypothalamus where it receives signals from the brain, gastrointestinal track and adipose tissue.

- Calories consumed by Americans increased 12% from 1971-74 to 1999-2002.

- Two-thirds of Americans are overweight, and more than one-third are obese. Seventeen percent of our children are obese and a higher percent overweight.
- Weight gain increases as patient's age. Despite food intake and energy expenditure (calories burned) varying less than ½ of 1%, the average person gains one pound per year making it difficult to perceive the specific cause or remedy for weight gain. A common finding is 20 pounds in twenty years with the person unable to know how it snuck up on him or her. Maintenance of weight within 20 pounds from the age of 21 to 65 years old requires matching intake and expenditure to within 0.2% variability (accuracy of 4-5 kcals per day).
- Muscle mass essentially determines resting energy expenditure (metabolism) and this declines at about 35 years old. Trained muscle consumes 9 kcals/lb./day and untrained muscle consumes 5-6 kcals/lb./day. If one eats the same amount every year and does not increase energy expenditure either through work or exercise, they will gain weight each year typically starting at 35 years old. Exercise is essential to maintain good health. Six pounds of muscle are lost per decade, metabolic rate decreases 3% per decade, and 16 pounds of fat are gained per decade.
- BMI gradually increases during most of adult life and reaches peak values at 50-59 years. After 60 years, mean body weight and BMI tend to decrease.
- The co-morbidities of obesity can be classified into two general categories, those relating to insulin resistance and cardio-metabolic disease and those relating to the mechanical or functional consequences of excess body weight.
- From a biomechanics viewpoint, 4 pounds of joint stress on our knees is decreased with every pound lost.
- The odds of sustaining musculoskeletal injuries is 15 percent higher for persons who are overweight and 48 percent higher for people who are obese, compared to persons of normal weight.
- It could be easily argued that weight loss medications should be considered for any overweight or obese patient with overt diabetes type 2 who fail to achieve moderate weight loss (10%) with lifestyle modification (Garvey, 2013). Only a minority of

patients achieve HgbA1c goals, blood pressure goals, lipid goals despite an increasing array of diabetic agents and newer types of insulin. A very common complication is the increased risk of infection with poor diabetic control.

- SSRIs (selective serotonin reuptake inhibitors) and TCAs (tricyclics) are associated with doubling the risk of type 2 diabetes in a dose-dependent manner. Antidepressant prescribing has risen nearly 400% since 1988.

- An important neurotransmitter is serotonin. It is made from the amino-acid tryptophan and a synonym is 5-hydroxytryptamine (5-HT). Serotonin is primarily found in the gastrointestinal tract, platelets, and the CNS. Approximately 90% of the body's serotonin is located in the GI tract where it regulates intestinal movement.

- The name serotonin comes from the discovery of a substance in the serum that increased muscular smooth muscle tone (serum + tone). Because serotonin regulates intestinal movement, this explains why nausea and diarrhea are common side effects and why the serotonin antagonist ondansetron (Zofran) is such an effective anti-emetic.

- Serotonin syndrome – fever, agitation, increased reflexes, tremor, sweating, dilated pupils, diarrhea. Predictable consequence of excess serotonin. Meds include selective serotonin reuptake inhibitors (SSRI), serotonin norepinephrine reuptake inhibitor (SNRI), tricyclic antidepressants (TCAs), tramadol, buspirone, ondansetron, dextromethorphan, metoclopramide, Monoamine oxidase inhibitor (MAOI), St John's wort, triptans. Treatment is discontinuing the drug. Benzodiazepines can be used for agitation and cyproheptadine (Periactin) is helpful due to being a serotonin antagonist.

- The weight change from medicines may not always be noticed since it occurs against a background of progressive weight gain in the normal population. Weight gain can also be dose related emphasizing the basic principle of always trying to use the lowest dose to achieve the desired result.

- The major issue with supplements is lack of quality control and lack of scientific evidence to support the claims. Many supplements are tainted with prescription medications and this is an illegal and dangerous practice. The three main categories of supplements prone to medical problems are those for sexual enhancement, weight loss, and sports performance/bodybuilding.

- A 10% weight reduction improves obstructive sleep apnea by 50%.
- Weight loss promotes so many positive benefits but one aspect that is probably overrated is blood pressure reduction.
- Weight loss in overweight and obese individuals to prevent elevated BP has been a nice recommendation that has been around for 50 years but has had limited successful impact (Kuller, 2009).
- The American Institute for Cancer Research reports that only half of all Americans are aware of the link between obesity and cancers. The following percentage of cancers are felt to be related to obesity; 38% breast cancer, 50% colon/rectal cancer, 69% throat cancer, 24% kidney cancers, and 19% pancreatic cancers. More than 60 diseases and 12 cancers are associated with obesity.
- Obesity disproportionately affects minorities, and people with low income and limited education. The obesity rates are 47.8% in blacks, 42.5% in Hispanics, 32.6% in whites and 10.8% in Asians. Black women suffer the highest rate at 54% with projections in 2030 of greater than 90% which is hard to believe.
- In 1998, the U.S. National Institutes of Health and the Centers for Disease Control and Prevention brought U.S. definitions in line with World Health Organization guidelines, lowering the normal/overweight cut-off from BMI 27.8 to BMI 25. This had the effect of redefining approximately 29 million Americans, previously healthy, to overweight. It is not clear where on the BMI scale the threshold for overweight and obese should be set. Because of this the standards have varied over the past few decades.
- BMI generally overestimates adiposity on those with leaner body mass (e.g., athletes) and underestimates excess adiposity on those with less lean body mass (elderly).
- Waist circumference is a good indicator of visceral fat, which poses more health risks than fat elsewhere. According to the US National Institutes of Health (NIH), waist circumference in

excess of 102 centimeters (40 in) for men and 88 centimeters (35 in) for (non-pregnant) women is considered to infer a high risk for type 2 diabetes, dyslipidemia, hypertension, and CVD. Waist circumference can be a better indicator of obesity-related disease risk than BMI.

- Increased medical risk starts at a BMI above 25 but weight loss programs suggest treatment at a BMI of 27 which corresponds to 20% above desirable weight. A BMI of 22 probably has the best medical/longevity statistics. The lowest mortality rates worldwide are those with a BMI of 20-22. The increased medical risk above a BMI of 25 goes back to 1983 Metropolitan Life Insurance data. Research shows reductions in blood pressure (probably overrated) glucose control and lipids consistently occur with 5% weight loss making 5% the traditional minimum benchmark for success.

- Multiple studies comparing diets do not show one diet to be superior than any other. Unfortunately, the usual pattern of weight loss with lifestyle intervention is maximum weight loss at 6 months, followed by plateau and gradual regain over time. 80% of patients will initially lose at least 10% weight but more than 95% of patients will regain all the lost weight or more within the next 2-5 years (Blackburn Course in Obesity Medicine, 2014).

- Only 10-17% of patients maintain 10% weight loss after one year.

- A 500-kcal deficit per day will result in a pound weight loss per week since 3,500 kcals equals one pound.

- Combining LCD (low calorie diet) with exercise produces greater weight loss, 10-15% more than LCD alone. Frequent monitoring of weight, consistent eating patterns, journaling food are very helpful.

- Obese people compared with metabolically healthy normal-weight individuals are at increased risk for adverse long-term outcomes even in the absence of metabolic abnormalities, suggesting that there is no healthy pattern of increased weight. An exception are overweight people greater than 70 years old with no chronic illnesses. The extra weight in this group is felt to be a sign of good health and they should not lose weight.

- The evidence to support the use of the major commercial and self-help weight loss programs is suboptimal (Tsai AG, 2005).
- Four popular weight loss diets include Adkins, South Beach, the Zone diet, and Weight Watchers. They produce at best only modest long-term benefits, with few differences across the four. Weight loss at 1 year is modest at 1.7-12 lbs. Longer term data out to 2 years, indicated that some of the lost weight was regained over time. Controlled trials are needed to assess the efficacy and cost-effectiveness of these interventions. The advertising claims of commercial programs are monitored by the Federal Trade Commission rather than the US Food and Drug Administration.
- Serious complications, including death, have been reported in obese persons who consumed very-low-calorie diets (800 kcals/day or less) without medical supervision. Medical supervision is critical to the safe use of very-low-calorie diets.
- A general principle used for children but applies well to adults is the 5-2-1-0 Rule. It stands for 5 vegetable servings, less than 2 hours' screen time, one-hour physical activity, and zero sugary drinks.
- Despite lack of scientific benefit, 50% of the United States population use supplements. In 1994, there were 4,000 supplements, and in 2012, more than 80,000 supplements. All weight loss supplements should be avoided since no legal ingredient in supplements has been proven to lose weight and most supplements lack quality control. Diet programs that sound too good and frequent the radio and newspaper with guarantees of quick weight loss should be avoided.
- It seems that curcumin has potential but does not have FDA approval for any disease process and therefore use is off label. It does seem to be very safe. Curcumin is just one of many compounds found in the bright yellow Indian spice Turmeric that belongs to the ginger plant family. It is the main spice used in curry.
- Diet soda using non-nutrient sweeteners promotes weight gain indirectly. Diet drinks increase the risk for diabetes type 2, metabolic syndrome and thus heart disease. They double the risk for going from normal weight to overweight and overweight to obesity. The sweet taste increases appetite

despite lack of calories. Artificial sweeteners do not give a satiety signal to the brain. The epidemic of obesity has coincided with the introduction of non-caloric sweeteners.

- People underestimate calories by 30-50%, overestimate physical activity by 50%.

- Quick-fix products and many diet plans are usually quackery and promise consumers what they want to hear: fast and effortless permanent weight loss. Unlike pharmaceuticals, diet products do not have to prove their effectiveness. For a diet to succeed it must be low in energy (low calories). Whether the diet is low fat, low carbs, high protein, high carbs has been shown in multiple studies to not be the key component. There is no necessity for carbohydrates in the human diet because metabolic pathways exist within the body to remove energy from dietary protein and fat. The human body does need fat and protein to survive. The idea of promising consumers quick fixes and promises is not new. An article April 8, 1911 in the British Medical Journal advertises the results of analyses of medicines for the reduction of obesity that stresses "My treatment allows you to eat what you like and drink what you like, without starvation diet or tiresome exercises."

- For a drug to be approved for weight loss, the FDA requires the drug be responsible for losing 5% or more body weight in at least 35% of people tested, the weight loss should be double the percentage which occurred in the placebo treated group and should last one year.

- The FDA's guidance statement to the pharmaceutical industry in 2009 mandated the demonstration of cardiovascular safety for all new glucose-lowering agents (DeFronzo, 2009).

- In 1947, the FDA approved methamphetamine (schedule 2 drug) for weight loss. In 1959 phentermine (schedule 4 drug) was approved. In 1973 with the country struggling with a long-running epidemic of amphetamine abuse (not phentermine abuse-big difference), the FDA limited the indication of all obesity drugs to short-term use (few weeks). Indiana does not restrict length of use for phentermine, but Ohio only allows use for 3 months.

- Studies up to eight years suggest long-term phentermine therapy is a safe and useful treatment for weight loss and weight maintenance. There are no published reports that orally administered phentermine has been associated with abuse or psychological dependence as defined by DSM-IV. Common side-effects include insomnia 1.1%, increased blood pressure 0.8%, nervous/shakiness 1%, palpitations 0.4% and the risk of abuse is 0.4 per 100,000. The risk of abuse with narcotics is 92.5 per 100,000 and 32.7 per 100,000 for anti-depressants. Abrupt cessation of phentermine after 90-day use or longer has resulted in no withdrawal symptoms or cravings. Intermittent usage or drug holidays is a viable and clinically effective use since the addictive potential is so low.

- There has been one case report in 2005 in Anesthesia Intensive Care where a woman had two perioperative hypertensive crises felt to be due to phentermine. Even though the half-life would indicate that phentermine is completely metabolized in a few days, the conservative recommendation based on this one case report is to hold phentermine one week before surgery (Stephens & Katz, 2005).

- Phentermine will cause a urine drug screen to be falsely positive for amphetamines with a confirmation test identifying phentermine. Phentermine is considered a performance enhancing medicine by the Olympic Committee since it is a beta-agonist and therefore not allowed in the Olympics. Beta-blockers are also not allowed but only in archery and shooting to lessen any tremor. Very common side effects are dry mouth, constipation and insomnia. No data is present in peer-reviewed medical literature to support that phentermine increases blood pressure or heart rate at a sustained elevated level. There have been no cases of valvular heart disease described with phentermine monotherapy use in over half a century (Connolly HM, 1997) (Roth, 2007) (Meltzer & Roth, 2013).

- By using the"12-week rule," we limit exposure to weight loss drugs and hopefully select out the subpopulation that has the best chance at long-term success. Most studies have shown that initial weight loss response at 12 weeks predicts later weight loss at 1 year and afterwards (Colman, et al., 2012) (Rissenen, Lean, Rossner, Segal, & Sjostrom, 2003) (Finer, Ryan, Renz, & Hewkin, 2005), Genetics plays an important factor in selecting out responders and non-responders. Based on my experience, phentermine works well. It is generic and costs about 20 dollars per month. The contraindications are unstable heart disease, untreated hyperthyroidism, unstable accelerated hypertension, drug addiction, pregnancy and unstable psychiatric illness.

- Physicians use insulin as a last resort for poor control rather than the logical next step in diabetes management. We need to emphasize insulin from the very first visit, not as a threat, but the realization that most patients with type 2 diabetes will eventually need insulin. Hopefully this will motivate them to improve diet and exercise. Many physicians exhibit inertia (a tendency to do nothing or to remain unchanged) when the time comes to starting insulin. Insulin is not the enemy; diabetes is the issue.

- Diabetic patients with no previous cardiovascular disease have the same long-term morbidity and mortality as nondiabetic patients with established cardiovascular disease. The 2000 OASIS study provided evidence for this foundation principle (Malmberg, et al., 2000).

- Secondary failure is a very important medical principle. A decline in a drug's effectiveness occurs due to disease progression. It is not a surprise that this happens because diabetes is a progressive beta-cell failure disease which will require more medicines to counteract decreasing beta-cell function.

- Despite a revolution of new diabetic medicines and new insulins over the last 2 decades, the majority of people with type 2 diabetes do not achieve the goals outlined by the American Diabetes Association, the American Association of Clinical Endocrinologists and the American College of Endocrinology. Only about 7% of patients reached these relatively modest targets for blood pressure (130/80 mmHg), LDL cholesterol (100 mg/dL), and HbA_{1c} (7%).

- Since 2005, more than 40 new medicines for the treatment of type 2 diabetes have been introduced on the market. These consist of 15 new active substances establishing three new classes of non-insulin products, and several new or modified insulin products and combinations.

- Remember the ABC's of diabetes care- A1c level, Blood pressure, Cholesterol.

- The main reason to start a statin is really to promote cholesterol plaque stability. By using this principle, one does not have to debate about whether to start a statin drug on a person with diabetes who has a very favorable lipid profile. The answer will always be yes unless statin intolerance is present.

- Insulin- works in everyone with diabetes but promotes weight gain. Insulin is the only drug that has long-term sustainability. Its effective longevity over several years of use is not debated like the majority of diabetic medicines. Insulin has the potential to achieve the desired goal in every patient.

- It is well known that too much sugar causes tooth decay, but it seems hard to convince patients that too much sugar causes the same decay in many important organs we have.

- Metformin has been associated with 39% relative risk reduction for MI and 36% reduction in all-cause mortality. Reduced the progression of diabetes by 31% over 4- year period. Metformin has also been used to prevent or ameliorate weight gain with atypical anti-psychotic agents and mood stabilizers.

- Complementary supplementation of cinnamon (500 mg TID) significantly reduced fasting insulin and insulin resistance in women with PCOS.

- Combination therapies are a promising new area in obesity treatment, similar to what occurs with diabetes and hypertension. Safety assessment is highly important due to the high number of potential users on a chronic basis.

- Resistance training with weights will not promote clinically significant weight loss but is very helpful for ADLs (activities of daily living) and helps maintain muscle mass. Statistics show 25% of individuals do no physical activity and 50% do insufficient physical activity.

- A dose-response relation appears to exist, such that people who have the highest levels of physical activity and fitness are at lowest risk of premature death. Having said that, less active men who participate in vigorous activity were more likely to have a myocardial infarction during exercise than the most active men. "You don't run before you walk."

- Bariatric surgery is the most successful tool for obesity treatment but is reserved for patients that are moderately or severely impacted by obesity and meet selection criteria. Most programs require failure from a medically supervised program for 6 months first. Indications for surgery are a BMI of 40 or greater or a BMI of 35 with co-morbidities. The FDA has approved gastric banding for a BMI of 30 with co-morbidities. Bariatric surgery has a 10-20% primary failure rate (no successful initial weight loss).

- Bariatric surgery has a mortality risk of less than 0.5%. Cohort studies show that bariatric surgery reduces all-cause mortality by 30% to 50% at seven to 15 years post-surgery compared with patients with obesity who did not have surgery. Dietary changes, such as consuming protein first at every meal, and regular physical activity are critical for patient success after bariatric surgery.

- Only one percent of medically eligible patients undergo bariatric surgery

- Bariatric surgery risk is divided into peri-operative (first 30 days) and long term. Pulmonary embolism is the most common reason for death. Peri-operative death is 1 in 500, anastomotic leak 1%, wound infection 2%, DVT/PE 2% and nausea/vomiting/dehydration about 20%. Long-term complications are peptic ulcer disease 3-5%, small bowel obstruction 1%, internal hernia 0.8%, surgical stenosis 2% and vitamin/nutrient deficiency 10-25%. Marginal ulcers occur in up to 20% of Roux-en-Y gastric bypass patients. Gallstone formation and kidney stone formation increase with any rapid weight loss. Most programs do not do prophylactic cholecystectomies.

- In general, about 60-70% of patients lose at least 50% excess weight at 10 years. Bariatric surgery is not only for adults but has been successful in adolescents. All organizations involved in bariatric surgery agree that 150 minutes per week (30 minutes 5x/week) is insufficient for prevention of weight regain after bariatric surgery. It needs to be 60-90 minutes per day.

- An uncommon statistic expressed is the five-fold increased successful suicide rate following gastric bypass surgery. This seems more realistic after realizing that 20-60% of bariatric surgery patients exhibit psychopathology. Mood disorders, anxiety disorders, and eating disorders can be aggravated with bariatric surgery. In general, about 60-70% of patients lose at least 50% excess weight at 10 years. Bariatric surgery is not only for adults but has been successful in adolescents. All organizations involved in bariatric surgery agree that 150 minutes per week (30 minutes 5x/week) is insufficient for prevention of weight regain after bariatric surgery. It needs to be 60-90 minutes per day.

- Bariatric surgery can be safe and effective for patients older than 60 years of age with a low morbidity and mortality; the weight loss and improvement in comorbidities in older patients are clinically significant.

- The Italian Society for Bariatric and Metabolic Surgery has extended the indications for bariatric surgery for morbidly obese patients up to 70 years of age.

- Outcomes and complication rates of bariatric surgery in patients older than 60 years are comparable to those in a younger population, independent of the type of procedure performed.

- Endoscopic sleeve gastroplasty (ESG), a minimally invasive same-day procedure reduces the gastric lumen to a size comparable to that of laparoscopic sleeve gastrectomy (LSG). ESG is a newer procedure.

- Weight loss after bariatric surgery did not improve self-esteem and marital satisfaction six months post operatively.

- Men who lost approximately one third of their weight after Roux-en-Y gastric bypass experienced significant increases in total testosterone and SHBG. They did not, however, report significant improvements in sexual functioning, relationship satisfaction, or mental health domains of quality of life. This pattern of results differs from that of women who have undergone bariatric surgery, who reported almost uniform improvements in sexual functioning and psychosocial status (Sarwer, et al., 2015).

- An estimated 10-30% of bariatric surgical patients regain their weight postoperatively starting as early as 18 months and as far out as 20 years.

- Phentermine and phentermine/topiramate in addition to diet and exercise appear to be viable options for weight loss in post-

Chapter 1: Highlight Reel

RYGB and LAGB patients who experience weight regain or weight loss plateau.

- A new idea with bariatric surgery is the principle that the metabolic changes that happen with surgery play a more important role than the conventional theory that bariatric surgery works by restricting oral intake (volume of stomach with sleeve is only 60-150 cc). Few patients become underweight after surgery unless a complication ensues. It would be common to expect some overshooting if the mechanism for weight loss were primarily mechanical/restrictive. The preponderance of evidence indicates that most bariatric procedures alter the physiology of energy balance and metabolic regulation, and that biological mechanisms largely account for the efficacy of these operations.

- Male hypogonadism is one of the many adverse consequences of overweight and obesity. Evidence indicates that testosterone deficiency induces increased adiposity while increased adiposity induces hypogonadism (Corona, et al., 2003).

- Early data suggest that targeted embolization of the arterial supply to the gastric fundus may provide a safe effective approach to weight loss in the obese patient. The blood supply to the stomach has adequate collateral flow to allow left gastric artery embolization. In terms of fat oxidation, we conclude that performing a low intensity aerobic exercise in a fasting [FAST] condition does not seem to offer an advantage, as compared with performing the same exercise under a feeding [FED] condition. Moreover, based on Cortisol (C) levels, we also concluded that if a primary goal is to burn fat while, simultaneously, maintaining muscle mass, performing a low intensity aerobic exercise under a fasting condition might not be the best choice.

- In some people, the reality may be to prevent more weight gain rather than weight loss. Although not as glamorous as weight loss, this could be very helpful for millions.

- There is moderate to low-quality evidence that high-dose antioxidant supplementation does not result in a clinically relevant reduction of muscle soreness after exercise of up to 6 hours or at 24, 48, 72 and 96 hours after exercise.

- This study found that low active, overweight women undertook significantly more physical activity when they had a daily 10,000 step goal using a pedometer, than when they were asked to achieve 30 minutes of walking/day. Therefore, we suggest that a public health recommendation of "10,000 steps/day", rather than the "30 min/day" could be applied to promote increased physical activity in sedentary middle-aged women.

- Fibromyalgia patients have a blunted surge response of beta-endorphins to exercise. This lower opioid tone (beta-endorphins are naturally occurring opioids) may be a key factor in the development of chronic allodynia (triggering of a pain response from stimuli which does not normally provoke pain) and the increased sensitization to peripheral stimuli seen in fibromyalgia patients.

- The human intestine contains approximately 100 trillion microorganisms comprising up to 1,000 different species of bacteria, yeasts, and parasites, weighting approximately 2 kg and carrying at least 100 times as many genes as the whole human genome. This microbiological population renews itself every 3 days and has an active biomass similar to that of a major human organ. We are the minority shareholders in our body.

- The human gastrointestinal tract harbors about 10^{14} bacterial cells, which is ten times the number of human cells in the body. Despite a high degree of interindividual variability in gut microbiota composition, there is a remarkable similarity in the basal gene metabolic activities across individuals.

- One hypothesis is obese and lean individuals have distinct different microbiota with measurable differences in their ability to extract energy from their diet and to store it in fat tissue. Microbiota alteration by using pro- and prebiotic dietary supplements is a potential nutritional target in the management of obesity and obesity-related disorders.

- There is increasing evidence that the gut microbiota plays a significant role in glucose homeostasis, the development of impaired fasting glucose, type 2 diabetes, and insulin resistance.

- There has been a long-standing understanding of the contribution of dysbiosis (abnormal changes in intestinal microbiota composition) to the pathogenesis of some diseases of altered intestinal health. The gut microbial ecosystem is arguably the largest endocrine organ in the body, capable of producing a wide range of biologically active compounds that, like hormones, may be carried in the circulation and distributed to distant sites within the host, thereby influencing different essential biological processes.

- Obesity can be considered a state of malnutrition by excess and also is a state of decreased immune function. (Obese patients have a diminished production of antibodies to vaccines, impaired wound healing from lower T and B cell proliferation.) Visceral fat is more detrimental than subcutaneous adipose tissue in triggering inflammation. Waist circumference is a measure of visceral fat and is more strongly associated with inflammatory markers than the BMI or total body fat. Waist circumference correlates better with morbidity and mortality than BMI and is a tool underappreciated (Cancello, et al., 2006).

- Two new terms are "FAT MASS DISEASE," which means healthy fat but just too much, and "ADIPOSOPATHY-SICK FAT DISEASE," which develops when fat cells enlarge and exceed the local environments ability to meet their metabolic demands. FAT MASS DISEASE turns to SICK FAT DISEASE when the balance between anti-inflammation and inflammation is disrupted towards inflammation. This imbalance of inflammatory and anti-inflammatory signals is called lipo-toxicity.

- Compared with no consumption, daily consumption of artificially sweetened beverages was associated with 2-fold higher risk of infant overweight at 1 year of age.

- Combining LCD (low calorie diet) with exercise produces greater weight loss, 10-15% more than LCD alone. Frequent monitoring of weight, consistent eating patterns, journaling food are very helpful.

- Whether the diet is low fat, low carbs, high protein, high carbs has been shown in multiple studies to not be the key component. There is no necessity for carbohydrates in the human diet because metabolic pathways exist within the body to remove energy from dietary protein and fat. The human body does need fat and protein to survive.

Obesity: A Clinical Review

- The idea of promising consumers quick fixes and promises is not new. An article April 8, 1911 in the British Medical Journal advertises the results of analyses of medicines for the reduction of obesity that stresses "My treatment allows you to eat what you like and drink what you like, without starvation diet or tiresome exercises."

- A dangerous practice is the "hCG diet." The human chorionic gonadotropin or "hCG diet" is such a diet, which after half a century still has no evidence to support its efficacy: in fact, all scientific publications subsequent to the original article counter these claims." (Butler & Cole, 2016)

- Don't focus on cutting out carbohydrates and/or fats... research points to the fact that calories are key

- Medications for obesity treatment must be considered for long-term use when evaluating their safety and efficacy. A lesson from the withdrawal of previous anti-obesity drugs is that serious adverse effects may become apparent only when a drug is used in larger populations or for longer periods of time than in preapproved trials. The Endocrine and Metabolic Drug Advisory Committee has recommended to the FDA that all new medications reviewed for an obesity indication undergo premarket testing to ensure they do not increase cardiac events.

- Phentermine has a half- life of 4-19 hours and is excreted by the kidney. It releases norepinephrine granules in the lateral hypothalamus with stimulation of beta-2 adrenergic receptors. Most doctors have used it for long-term weight loss for years and it is by far the most popular and successful medicine for this for decades. From 2008-2011, 25.3 million scripts were written for an estimated 6.2 million people (Hampp, Kang, & Borders-Hemphill, 2019) In Europe, weight loss medicines don't exist due to the belief that obesity is more a lifestyle than a disease. Phentermine, Belviq, Qysmia and Contrave are not approved in Europe.

- Studies up to eight years suggest long-term phentermine therapy is a safe and useful treatment for weight loss and weight maintenance. There are no published reports that orally administered phentermine has been associated with abuse or psychological dependence as defined by DSM-IV.

Intermittent usage or drug holidays is a viable and clinically effective use since the addictive potential is so low.

- Greater weight loss without increased risk of incident CVD or death was observed in patients using phentermine monotherapy for longer than 3 months.

- The doses ranged from 18.75 to 112.5 mg/day. This study provides evidence of the long duration and high dose of phentermine that some patients have received without trouble.

- There has been one case report in 2005 in Anesthesia Intensive Care where a woman had two perioperative hypertensive crises felt to be due to phentermine. Even though the half-life would indicate that phentermine is completely metabolized in a few days, the conservative recommendation based on this one case report is to hold phentermine one week before surgery.

- Because of the half-life of phentermine, we recommend discontinuing phentermine for at least 4 days prior to surgery.

- Phentermine will cause a urine drug screen to be false positive for amphetamine with a confirmation test identifying phentermine. Amphetamines are 10-fold as potent as phentermine in maintaining self-administration behavior in baboons, and phentermine has been demonstrated to decrease self-administration behavior in baboons (Hendricks & Greenway, 2011). Baboons were chosen over politicians in these studies due to less innate erratic behavior.

- Phentermine is considered a performance enhancing medicine by the Olympic Committee since it is a beta-agonist and therefore not allowed in the Olympics. Beta-blockers are also not allowed but only in archery and shooting to lessen any tremor.

- Very common side effects are dry mouth, constipation and insomnia. No data is present in peer-reviewed medical literature to support that phentermine increases blood pressure or heart rate at a sustained elevated level.

- The most obvious effect was appetite and hunger suppression. The second effect was more subtle and variously described as improved or stronger control of eating, diminution or absence of food cravings or improved ability to follow their eating plan.

- There have been no cases of valvular heart disease described with phentermine monotherapy use in over half a century (Connolly HM, 1997) (Roth, 2007) (Meltzer & Roth, 2013).
- Simply stated phentermine does not cause pulmonary hypertension. We will catch a whole bunch of people with pulmonary hypertension by thinking of obstructive sleep apnea (Rich, Rubin, Walker, Schneeweiss, & Abenhaim, 2000).
- One of the most difficult issues with improving management of diabetes is called clinical inertia. Clinical inertia is defined as lack of treatment intensification in a patient without good clinical reason. Recent work suggests that clinical inertia related to the management of diabetes, hypertension, and lipid disorders may contribute to up to 80% of heart attacks and strokes. The median time from initiation of basal insulin to treatment intensification was 4.3 years. Using a threshold HbA1c equal to or greater than 8.0% showed a median time to intensification of 3.2 years.
- A rough but accurate estimate is a 5-lb. weight gain for every 1% decrease in HgbA1c level. This is a very important clinical concept. For example, most diabetic medicines will decrease HgbA1c by about a point except for insulin. If I have a person with a HgbA1c level of 10% I know that it will take several medicines to bring his sugars under control. I can start him on insulin and he will gain a lot of weight, or I can try metformin and an SGLT-2 agent while working on diet and exercise.
- 1500 rule-tool used to assess how much one unit of insulin will decrease a person's sugar. For example, a person takes 50 units of insulin per day. 1500 divided by 50 equals 30. One unit of insulin will decrease the person's sugar by 30 mg/dl.
- Despite a revolution of new diabetic medicines and new insulins over the last 2 decades, the majority of people with type 2 diabetes do not achieve the goals outlined by the American Diabetes Association, the American Association of Clinical Endocrinologists and the American College of Endocrinology.
- Elevated HbA1c $\geq 8.6\%$ caused a four-fold increase in CABG mortality. Postoperative complications such as renal failure (RF), cerebrovascular accident (CVA), and DSWI (deep sternal wound infection) occurred more frequently at HbA1c $\geq 8.6\%$.

Chapter 1: Highlight Reel

- "RULE OF 6"-each doubling of the statin dose produces an average additional decrease in LDL of about 5-6%. I typically do not see this when I increase from 40 mg to 80 mg atorvastatin.

- Oral hypoglycemic agents and warfarin account for nearly half of adverse drug events leading to the emergent hospitalization of elderly (Budnitz & Richards, 2011).

- Metformin has been associated with 39% relative risk reduction for MI and 36% reduction in all-cause mortality. Reduced the progression of diabetes by 31% over 4- year period. Metformin has also been used to prevent or ameliorate weight gain with atypical anti-psychotic agents and mood stabilizers (Hasnain, Vieweg, & Fredrickson, 2010).

- One million to three million islets of Langerhans (pancreatic islets) form the endocrine part of the pancreas, which is primarily an exocrine gland. The endocrine portion accounts for only 2% of the total mass of the pancreas. Within the islets of Langerhans, beta cells constitute 65–80% of all the cells.

- Beta cells in the islets of Langerhans release insulin in two phases. The first phase consists of a brief spike lasting 10 minutes followed by the second phase, which reaches a plateau at 2-3 hours. It is widely thought that diminution of first-phase insulin release is the earliest detectable defect of beta-cell function in individuals destined to develop type 2 diabetes and that this defect largely represents beta-cell exhaustion after years of compensation for antecedent insulin resistance (Gerich, 2002). Even during digestion, in general, one or two hours following a meal, insulin release from the pancreas is not continuous, but oscillates with a period of 3–6 minutes, changing from generating a blood insulin concentration more than about 800 pmol/l to less than 100 pmol/l. This oscillation avoids downregulation of insulin receptors in target cells, and to assist the liver in extracting insulin from the blood (Hellman, Gylfe, Grapengiesser, Dansk, & Salehi, 2007). This oscillation is important to consider when administering insulin-stimulating medication, since it is the oscillating blood concentration of insulin release, which should, ideally, be achieved, not a constant high concentration.

Obesity: A Clinical Review

- The body's blood sugar range is carefully controlled in a healthy individual, which will usually measure 80 mg/dl in the blood. So, how much actual sugar (or glucose) is in the body? This amounts to 4 grams of sugar (16 kcals) in the blood, which is less than a teaspoon of sugar! The American Diabetes Association draws the line between a healthy individual and someone being pre-diabetic at 100 mg/dl. This 100 mg/dl is about 1 teaspoon. For someone to be diagnosed as diabetic, her fasting blood sugar is over 126 mg/dl. or about 1 ¼ teaspoons. The difference between being healthy and being diagnosed as diabetic is a quarter of a teaspoon of sugar. If one eats something with 400 kcals and 50% are carbohydrates (200 kcals or 50 grams of glucose), then your body is exposing itself to greater than 10x the amount of sugar in your bloodstream at that time.

- Insulin is the only drug that has long-term sustainability. Its effective longevity over several years of use is not debated like the majority of diabetic medicines.

- North America accounts for 7% of diabetes in the world and pays 52% of the cost of insulin in the world.

- The secretion of insulin and glucagon into the blood in response to the blood glucose concentration is the primary mechanism responsible for keeping the glucose levels in the extracellular fluids within very narrow limits at rest, after meals, and during exercise and starvation (Koeslag, Saunders, & Terblanche, 2003).

- Metformin is effective in reducing body weight of simple obesity patients, and metformin does not induce hypoglycemia as a side effect. Homer Simpson stated "Donuts, what can't they do"! My quote is "Metformin, what can't it do"!

- The apparent reductions in all-cause mortality and diseases of ageing associated with metformin use suggest that metformin could be extending life and health spans by acting as a geroprotective agent.

- Combination therapies are a promising new area in obesity treatment, similar to what occurs with diabetes and hypertension. Safety assessment is highly important due to the high number of potential users on a chronic basis (Halpern & Mancini, 2017).

Chapter 1: Highlight Reel

- With most adults spending at least half of their life working, the workplace is an important setting for promoting mental health and well-being change. 10,000 step challenges may significantly and meaningfully improve mental health and well-being through simple and inexpensive work-based interventions (Hallam, Bilsborough, & de Courten, 2018).

- A public health recommendation of "10,000 steps/day", rather than the "30 min/day" could be applied to promote increased physical activity in sedentary middle-aged women (Pal, Cheng, & Ho, 2011).

- Preliminary evidence suggests that a goal of 10000 steps/day may not be sustainable for some groups, including older adults and those living with chronic diseases. Another concern about using 10000 steps/day as a universal step goal is that it is probably too low for children, an important target population in the war against obesity.

- The ability to walk ≥100 steps/minute (equal to 3 mph which is normal walking speed) predicts a reduction in mortality among a sample of community-dwelling older adults (Brown, Harhay, & Harhay, 2014).

- It seems that curcumin has potential but does not have FDA approval for any disease process and therefore use is off label. It does seem to be very safe. Curcumin is just one of many compounds found in the bright yellow Indian spice Turmeric that belongs to the ginger plant family. It is the main spice used in curry.

- Whey proteins appear to be the most extensively researched for pre/post resistance exercise supplementation, possibly because of their higher EAA (essential amino acid) and leucine content, solubility, and optimal digestion kinetics. These characteristics yield a high concentration of amino acids in the blood (aminoacidemia) that facilitates greater activation of muscle protein synthesis and net muscle protein increase, in direct comparison to other protein choices. The addition of creatine to whey protein supplementation appears to further augment these adaptations.

- Pooled results of multiple studies using meta-analytic and other systematic approaches consistently indicate that protein supplementation (15 to 25 g over 4 to 21 weeks) exerts a positive impact on performance.

- Resistance training with weights will not promote clinically significant weight loss but is very helpful for ADLs (activities of daily living) and helps maintain muscle mass. Statistics show 25% of individuals do no physical activity and 50% do insufficient physical activity.

- Exercise is so effective that it should be considered as a drug. As with any drug, dosing is very important. More attention needs be paid to the dosing and to individual variations between patients. The philosopher Plato (427-347BC) said "Lack of activity destroys the good condition of every human being while movement and methodical physical exercise saves and preserves it." (Vina, Sanchis-Gomar, Martinez-Bello, & Gomez-Cabrera, 2012)

- A dose-response relation appears to exist, such that people who have the highest levels of physical activity and fitness are at lowest risk of premature death (Warburton, Nicol, & Bredin, 2006). Having said that, less active men who participate in vigorous activity were more likely to have a myocardial infarction during exercise than the most active men (Thompson, et al., 2007). "You don't run before you walk."

- The number of orthopedic surgical treatments requiring hospitalization dramatically increase after the age of 50 years. While physical interventions are effective in people with mild to moderate disability, their utility is limited in people with severe disability, emphasizing the importance of early detection of the locomotive syndrome and early intervention. (Nakamura & Ogata, 2016). If you wait too long, games over.

- 90-day surgical complications increased with every BMI category. For mortality and periprosthetic fractures there was a higher risk only for patients with BMI ≥40.

- BMI increases the risk of revision rates in a liner trend. Therefore, the authors believe that patients with a BMI >40 kg/m² should be sent to obesity medicine physicians in order to decrease body weight prior to elective surgery (Jeschke, et al., 2018).

- Patients with a BMI > 40 kg/m carried a threefold higher risk for total joint infections and for these patients, the risks of surgery must be carefully weighed against its benefits (Shohat, Fleischman, Tarabichi, Tan, & Parvizi, 2018).

- Being obese but "physically fit" helps but does not protect one from the increase in mortality with obesity compared to non-obese people. This provides evidence against "fat but fit."

- The obesity paradox is the concept that obesity may be protective and associated with greater survival in certain groups of people. A person that can maintain excess weight under the increased stressed environment of obesity may have a survival advantage over someone of normal weight but the key point to me is the survival advantage is short-term and not long-term. Essentially, the person is running a race all the time and passing a stress test daily.

- Data suggest that age and vigorous exercise interact with each other in affecting men's adiposity and are consistent with the proposition that vigorous physical activity must increase with age to prevent middle-age weight gain

- The anti-depressant bupropion works by increasing dopamine and norepinephrine neurotransmission which energizes a person to help with depression. Bupropion (SNRI) has been shown to induce significant weight loss via selective inhibition of dopamine. The anti-platelet drugs ticlopidine (Ticlid) and clopidrogel (Plavix) can increase bupropion levels.

- In representative surveys in the USA, overweight and obese individuals were consistently more likely to report subjectively perceived discrimination in the work place. A common judgmental bias is the halo effect. The halo effect refers to the phenomenon that a single person's outstanding characteristic influences the total judgment of that person. Body weight is an early perceptible personal characteristic and can serve as an outstanding attribute for a halo effect. As obesity often is associated with laziness and low self-discipline, it is well conceivable that this primary impression and judgment serves as the basis of a halo effect and extends to other characteristics to be evaluated, such as work-related abilities and qualities.

- Eating disorders, such as binge eating disorder (BED), bulimia nervosa (BN) and anorexia nervosa (AN), are often stigmatized as a lifestyle choice and their pathologies are frequently trivialized.

- The prevalence is 0.6% for anorexia nervosa (AN), 1.0% for bulimia nervosa (BN), and 2.8% for binge-eating disorder (BED). Women are more at risk and midlife women have an estimated lifetime prevalence of 15.3% for an eating disorder.
- Lisdexamfetamine dimesylate (Vyvanse) is the first medication with United States Food and Drug Administration approval for the treatment of Binge-Eating Disorder (BED).
- In clinical trials, lisdexamfetamine dimesylate (Vyvanse) demonstrated statistical and clinical superiority over placebo in reducing binge eating days per week at doses of 50 and 70 mg daily. Commonly reported side effects include dry mouth, insomnia, weight loss, and headache, and its use should be avoided in patients with known structural cardiac abnormalities, cardiomyopathy, serious heart arrhythmia or coronary artery disease. As with all CNS stimulants, risk of abuse needs to be assessed prior to prescribing. The Drug Enforcement Agency (DEA) has classified lisdexamfetamine dimesylate as a Schedule II controlled medication
- Data suggest that at the 50 mg dose, lisdexamfetamine has low abuse potential.
- Fluoxetine (Prozac) was FDA approved for the treatment of major depressive disorder in 1987 and is also approved for obsessive compulsive disorder and acute treatment of panic disorder with or without agoraphobia. Fluoxetine was approved for acute treatment and maintenance of Bulimia Nervosa (BN) in 1994.
- The effectiveness of fluoxetine to treat BN has been determined by several randomized placebo-controlled studies.
- Use of an intragastric balloon (IGB), has a long history of early enthusiasm and late disappointment, successes and failures.
- ORBERA (intragastric balloon-IGB), was FDA approved in the summer of 2015.
- Many published results have revealed an average of between 55.6% and 32.1% loss of excess body weight at 6 months after treatment, or around 25% at 1 year.
- It is also recommended that the balloon be left in place within the stomach for a maximum of 6 months while the patient is

enrolled in a medically supervised weight loss program and receives proton pump inhibitors (PPIs).

- Balloon insertion should be carefully considered in cases of a large hiatus hernia, inflammatory bowel disease, increased risk of upper gastrointestinal bleeding, pregnancy, and uncontrolled psychiatric disease or drug/alcohol abuse. Previous bariatric or gastric surgery is also considered a contraindication, although the absolute contraindication is reserved strictly for partial gastrectomy cases.

- The relatively recent FDA approval for use of the Orbera IGB in the United States has led to increased reports of deaths in obese individuals with a balloon in their stomach.

- Individual doctors or even institutions without experience, accreditation or the ability to resolve obesity-related or bariatric surgery-related complications must not undertake such procedures.

- Apollo manufacturers in the United States, since FDA approval, report about 5000 balloons sold between July 2015 and August 2017; the American Society for Metabolic and Bariatric Surgery reports 5744 balloons had been inserted in 2016, while facilities accredited to perform the procedure have placed only 1003 of the devices. Who has placed the other 4741 devices in the United States?

- When a "balloon" patient comes to an emergency department complaining of severe abdominal pain, gastric perforation needs to be ruled out. Should the suspicion arise, the patient should not be allowed to leave without a computed tomography scan, and this makes the difference.

- Sumo wrestlers share many similarities to NFL lineman, they are massive people with great strength, dedication, discipline and athleticism. Unfortunately, their large size hurts them mechanically and metabolically with time. They put their career over health. The average lifespan for an NFL lineman is about 55 years. Chronic diseases such as hypertension, type 2 diabetes, obstructive sleep apnea and joint replacements are very common. Sumo wrestlers are a great example of the general principle that there are no healthy excess weight situations.

Obesity: A Clinical Review

- Obesity is a disease that can be fatal. Why the insurance companies will charge extra or not even give insurance to people that are grossly obese and then turn around and refuse to pay for an operation that treats that condition is beyond me. This is not cosmetic surgery. This is a disease. It is potentially lethal. (Dr Edward Mason "the Father of Gastric Bypass Surgery said in 1977).
- Edward H. Rynearson, M.D in 1940 said "Obesity is a menace by tending to promote diabetes, hypertension, cardiac failure, cholelithiasis, varicosities, sterility, arthritis, sweating, faulty gait, faulty posture, hernia, and by increasing the risks and difficulties during any operation" "If we are agreed that the use of a weight reduction diet is the best method for treating obesity, how shall we plan this diet? First of all, let us eliminate the fad diet from further discussion. These diets are often inadequate in proper food constituents. Great harm may follow the unwise adherence to an unscientific diet. Some obese patients will lose weight satisfactory simply by eliminating from the diet those foods which are rich in fat and carbohydrate."
- Marie M. Alexander and Fredrick J. Stare wrote in 1967 "every patient's temptation is to follow the line of least resistance, to try the latest craze of capsule, drug or gimmick that is guaranteed to eliminate quickly and easily every surplus pound and inch. Constantly tempted by advertisements and advice, by unscrupulous publications and alluring promises, Mrs. And Mr. American waste valuable dollars and invaluable time in the pursuit of slimness through get-thin-quick drugs and dreams. The physician has to doff the robes of medicine and don the flannels of Madison Avenue. He has to be a counter-salesman, battling all the sources of misleading misinformation with convincing, correct, information. He has to prove to his patient that "reducing" foods do not reduce, that there are no "fattening" foods or "slimming" foods, just too much food.
- Definitions of terms used to describe different types of eating patterns.
- **Intermittent Fasting (IF)** - fasting for varying periods of time, typically for 12 hours or longer.

Chapter 1: Highlight Reel

- **Calorie Restriction (CR)** - a continuous reduction in caloric intake without malnutrition.
- **Time Restricted Feeding (TRF)** - restricting food intake to specific time periods of the day, typically between an 8 – 12 hours each day.
- **Alternate Day Fasting (ADF)** - consuming no calories on fasting days and alternating fasting days with a day of unrestricted food intake or "feast" day.
- **Alternate Day Modified Fasting (ADMF)** - consuming less than 25% of baseline energy needs on "fasting" days, alternated with a day of unrestricted food intake or "feast" day.
- **Periodic Fasting (PF)** - consists of fasting only 1 or 2 days/week and consuming food ad libitum on 5 to 6 days per week.
- An estimated 11% of all neonatal deaths can be attributed to the consequences of maternal overweight and obesity.
- Many of the pregnancy risks have been found to depend linearly on the BMI. The probability of conception declines linearly, starting from a BMI of 29, by 4% for each additional 1 of BMI.
- Super-obesity, defined as body mass index 50 kg/m^2 or greater, is the fastest-growing obesity group in the United States. Currently, 2% of pregnant women in the United States are superobese, and 50% will deliver via cesarean delivery. Super-obese are twice normal weight.
- Superobese women have a 30% to 50% risk of wound complications, a 20% risk of neonatal intensive care unit admission, and a 1% to 2% risk of maternal intensive care unit admission. Preoperative cefazolin with a 3-g dose, chlorhexidine skin preparation, and availability of adequate personnel for patient transfers are important evidence-directed approaches to reducing maternal and personnel morbidity (Smid M. , Dotters-Katz, Silver, & Kuller, 2017)
- Regarding cardiac surgery (CABG, MVR, AVR), morbidly obese patients incurred nearly 60% greater observed mortality than normal weight patients. Morbidly obese patients had

greater than 2-fold increase in renal failure and 6.5-fold increase in deep sternal wound infection. The risk-adjusted odds ratio for mortality for morbidly obese patients was 1.57 compared to normal patients.

Chapter 2: Obesity is a disease

"The future ain't what it used to be." Yogi Berra

On June 21, 2013, the American Medical Association declared obesity a disease. In 1995, the FDA expressed obesity as a chronic disease, but nothing happened officially until 2013. A great deal of debate was involved in classifying obesity a disease. A disease is defined as an impairment of normal functioning of some aspect of the body which has characteristic signs or symptoms and causes harm or morbidity.

Obesity can be defined in many ways. Some definitions include the following:

1. Excessive fat accumulation that presents a risk to health.
2. Hormonal disease impairing function of appetite regulation, energy balance, and endocrine function.
3. BMI greater/equal to 30.
4. Excessive fat accumulation with or without inflammation.
5. Heterogenous disease of excess adipocytes (adipose cells).
6. Chronic relapsing, stigmatized, neurochemical disease.

Clearly obesity is a chronic disease. We see people go from obese children to obese adults. Despite being a chronic disease, it is not treated like one. In 2011, approximately 2.74 million patients were estimated to use obesity drugs in US, a small number given the high prevalence of obesity. Some reasons are:

1. Cultural conviction that medications are inappropriate for obesity management.
2. The history of medications for obesity has been clouded by complications and failures.

3.   Worry about abuse, dependency, and addiction.
4.   Concern that a pill becomes an excuse for poor life choices. Europe has not approved Qysmia (phentermine/extended release topiramate), Contrave (bupropion/naltrexone), Belviq (lorcaserin), or phentermine for weight loss which are approved in the United States.

It is non-scientific to think that once weight is lost that weight will stay off. We do not stop a hypertensive medicine when blood pressure is improved. We give medicines to establish control of a disease and many times continue the medicine to sustain that control. It is a therapeutic misunderstanding that once a patient has reached his weight loss goal, the medicine can be discontinued. A maintenance phase is then instituted which may mean using a lower dose, having medication holidays, or sometimes just the idea of having something to aid a person provides adequate support. Albert Einstein said, "Insanity is defined as expecting different results from doing the same thing." Several states allow weight medicines to be prescribed for only 3 months. They must have not received the Einstein memo. The three-month limitation was brought about due to the amphetamine abuse scandal in the 1970s. By declaring obesity a disease, the medical community started to remove the stigma and prejudice away from having obesity. It removed some of the barriers to treatment but not the personal responsibility. Medicare will pay now for 22 visits per year for obesity and many insurance companies do the same. Hopefully by declaring obesity a disease, it will decrease the frequency of insurance companies denying payment for obesity drugs and bariatric surgeries. It should also protect doctors more from legal issues stemming from off-label use and broaden the number of physicians that are comfortable with trying obesity medicines for their patients.   Obesity medicines have been stigmatized by past complications and failures. It is important to review each medicine individually for its benefits and/or dangers and not stereotype them. **A lesson from the withdrawal of previous anti-obesity drugs is that uncommon but serious adverse effects may become apparent only when a drug is used in larger populations or for longer periods of time than in short small clinical trials.** Medications for obesity must be viewed through the lens of long-term use when evaluating their safety and efficacy

Chapter 2: Obesity is a disease

(Yanovski & Yanovski, 2014). Now, any medication has to be evaluated in regard to cardiovascular safety. Remember, as the famous deceased astrophysicist Carl Sagan used to describe the universe as dealing with billions and billions the potential number of people with unhealthy weight is also in the billions.

People who suffer from obesity are discriminated against daily. A 2004 study revealed that greater than one third of obese patients are willing to risk death to lose 10% of body weight (Blackburn Course in Obesity Medicine, 2014). People look at them with low expectations. The great philosopher Hippocrates wrote "Sudden death is more common in those who are naturally fat than in the lean." The life expectancy for a 20-year-old with severe obesity is 13 years shorter than a healthy weight male of the same age (Blackburn Course in Obesity Medicine, 2014). Obese people are stigmatized in employment, education and entertainment. Research studies reveal obese children have a similar quality of life as children diagnosed with cancer (Blackburn Course in Obesity Medicine, 2014). Many obese children are exposed to bullying and teachers have lower expectations for overweight kids. Kindergarteners would rather sit next to a child with a physical handicap than a child with obesity (Blackburn Course in Obesity Medicine, 2014). It has been documented that doctors are the second most common source of stigma only to be behind family members despite 51% of primary care practitioners being overweight or obese themselves. Obese patients prefer terms like excess weight, unhealthy weight, elevated BMI, or unhealthy BMI. They don't like descriptions like heavy, fat, excess fat, fatness, big-boned, obese, or morbidly obese. Many are embarrassed with their weight and do not like being weighed in front of others. Stereotypes of SLOTH (apathy, laziness) and GLUTTONY (overindulgence, overconsumption), ("two of the seven deadly sins"), have been used to label them. This negative attitude diminishes our ability to help. We prejudge and stereotype. Our advice to them is "EAT LESS, MOVE MORE" but this advice is often not taken. Sometimes messages that have the best intentions are not accepted well. A good example is a study conducted at Bryn Mawr College in 2018 entitled "**Don't Say That to ME: Opposition to Targeting in Weight-Centric Intervention Messages."** Bryn Mawr is a very small elite all-woman's college in Pennsylvania. The College targeted overweight students to offer a free fitness and nutrition program. Unfortunately, it was met with accusations of fat-shaming and not accepted well.

Our knowledge regarding weight balance is increasing yearly, but we still lack understanding in many details. Thus, "EAT LESS, MOVE MORE" is still advocated. **Most weight loss studies do not involve minorities, and this is a shortcoming that needs to be addressed in the clinical environment.** Obesity is more prominent in minorities and plays a large role in the obesity epidemic and minorities need to be included in studies and trials.

Along with environment, more than 100 genes are linked to obesity and the large number of hormones involved is intricate enough to compete with our present tax system. It's like going to Starbucks coffee shop without knowing the coffee dialect. Distinct phenotypes of diet sensitive and diet resistant obesity have been noted at the clinical level, transcription level, and cellular level. There are inherent biological factors underlying diet response. Weight loss is an inheritable response.

A simple anecdotal observation will help understand that obesity is complicated and requires openness and objectivity in treating this newly designated disease. Most people, both doctors and non-professionals, would agree that people with grey hair have more heart disease and cancer then people without grey hair. Therefore, grey hair must cause heart disease and cancer and the best treatment for these ailments would be simply cutting grey hair. We know this is not true but sometimes we think this way towards obesity. We look for simple solutions to complicated questions. It is not just overeating and being lazy. Many overweight people with difficulty losing weight have varying degrees of leptin resistance and other metabolic perturbations. Leptin resistance will be discussed later. Remember, the American Medical Association officially recognized obesity as a disease in 2013 to draw attention, promote understanding and prevention. Being mindful towards obesity is my favorite new word.

Three New Perspectives on the Perfect Storm: What's Behind the Obesity Epidemic?

Chapter 2: Obesity is a disease

- According to statistical forecasts, by 2030, 51% of the US population will have obesity. Overweight and obesity occur when energy intake exceeds energy expenditure over an extended period.
- As Joslin described almost a century ago, genetics probably loads the gun, while lifestyle in our obesogenic environment pulls the trigger for the spreading of the obesity epidemic.
- In this issue of Obesity, we asked three groups of investigators to provide us with their personal view (Perspectives) on the respective roles of the food environment, the decrease in physical activity, and other environmental and/or behavioral factors in triggering the obesity epidemic.

In the first perspective, Hall concludes that the overall caloric content, rather than changes in a single macronutrient, is to blame for the overall population weight gain. More specifically, he hypothesizes that the changes in the quantity and quality of the food supply in conjunction with a drastic increase in the consumption of highly processed, palatable, and cheap food (with high amounts of sugar, fat, salt, and flavor additives) have triggered overconsumption of calories. The traditional normative eating behaviors have progressively switched from time-consuming home meal cooking to more ubiquitous snacking and eating of large-portion-size meals, often at restaurants.

In the second Perspective, Church and Martin remind us that formal exercise (regular recreational exercise) has not changed over the past few decades but occupational activity has. Indeed, by 2006, only 20% of American jobs required high levels of physical activity, thus representing a huge drop from the 1960s when more than 50% of jobs required levels of physical activity that met the current daily physical activity goals.

Finally, in the third Perspective, Davis, Plaisance, and Allison update the list of other environmental and behavioral factors. They propose that poor sleep hygiene, decreased cigarette smoking as behavioral factors and environmental factors, such as increased atmospheric levels of CO_2, living in thermoneutrality most of the year, spending countless hours in front of electronic screens, being exposed to chemicals known to disrupt endocrine functions, and increased consumption of medications, can all tip the energy balance equation in an unhealthy direction. Finally, they add an unhealthy microbiome and economic disparity to the long list of weight gain drivers (Ravussin & Ryan, 2018).

Physician weight loss advice and patient weight loss behavior change: a literature review and meta-analysis of survey data.

- We performed a systematic review and meta-analysis of published studies of survey data examining provider weight loss counseling and its association with changes in patient weight loss behavior.
- PCP advice on weight loss appears to have a significant impact on patient attempts to change behaviors related to their weight. Providers should address weight loss with their overweight and obese patients (Rose, Poynter, Anderson, Noar, & Conigliaro, 2013).

Effects of medical trainees' weight-loss history on perceptions of patients with obesity.

- Medical professionals often express weight-biased attitudes. Prior research suggests that people who overcome a challenge are critical of individuals who struggle to overcome the same challenge. Thus, medical trainees who have successfully achieved and maintained weight loss may express greater weight bias and more critical attitudes toward patients with obesity who fail to overcome these challenges.
- An online survey was completed by 219 medical students and internal medicine residents. Weight-biased attitudes were assessed before they were randomly assigned to read one of three patient vignettes in which the patient lost no weight, lost/regained weight, or lost/maintained weight. Medical trainees' personal success with weight loss and maintenance may negatively affect their perceptions of patients

with obesity who struggle with weight management (Pearl & Wadden, 2017).

Mortality of the Severely Obese: A Population Study.

- Patients who are severely obese [body mass index (BMI) ≥35kg/m] are at increased risk of all-cause mortality as a result of metabolic sequelae including hyperlipidemia, hypertension, and diabetes.
- Bariatric surgery has been shown to reduce the severity of the metabolic complications of obesity.
- A case-controlled analysis of patients with a BMI of 35kg/m or more from the UK database of primary care clinics.

Results:
A total of 187,061 records were identified. Median follow-up time was 98.0 months. A total of 8655(4.6%) died during the study period. The median time from baseline obesity diagnosis until death was 137.0 months.

Multivariate analysis found bariatric surgery to be associated with reduced risk of all-cause mortality (HR: 0.487; $P < 0.001$). The following were associated with increased risk of death:

- male sex (HR: 1.805; $P < 0.001$)
- BMI of 60 or greater (HR: 2.541; $P < 0.001$)
- hypertension (HR: 2.108; $P < 0.001$)
- diabetes (HR: 2.766; $P < 0.001$)
- hyperlipidemia (HR: 1.641; $P < 0.001$).

Bariatric surgery was shown to be associated with reduced risk of all-cause mortality. Improving access to bariatric surgery and public health campaigns can improve the prognosis of severely obese patients (Moussa, et al., 2019).

Chapter 3: Stereotype

A widely held but fixed and oversimplified image or idea of a particular type of person or thing.

The following are excerpts of medical journals discussing obesity and treatment. Stereotyping and discrimination have been around since man and woman evolved into a walking, talking species.

1880

Post-Mortem in a Case of Extreme Obesity

"W. S., aged 50 years, was an over-looker of the cotton factories, but owing to the increasing bulk he had been obliged to give up his situation. He was not a tall man but was extremely fat. He was very lazy; everything in the shape of movement was a trouble to him. He was a perfect glutton. On the evening before his death he ate six eggs and two tea-cakes; and on one occasion-four months before his death, Dr Smith's assistant found him demolishing two loaves of bread, two bottles of porter, half-dozen onions and half a pound of butter. The usual thing was to find him asleep in his chair since he could not sleep in his bed. Autopsy showed the heart is very much enlarged -resembling in appearance to that of an ox. It weighed nearly three and a half times normal size." (Oliver, 1880)

1890

The Treatment of Obesity

"Frequently, the practicing physician is called upon to treat obesity in women where this morbid condition constitutes a most tiresome infirmity and is a complication of most of the affections of the feminine sex." (The Treatment of Obesity, 1890)

1891

Obesity: Its Causes and Treatment.

"Consequently, the adult man or woman who is "putting on flesh" is not generally to be congratulated. Fat people are less able to resist the attacks of disease or the shock of injuries and operations than the moderately thin. In ordinary every-day life they are at a decided disadvantage; their respiratory muscles cannot so easily act; their heart is often handicapped by the deposit on it; and the least exertion throws them into a perspiration. This last fact is curiously misunderstood; it is almost universally looked upon as an actual "melting" of the subcutaneous fat and is considered to be nature's method of getting rid of the superfluity."

"In endeavouring to ascertain the reason why some people are corpulent and others not, we must realize at once that the condition is markedly hereditary. As one breed of pigs is noted for the ease with which it fattens, so with men."

"Diminished mental activity is both a cause and a consequence of corpulency. People whose circumstances are too easy, and those whose intellects are clouded or apathetic frequently become stout. Exercise must next be considered. The easy-going man is too frequently lazy and unwilling to use his muscles; the fidgety man is continuity "on the go"; the one gets stout, the other thin."
(Obesity: Its Causes and Treatment., 1891)

1908

An advertisement for Marmola, found in the November 21, 1908 issue of the British Medical Journal, which claimed to cure obesity by prescription. It was patented in 1907 before being discontinued amid a fraud investigation in 1935.

Is Fatness a Social Offence?

"The female form, being capable of expressing a supreme degree of grace, should be an inspiration in our daily lives and lead up to higher ideals of beauty," said an art lecturer lately. Therefore, the fat woman is an enemy to the artistic uplift, for she is entirely too heavy for any wings of fancy to raise. Why should any woman remain fat when it is so easy to reduce one's flesh? A woman may take but little exercise and enjoy the best of food, and still preserve a beautiful figure."

Every over-fat person should try it. It's quite harmless, and will take off as much as a pound of fat a day. With a chemist's handy, anyone can have a good figure at a reasonable cost."

1928

The Radical Cure of Simple Obesity by Dietary Measures Alone

A question/answer session expressed a question by Dr. George Draper: I would like to ask Dr Evans whether he noticed any change in the psychological aspect of these patients, whether their psychopathy changes in any way. There are often in these people unusual expressions of fantasy and they have numerous tendencies, but the most important thing is that these are the people that have kleptomania and other manias. I would like to know whether, with the reduction of weight, these vagaries of a psychic aspect change, and whether there is any dysfunction of the pituitary gland.

No real reply to the question occurred but Dr Evans stated "In regard to patients who said they were light eaters-they all thought they were, but were not. Several obese patients in the metabolism ward now were given free choice of food for a week before the limited diets were begun. They all ate more than most of you in this room, while maintaining they did not eat much." (Evans, 1928)

1934

ON THE CONTROL OF OBESITY

"All who have conducted post-mortem examinations will testify to the deplorable condition of the heart in the fat person."

"The fat person, as a rule, avoids effort, mental and physical, his critical facilities are dulled, and a tendency to laugh rather than to grumble shows his bias towards taking the easier path."

"Loss of sexual attraction is an important consideration in keeping the population from obesity.

Until recent years we have seen the younger females abolishing so far as possible every typical feminine curve. The explanation of this remarkable state of affairs is to be found in the increase of frankly or potentially homosexual males; who arose from a childhood spent during the war, when they were subjected purely to feminine influence. We see now how cause and effect are on the wane."

"We recall the unpleasant body odor of the fat person, we need no more to convince us that obesity, if avoidable, is disgusting." (Douthwaite, 1934)

1940

Obesity

"Why should so much attention be given to the possibility of hypothyroidism as the cause of obesity when so few patients with true myxedema are obese?"

"Obesity is a menace by tending to promote diabetes, hypertension, cardiac failure, cholelithiasis, varicosities, sterility, arthritis, sweating, faulty gait, faulty posture, hernia, and by increasing the risks and difficulties during any operation"

"If we are agreed that the use of a weight reduction diet is the best method for treating obesity, how shall we plan this diet? First of all, let us eliminate the fad diet from further discussion. These diets are often inadequate in proper food constituents and have nothing to recommend them. Great harm may follow the unwise adherence to an unscientific diet. Some obese patients will lose weight satisfactory simply by eliminating from the diet those foods which are rich in fat and carbohydrate." (Rynearson & Sprague, 1940)

1951

Weight Control: A Simplified Concept

"In all but a very small percentage of overweight people, the condition is brought about through a combination of overeating and inactivity. Each generation has to discover these basic facts. Each generation exhibits some new concept of obesity which represents an attempt to avoid the harsh fact that only by prolonged re-education of obese people can normal eating patterns be restored and obesity ended. The prevalence of obesity is high. In 1939, a study of physical impairments among 10,000 unselected examinees for life insurance disclosed that approximately 28 percent of this group were 10 percent or more overweight. Obesity was the most frequent physical abnormality found.

The prevalence of serious obesity (10% above average weight for sex and height) tends to increase directly with age. Dublin first reported this fact in 1925 after physical examinations of 16,662 male policyholders in the Metropolitan Life Insurance Co. The prevalence at age 25 was found to be 4.9 percent, and at age 55 it had increased to 19.8 percent. Study after study has shown that the mortality rates among people are higher than among people of normal weight. Overweight tends to shorten life. As early as 1930, Dublin had shown that 50 pounds of excess weight at age 50 increased the death rate by 56 percent – 1 percent per pound – and that in those who were 100 pounds overweight the death rate was increased more than 100 percent.

In an article entitled, "Psychological Aspects of Obesity," Hilde Bruch makes this illuminating observation, "In those happy-go-lucky fat people whom I have had the opportunity to observe, the joviality and often boisterous cheerfulness was nothing but a thin veneer put on for the benefits of the public, a compensatory defense against underlying feelings of unhappiness and futility" In other words, fat people simply are not happy. They employ a camaraderie reactive defense mechanism unconsciously designed to mask their underlying tenseness, frustration, and uncertainty. (Chapma, 1951)

1967

Overweight, Obesity and Weight Control

"Every patient's temptation is to follow the line of least resistance, to try the latest craze of capsule, drug or gimmick that is guaranteed to eliminate quickly and easily every surplus pound and inch. Constantly tempted by advertisements and advice, by unscrupulous publications and alluring promises, Mrs. And Mr. American waste valuable dollars and invaluable time in the pursuit of slimness through get-thin-quick drugs and dreams. The physician has to doff the robes of medicine and don the flannels of Madison Avenue. He has to be a counter-salesman, battling all the sources of misleading misinformation with convincing, correct, information. He has to prove to his patient that "reducing" foods do not reduce, that there are no "fattening" foods or "slimming" foods, just too much food." (Alexander & Stare, 1967)

1985

Social and psychological consequences of obesity.
The strong prejudice in this country against obese persons is
evident in children as young as 6 years of age. There
is discrimination against obese persons in both academic and work
settings. Despite this discrimination, overweight persons in the
general population show no greater psychological disturbance than
do non-obese persons. Similarly, obese patients seen for medical or
surgical procedures generally show no more psychopathology than
do non-obese patients. Serious psychiatric disturbances associated
with obesity include disparagement of body image and negative
emotional reactions to dieting. Dieting may also be responsible for
the increased incidence of bulimia observed in this country in
recent years. Women, adolescent girls, and the morbidly obese
appear to suffer the most deleterious consequences of society's
contempt for the obese. (Wadden & Stunkard, 1985)

1990

Morbidly obese patients' perceptions of
social discrimination before and after surgery for obesity.
Morbidly obese patients' perceptions of obesity-related prejudice
and discrimination were assessed before and 14 months after
operation for obesity. Preoperatively, the 57 consecutive patients
perceived overwhelming prejudice and discrimination at work,
within the family, and in public places. After a weight loss of more
than 45.5 kg (100 lb), these patients perceived little or no prejudice
or discrimination. (Rand & Macgregor, 1990)

2002

[Bariatric surgery -- stereotypes and paradigms].
Many physicians regard obesity as a sin and treat fat patients with
disdain befitting a moral leper. Non-bariatric physicians, being a
product of our culture, seem more likely to have
an obesity paradigm close to that of the public. Many insurers reject
patients from bariatric surgery believing that obesity is totally the
fault of a fat person. These medical experts do not
accept obesity as a disease (which the World Health Organization

does) and therefore social courts also reject applications of patients who want to undergo bariatric surgery. Morbid obesity is a multifactorial problem with genetic, biochemical, hormonal, environmental, behavioral and cultural elements. It is recognized as an extreme health hazard which is rarely the result of an aberrant moral problem or true addictive behavior. We need to change effectively the negative paradigms towards obesity and its surgery. The existing prejudices are not acceptable. (Hell & Miller, 2002)

2010

Weight Bias in Work Settings – a Qualitative Review

Research has consistently shown that physical appearance plays a role in the work place, even in professions which do not deal with physical appearance themselves and where performance is unrelated to bodily characteristics. The attractiveness bias for job-related outcomes where individuals benefit from their physical appearance is well-documented. Physical appearance can contribute to biased attitudes or treatments in terms of stereotypes, discrimination or stigmatization

In representative surveys in the USA, overweight and obese individuals were consistently more likely to report subjectively perceived discrimination in the work place. A common judgmental bias is the halo effect. The halo effect refers to the phenomenon that a single person's outstanding characteristic influences the total judgment of that person. Body weight is an early perceptible personal characteristic and can serve as an outstanding attribute for a halo effect. As obesity often is associated with laziness and low self-discipline, it is well conceivable that this primary impression and judgment serves as the basis of a halo effect and extends to other characteristics to be evaluated, such as work-related abilities and qualities.

There is strong evidence for an income disadvantage for obese women in western societies. This gender difference suggests that socioeconomic status is more independent of body weight in men than in women. A possible explanation for this circumstance can be seen in the ideal of beauty in today's western societies and the interpretation of overweight. The beauty ideal puts more pressure on women to be slim than on men. Thus, women might be penalized earlier by society for being overweight. (Giel, Thiel, Teufel, Mayer, & Zipfel, 2010)

2019

The association of mobility disability and obesity with risk of unemployment in two cohorts from Sweden.

- People with mobility disability (MD) or obesity often have more health problems and are less able to participate in work than individuals without these conditions.
- The study included two Swedish population-based cohorts, a national cohort (n = 39,947) and a regional cohort (n = 40,088).
- In summary, the groups with MD and the obese group without MD had a higher risk of becoming unemployed than the reference group. The obese group with MD did not differ from the groups with MD only or obesity only in terms of unemployment risk.
- People with MD and/or obesity are vulnerable groups at risk of prolonged unemployment during their working life in a country with a highly developed welfare system. (Norrback, Tynelius, Ahlstrom, & Rasmussen, 2019)

Chapter 4: Basic Ideas

"A nickel ain't worth a dime anymore" Yogi Berra

There are many principles we do know about weight/energy balance. "Humans have evolved elaborate and complex genetic and physiological systems to protect against starvation and defend stored body fat." (Bellisari, 2008)
Because our evolutionary make-up cannot differentiate starvation from voluntary weight loss, the human body does not like change. Our body treats weight loss as a non-physiologic, non-steady state which turns on alarms to correct this deviation. Our body gets used to a certain set-point and will trigger hormones to get back to a safe set-point. These counter-regulatory mechanisms and hormones promote hunger. Our voluntary response to hunger determines success or failure. One theory is obese patients have a higher set point than non-obese patients making weight loss harder for them. A higher set point is a theory dating back several decades stating that our bodies are programmed to live within a certain weight range and any deviation from that elicits a dramatic revolution to get back to that level. Unfortunately, **it is felt that obese individuals were born with a maladaptive set point that protects a medically unhealthy body weight, hence obesity is a congenital disease and not simply a lifestyle.** Clinically, set point theory is not very helpful and does not seem to have strong basic science evidence supporting or refuting it.
Research has shown obese patients need more dopamine in response to eating, consequently it takes more food to satisfy them. Dopamine levels increase 50% with food, 100% with sex, 350% with cocaine, and 1200% with methamphetamines (Blackburn

Course in Obesity Medicine, 2014). Dopamine is an addictive substance. It is one of the brain's pleasure chemicals similar to endorphins.

Many weight-loss drugs work on the dopamine/ norepinephrine/epinephrine neurotransmitter systems. Many psychiatric medicines work on this system also but in a different manner which helps explain why many psychiatric medicines have weight gain as a major side-effect. Body weight is regulated in the hypothalamus where it receives signals from the brain, gastrointestinal track and adipose tissue.

Twin studies point towards an obesity inheritance pattern of 60-70 %. Twin studies suggest that genetics at birth can predict 25% of lifespan thus showing how important our reaction to the environment is. If obesity was totally genetic, you would not have seen the epidemic in obesity develop in the last 20-30 years since genetics do not evolve that rapidly. Environment must account for the rest since genes do not contribute 100%. "A novel social network analysis of Framingham Heart Study revealed that males had a 100% increase in the chance of becoming obese if their male friend became obese, whereas this same effect of friendship on obesity was not significant among females." (Kanter & Caballero, 2012) Other data from the Framingham Study indicate that people who were obese at age 40 years died 6 to 7 years earlier than normal-weight peers (Peeters, et al., 2003) The life expectancy in severely obese individuals is even worse. Median survival is decreased 8 to 10 years (Whitlock, et al., 2009). Compared with normal-weight individuals, obese individuals have a 30% greater chance of mortality from surgery and a 50% increase in the risk of major complications from surgery (Hruby & Hu, 2015). This is a comparison. It is not stating that obese individuals have a 30% mortality rate from surgery.

In Jamaica, obesity is more culturally acceptable among women because excess weight gain is associated with maternity and nurturing. In East Asia and the Pacific, a larger body type is accepted and still may be culturally associated with a greater socioeconomic status. **Globally, more women are <u>obese</u> than men. In developed countries, more men are <u>overweight</u> than women.** All income groups have a greater overall prevalence of female obesity compared with male obesity. Alcohol intake is perceived either as a cause of or associated with excess weight gain in men but not women (Kanter & Caballero, 2012).

Industrialization has provided access to great quantities of food, especially calorie dense foods, along with labor saving machines and multiple transportation devices. Technology has made our lives easier and less time is needed on basic survival needs such as food gathering and shelter. The masses no longer walk to places or engage in heavy labor. Television and home computers have increased sedentary behavior. We have moving walkways at airports, electric knifes, electric toothbrushes and remote controls. I don't know if my kids would know how to change the channels on an old TV that does not work by remote control. The number and quantity of food choices have skyrocketed. Just think of all the variety of cereals, cookies, ice cream flavors and sodas available now compared to 30 years ago.

Calories consumed by Americans increased 12% from 1971-74 to 1999-2002. I remember how exciting it was when "cookies and cream ice cream" came out and I was amazed to see the embossing of the OREO logo in cookie parts embedded in the ice cream. Also, larger portion sizes and larger packaging promote larger consumption as the "norm." The picture of Americans and others worldwide has changed. Affluence has a price on our health. Between 1980 and 2008, age-standardized BMI for men increased in every region apart from Central Africa and South Asia, with USA and UK being highest. **Contrary to conventional wisdom, the obesity epidemic is not restricted to developed societies only.**

Two-thirds of Americans are overweight and more than one-third are obese. Seventeen percent of our children are obese and a higher percentage are overweight. The famous Pima Indians in Mexico had an average BMI of 25 and were relatively free of obesity and diabetes in the past. They were a self-sufficient farming people. The modern-day Pima Indians in Arizona have an average BMI of 32 and struggle with obesity, diabetes and alcoholism. Their traditional subsistence diet has been replaced by food laden with processed flour, sugar and lard (essentially chocolate muffins). Their environment has changed and so has ours and neither group has adapted well.

Weight gain increases as patient's age. Despite food intake and energy expenditure (calories burned) varying less than ½

of 1%, the average person gains one pound per year making it difficult to perceive the specific cause or remedy for weight gain. A common finding is 20 pounds in twenty years with the person unable to know how it snuck up on him or her. Maintenance of weight within 20 pounds from the age of 21 to 65 years old requires matching intake and expenditure to within 0.2% variability (accuracy of 4-5 kcals per day). A person's basal metabolic rate decreases with age along with a decrease in muscle mass and an increase in adipose tissue especially around internal organs (visceral fat). This downhill slide starts at about 30-35 years of age. I tell patients that they are invincible till 35 than our bodies start to fail.

Muscle mass essentially determines resting energy expenditure (metabolism) and this declines at about 35 years old. Trained muscle consumes 9 kcals/lb./day and untrained muscle consumes 5-6 kcals/lb./day. If one eats the same amount every year and does not increase energy expenditure either through work or exercise, they will gain weight each year typically starting at 35 years-old. Exercise is essential to maintain good health. Six pounds of muscle are lost per decade, metabolic rate decreases 3% per decade, and 16 pounds of fat are gained per decade. A few general estimates are;

1. 6-8% muscle mass loss before 50 years.
2. 8-10% muscle mass loss after 50 years and before 70 years.
3. 15% loss after 70 years and continues every decade. About 14% of people 65-75 years old require help in basic ADLs, a proportion that increases to 45% in people over 85.
4. Muscle mass loss is greater in men as compared to women.

As someone loses weight the calorie needs to maintain that weight decrease thus making it harder to lose more weight. Basal metabolic rate is analogous to gasoline in a vehicle. A large truck requires more gas to drive than a subcompact car. If you lose 30 pounds it takes less energy to take care of the smaller body mass. BMI gradually increases during most of adult life and reaches peak values at 50-59 years. After 60 years, mean body weight and BMI tend to decrease.

Basal Metabolic Rate (BMR) decreases as we get older. Basal metabolic rate consists of the processes that the body needs to function. It is the amount of energy per unit time that a person needs to keep the body functioning at rest. Some of those processes are breathing, blood circulation, controlling body temperature, cell growth, brain and nerve function, and contraction of muscles. It is the amount of energy we consume in 24 hours if we sat on the couch in a comfortable temperature environment without eating or doing any activity. Basal metabolic rate is our "couch-potato rate."

The following calculation demonstrates why weight loss is hard.

A typical person roughly needs 12 kcals per pound for basal metabolic rate and a person's body adapts to weight loss by decreasing BMR by 6.8 kcals per pound of lost weight. Our body adapts to the weight loss by decreasing the basal metabolic rate as a survival tool.

If a 200-lb. person loses 50 lbs. what happens to his BMR? 200 lbs x 12 kcals/lb = 2400 kcals. He loses 50 lbs. 50 lbs x 6.8 kcals/lb = 340 kcals.

His new BMR is 150 lbs. x 12 kcals/lb. =1800 kcals minus 340 kcals =1460 kcals. The person's BMR goes from 2400 kcals to 1460 kcals, instead of 1800 kcals. This is one reason why patient's plateau. A person is following the same diet but the weight does not decrease because his metabolic needs have decreased substantially. Exercise/physical activity needs to increase to burn calories to continue to lose weight. Weight loss gets harder as you lose more and more weight.
If you lose 11 lbs. metabolism slows 75kcals/day.
If you lose 22 lbs. metabolism slows 150kcals/day.
If you lose 50 lbs. metabolism slows 340kcals/day.

Untreated obesity is disease promoting.
The co-morbidities of obesity can be classified into two general categories, those relating to insulin resistance and cardio-metabolic disease and those relating to the mechanical or functional consequences of excess body weight.
From a biomechanics viewpoint, **every pound lost lessens 4 pounds of joint stress on our knees**. When you walk across level ground, the force on your knees is equivalent to 1 ½ times your

body weight. A 200-lb man will put 300 pounds of pressure on his knees with each step. Add incline, and the pressure is even greater: the force on each knee is 2-3 times your body weight when you go up and down stairs, and 4-5 times your body weight when you squat to tie a shoelace or pick up an item you dropped. This is why elderly people have such trouble with many ADLs and again stresses the importance of regular physical activity.

Laura Gilbert in the spring of 2014 wrote an article entitled **"The Effects of Obesity on Human Ambulation"** and noted that the body is not intended to bear excess weight (Gilbert, 2014). Subjects that carried a backpack containing 40% of their weight while walking decreased their length of stride and increased the frequency of their stride. The body compromises its walking mechanics when stressed. For all major lower extremity joints, obese individuals have 7 times higher risk of developing osteoarthritis (Ackerman & Osbourne, 2012). When comparing obese to non-obese individuals, the recovery time for obese individuals after a surgical procedure is longer, and in some surgeries, excess adipose tissue hinders the ability of the surgeon to perform. Obesity is a contraindication for a bilateral total knee replacement, and a BMI of greater than 32 has a predicted higher failure rate for minimally invasive surgeries such as knee arthroplasty. The surgical infection rate in several operations increases from 0.37% in normal weight individuals to 4.44% in obese individuals. The need for a total knee arthroplasty is estimated to be at least 8.5 times higher among patients with a BMI greater than or equal to 30. Many orthopedic surgeons require a BMI below 40 for surgery due to the increased risk. **The odds of sustaining musculoskeletal injuries is 15 percent higher for persons who are overweight and 48 percent higher for people who are obese, compared to persons of normal weight.**

Increased risk is noted in a 2016 study in the Journal of Neuroscience, entitled **Impact of obesity on lumbar spinal surgery outcomes:**

Controversy exists regarding the effect of obesity on surgical outcomes and complications following spinal surgery. Significant differences between obese and non-obese patients were found for operation time, blood loss, surgical site infections and nerve injury. Deep vein thrombosis, dural tear, revision surgery, and mortality were not significantly different between the two groups. The results of this meta-analysis should be interpreted with caution due to heterogeneity amongst the included studies (Cao, Kong, Meng, Zhang, & Shen, 2016).

It could be easily argued that weight loss medications should be considered for any overweight or obese patient with overt diabetes type 2 who fail to achieve moderate weight loss (10%) with lifestyle modification (Garvey, 2013). Only a minority of patients achieve HgbA1c goals, blood pressure goals, lipid goals despite an increasing array of diabetic agents and newer types of insulin. A very common complication is the increased risk of infection with poor diabetic control. The 2017 Circulation article **Glycated Hemoglobin and Risk of Sternal Wound Infection After Isolated Coronary Surgery** looked at preoperative HbA1c levels and sternal wound infection in 2,130 patients undergoing isolated CABG. **A HgbA1c level of greater than 8.6% was associated with the highest risk of sternal wound infection (20.6% vs 4.6%)** (Gatti, et al., 2016).

What Matters in Weight Loss? An In-Depth Analysis of Self-Monitoring.

The purpose of this study was to analyze the contribution of self-monitoring to weight loss in participants in a 6-month commercial weight-loss intervention administered by Retrofit.
Methods:
A retrospective analysis was performed using 2113 participants enrolled from 2011 to 2015. Participants were males and females aged 18 years or older with a starting body mass index of ≥25 kg/m2.
Results:
Participants lost a mean -5.58% of their baseline weight with 51.87% (1096/2113) losing at least 5%. The following measures were significant predictors of weight loss at 6 months:

- Weighing in at least three times per week
- Having a minimum of 60 highly active minutes per week
- Food logging at least three days per week
- Having 64% (16.6/26) or more weeks with at least five food logs were associated with clinically significant weight loss (Painter, et al., 2017).

Chapter 5: Common Medicines and Weight Gain

"A spoonful of sugar makes the medicine go down."
No one said the medicine causes weight gain?

Many common medicines that are prescribed regularly promote weight gain. As more medicines are available to treat medical issues the number that cause weight gain will clearly increase. Medicines that are used for chronic conditions such as type 2 diabetes, hypertension, depression, bipolar disorder, auto-immune disorders, etc. require long-term use making it even more important to appreciate the potential side effects. Some of the most popular include insulin, B-blockers, anti-psychotics, narcotics, anti-depressants, and anti-anxiety medicines. For example, paroxetine (Paxil) promotes large weight gain and sertraline (Zoloft) is weight neutral. **SSRIs (selective serotonin reuptake inhibitors) and TCAs (tricyclics) are associated with doubling the risk of type 2 diabetes in a dose-dependent manner.**
Antidepressant prescribing has risen nearly 400% since 1988. Adult obesity rates have doubled since 1980 from 15 to 30%, while childhood obesity rates have more than tripled. **Prevalence of major depressive disorder (MDD) is 16.2% in women which is twice the rate for men.** From 2005-2008 antidepressants were the third most prescribed class of drugs for people aged 18-44 years old. Cortisol levels are often increased in the plasma of MDD patients and antidepressant treatment downregulates the HPA (hypothalamic-pituitary-adrenal) axis response (Wong & Licinio,

2004). **Most drugs used in depression and in obesity predominately affect either serotonin or norepinephrine.** Women with a history of MDD have twice the chance of developing metabolic syndrome than women without such history (Kinder, Carnethon, Palaniappan, King, & Fortmann, 2004). Chronic stress is a state where there is persistent activation of the HPA axis which occurs not only in MDD but also in obesity (Björntorp, 2001). The simultaneous activation of inflammatory pathways by depression and by obesity can only be detrimental. Antidepressants first came out in the 1950s by accident when MAOI (monoamine oxidase inhibitors) being used to treat tuberculosis showed anti-depressant-like effects by preventing monoamine depletion in the brain. Since then, it has been hypothesized that a depletion in other neurotransmitters such as norepinephrine, dopamine and serotonin contribute to MDD. There are different classes of antidepressant drugs that work by modulating neurotransmitter levels in the brain. Older generation antidepressants include MAOIs and tricyclics (TCAs), whereas newer types of antidepressants have greater specificity and include selective reuptake inhibitors (selective serotonin reuptake inhibitor-SSRIs), serotonin and norepinephrine reuptake inhibitors (SNRIs), and norepinephrine and dopamine reuptake inhibitors.

1. Tricyclic anti-depressants (imipramine, amitriptyline, nortriptyline, trimipramine, protriptyline, iprindole) inhibit serotonin and norepinephrine reuptake. TCAs have multiple nonspecific actions that are associated with side effects. They include anticholinergic, alpha-1 adrenergic antagonistic and antihistaminergic activities. **TCA-induced weight gain is one of the main reasons for the discontinuation of treatment within 1 month (Berken, Weinstein, & Stern, 1984).** In this study, low to moderate doses of the TCAs amitriptyline (150 mg per day), nortriptyline (50 mg per day), and imipramine (80 mg per day) were associated with a mean weight gain of 1.3-2.9 pounds per month, and the trend of weight gain remained linear overtime. Since the FDA approval of fluoxetine (Prozac) in 1988, SSRIs have been the most prescribed antidepressants on the market. They act by inhibiting serotonin (5-hydroxytryptamine, 5HT) uptake.

2. The Canadian National Population Health Survey (NPHS) is a longitudinal study that has found that SSRIs and the SNRI

venlafaxine are associated with significant weight gain (Patten 2009). A long-term comparison study investigated the effects of different types of SSRI on weight gain in patients with panic disorder. It showed the following in a 1-year period (Dannon, et al., 2007).

Medication	Weight Gain kg (avg)	Weight Gain lbs (avg)
Paroxetine (Paxil)	8.2 kg	18.0 lbs
Fluoxetine (Prozac)	5.2 kg	11.4 lbs
Citalopram (Celexa)	6.9 kg	15.2 lbs
Fluvoxamine (Luvox)	6.3 kg	13.9 lbs

SSRIs are useful for the treatment of obese patients with binge eating disorder, given SSRIs anti-impulsive action. **Weight gain is one of the most undesired effects of treatment, and one of the major reasons for discontinuing treatment within the first 2 months of treatment initiation (Uher, et al., 2011). Carbohydrate craving is an important feature and complication of the treatment of depression and is often ignored.** Eight of 18 patients had significant increase in carbohydrate craving together with weight gain shortly after initiation of treatment (Bouwer & Harvey, 1996).

Another important neurotransmitter is serotonin. It is made from the amino-acid tryptophan and a synonym is 5-hydroxytryptamine (5-HT). **Serotonin is primarily found in the gastrointestinal tract, platelets, and the CNS. Approximately 90% of the body's serotonin is located in the GI tract where it regulates intestinal movement. The name serotonin comes from the discovery of a substance in the serum that increased muscular smooth muscle tone (serum + tone). Because serotonin regulates intestinal movement, this explains why nausea and diarrhea are common side effects and why the serotonin antagonist ondansetron (Zofran) is such an effective anti-emetic.** Serotonin is stored in platelets and is released when platelets bind to a clot. When a patient has heparin-induced thrombocytopenia the gold standard is to measure a serotonin release assay.

The neurotransmitter, serotonin, is released from synaptic vesicles into the synaptic cleft where it interacts with a receptor on the nerve ending of adjacent neurons. Various agents can inhibit the uptake and thus prolong the effects of serotonin. These agents include cocaine, tricyclic anti-depressants, selective serotonin reuptake inhibitors (SSRIs) and dextromethorphan (an anti-tussive). A new medicine called "Nuedexta" combines low dose dextromethorphan (nonselective serotonin reuptake inhibitor) and low dose quinidine to help with people who suffer from brain injury or other neurological diseases who have involuntary, sudden inappropriate outbursts of crying or laughing.

When we smell food, dopamine is released to increase our appetite. As food enters our gut serotonin is released from our GI tract providing negative feedback to dopamine to signal satiety and decrease appetite. Drugs that block the serotonin receptors (anti-depressants) prevent this satiety signal and thus promote weight gain.

Too much serotonin can cause troubles. Tramadol (Ultram), a common schedule 4 pain medicine, has much less additive potential compared to schedule 2 drugs such as hydrocodone, hydromorphone, or oxycodone. Tramadol is an opioid pain medicine that also increases serotonin by inhibiting the uptake of serotonin/norepinephrine. This is important because many people that are prescribed tramadol also take antidepressants that work by increasing serotonin as the mechanism of action. Most people who develop serotonin syndrome are taking two medicines that increase serotonin. The weight loss medicine lorcaserin (Belviq) is a selective serotonin 2C receptor **agonist** and thus promotes satiety. **Serotonin syndrome – fever, agitation, increased reflexes, tremor, sweating, dilated pupils, diarrhea. Predictable consequence of excess serotonin. Meds include selective serotonin reuptake inhibitors (SSRI), serotonin norepinephrine reuptake inhibitor (SNRI), tricyclic antidepressants (TCAs), tramadol, buspirone, ondansetron, dextromethorphan, metoclopramide, Monoamine oxidase inhibitor (MAOI), St John's wort, triptans. Treatment for serotonin syndrome is discontinuing the drug. Benzodiazepines can be used for agitation and cyproheptadine (Periactin) is helpful due to being a serotonin antagonist.**

Another good example of how anti-depressants and weight loss medications share common pathways is mirtazapine (Remeron-

SNRI). Mirtazapine has been associated with weight gain and this feature is used many times in prescribing it. Many debilitated patients are specifically given mirtazapine due to its weight gain side effect. It works by blockade of alpha 2-adrenergic receptors and histamine receptors. Histaminergic cell bodies are part of the hypothalamus which we know is intricately involved in appetite and feeding control. Histaminergic receptors have been shown to interact with orexigenic neuropeptides such as orexin A, NPY, and ghrelin. Anti-histaminergic effects of mirtazapine were associated with enhanced appetite by activation of ghrelin and NPY. Anti-histamines which we use daily promote weight gain. Clinical doses of mirtazapine block both 5HT2 and 5HT3 receptors. 5HT2 receptors have an essential role in appetite, and antagonizing 5HT2 results in weight gain. Orexigenic and anorexigenic neuropeptides are constantly orchestrating are responses to food and attempts at dieting. This is why obesity is complicated to understand and treat (Lee, Mastronardi, Licinio, & Wong, 2016).

Antidepressant utilisation and incidence of weight gain during 10 years' follow-up: population-based cohort study

- Between 1975 and 2014 the global prevalence of obesity increased from 3.2% to 10.8% for men and from 6.4% to 14.9% for women. The United States and United Kingdom have among the highest rates of obesity in the world: 69% of US adults are overweight or obese and 36% are obese, and 61% of UK adults are overweight or obese. Once obesity is established, it is difficult to achieve substantial and sustained weight loss.
- Antidepressants are increasingly being prescribed. In a primary care population 23% of 1.5 million participants were prescribed an antidepressant on at least one occasion between 1995 to 2011.
- We carried out a population-based cohort study in the UK Clinical Practice Research Datalink (CPRD). This included 294 719 (93.7%) participants.
- Among 294 719 participants, 53 110 (18.0%) were prescribed antidepressants, 22.4% women and 13% men. Antidepressant use was least in those of normal body weight (13.9%) and increasing with BMI up to 26.5% in

those with a BMI of ≥45. Antidepressant use was greater in patients with comorbidity, co-prescriptions, current smoking and lower socioeconomic level.

- NNH (number needed to harm) of 59 patient years treated with antidepressants for one episode of weight gain.
- During the second year of treatment, the risk of one additional episode of ≥ 5% weight gain may be expected for every 27 patients treated.

Discussion

- Considering the entire period of follow-up (10 years), participants who were prescribed an antidepressant had an increased risk of ≥5% weight gain. The risk of weight gain was substantially increased during the second and third years of treatment with the risk of weight gain for at least the first five years of treatment.
- Less than 12 months' use of antidepressants did not appear to be associated with weight gain. Mirtazapine was associated with the highest incidence rate ratio of weight gain.

Initiation of antidepressant drugs shows a strong temporal association with weight gain, which is greatest during the second and third years of treatment. During the second year of treatment, the risk of ≥5% weight gain is 46.3% higher than in a general population comparison group. (Gafoor, Booth, & Gulliford, 2018)

Other potential weight-gaining medicines include beta-blockers, alpha blockers, steroids, anti-histamines, narcotics, and neuropathy medicines like gabapentin (Neurontin) and pregabalin (Lyrica). The bipolar medicine, Lithium, causes a 10 kg gain or more over the course of treatment in over 20% of patients. Beta-blockers are lipogenic, decrease basal metabolic rate, promote fatigue, depression, aggravate glucose and should not be used for primary cardiac prevention since effect is similar to placebo. Most drugs will have the most marked effect early in treatment reaching a plateau by 6-12 months. **The weight change from medicines may not always be noticed since it occurs against a background of progressive weight gain in the normal population.** It is always important to look at medicines routinely to evaluate the risk/benefit ratio of each of them. **Compliance may worsen if the person notices a lot of weight gain.** This can be detrimental especially with anti-psychotic medications. **Weight gain can also be dose related emphasizing the basic principle of always trying to use the lowest dose to achieve the desired result.** Just as the amount of food we consume has increased over the last decades the number of prescription drugs, non-prescription drugs, and supplements we consume has increased too. Supplements are used frequently. Good judgement is necessary in providing guidance to patients. **The major issue with supplements is lack of quality control and lack of scientific evidence to support the claims. Many prescription medications are found unlabeled in supplements.** An overriding majority of doctors would suggest avoiding all weight loss supplements. A middle of the road approach recommends asking the local pharmacist about the medicine before purchasing it. 50% of the US population use supplements and the number has increased from 4,000 supplements in 1994 to 80,000 supplements in 2012. **A supplementary group that is beneficial are pro-biotics, prebiotics, and fish oils.** In 2002, the FDA approved a qualified health claim for EPA and DHA omega-3 fatty acids in dietary supplements. Evidence from prospective secondary prevention studies suggest that EPA and DHA supplementation ranging from 0.5 to 1.8 gm/day significantly reduces subsequent cardiac and all-cause mortality (Lee, Mastronardi, Licinio, & Wong, 2016). Another class of medicines that aggravate obesity are narcotics. Narcotics are not only dangerous but sometimes nonproductive. A 2016 article by C Stephan, MD and Fereydoun D Parsa, MD expresses helpful information:

Avoiding Opioids and Their Harmful Side Effects in the Postoperative Patient: Exogenous Opioids, Endogenous Endorphins, Wellness, Mood, and Their Relation to Postoperative Pain.

The primary advantage of eliminating the use of opioids for postoperative pain control appears to be avoidance of the common negative side effects of opioid analgesics. In addition, patients who do not use opioids are often more pleased with their overall postsurgical wellness in our experience. We believe that the profound impact of beta-endorphins are often underscored in the literature. Based on our research, the following guidelines should be implemented to achieve adequate opioid- free postoperative pain control:

1. The patient must be provided adequate preoperative verbal and written education concerning the rationale for eliminating the use of opioids in the perioperative period.
2. The preoperative and intraoperative use of local anesthetic is strongly recommended.
3. Preoperative use of gabapentin and celecoxib (in appropriate-risk patients) is advised.
4. The practitioner should avoid intraoperative use of opioids to preserve the effects of endogenous beta-endorphins.
5. Avoidance of postoperative opioid use is strongly recommended.

(Stephan & Parsa, 2016)

Antipsychotic drugs have significant metabolic side effects such as weight gain and disturbed glucose metabolism.

A study by Ebdrup BH, et al. in September 2014 in Clinical Psychiatry **"Glucometabolic hormones and cardiovascular risk markers in antipsychotic-treated patients"** looked at 50 nondiabetic men treated with anti-psychotic medication and 93 men with similar measurements but not treated with anti-psychotic medicines.

- Mean age was 33 years old, BMI 26, HbA1c 5.7%, waist circumference 43.6 inches.
- Fasting samples along with samples 90 minutes after ingestion of a standardized liquid meal (542 kcals).
- Patients on anti-psychotic medicines had elevated levels of C-reactive protein, proinsulin, C-peptide, and GIP.

The conclusion was that nondiabetic antipsychotic-treated patients display emerging signs of dysmetabolism and a compromised cardiovascular risk profile. Metabolic screening is important in psychiatric practice (Ebdrup, et al., 2014).

Withdrawal Symptoms after Serotonin-Noradrenaline Reuptake Inhibitor Discontinuation: Systematic Review.

Serotonin-noradrenaline reuptake inhibitors (SNRI);

- duloxetine (Cymbalta)
- venlafaxine (Effexor XR)
- desvenlafaxine (Pristiq)
- milnacipran (Savella)
- levomilnacipran (Fetzima)
- Their discontinuation has been associated with a wide range of symptoms. The aim of this paper is to identify the occurrence, frequency, and features of withdrawal symptoms after SNRI discontinuation.

Results:

- Withdrawal symptoms occurred after discontinuation of any type of SNRI. The prevalence of withdrawal symptoms varied across reports and appeared to be higher with **venlafaxine (Effexor).** Symptoms typically ensued within a few days from discontinuation and lasted a few weeks, also with gradual tapering. Late onset and/or a longer persistence of disturbances occurred as well.

Conclusions:

- Clinicians need to add SNRI to the list of drugs potentially inducing withdrawal symptoms upon discontinuation, together with other types of psychotropic drugs. The results of this study challenge the use of SNRI as first-line treatment for mood and anxiety disorders (Fava, et al., 2018).

Validating pre-treatment body mass index as moderator of antidepressant treatment outcomes: Findings from CO-MED trial.

- Currently, there are no valid clinical or biological markers to personalize the treatment of depression. Recent evidence suggests that body mass index (BMI) may guide the selection of antidepressant medications with different mechanisms of action.

Methods:

- Combining Medications to Enhance Depression Outcomes (CO-MED) trial participants with BMI measurement (n =

662) were categorized as normal- or underweight (<25), overweight (25-<30), obese I (30-<35), and obese II+ (≥35).

- Evaluate if BMI differentially predicted response to antidepressant escitalopram (SSRI) monotherapy, bupropion-escitalopram combination, or venlafaxine-mirtazapine combination, after controlling for gender and baseline depression severity.

Results:

- Remission rates among the three treatment arms differed on the basis of pre-treatment BMI (p = .046).
- Normal- or under-weight participants were less likely to improve with the bupropion-SSRI combination (26.8%) than SSRI monotherapy (37.3%),) or venlafaxine-mirtazapine combination (44.4%.
- Obese II+ participants were more likely to improve with bupropion-SSRI (47.4%) than SSRI monotherapy (28.6%) or venlafaxine-mirtazapine combination (37.7%). Remission rates did not differ among overweight and obese I participants.

Conclusions:

- Antidepressant selection in clinical practice can be personalized with BMI measurements. Bupropion-SSRI combination should be avoided in normal- or under-weight depressed outpatients as compared to SSRI monotherapy and venlafaxine-mirtazapine combination and preferred in those with BMI≥35 (Jha, et al., 2018).

Another class of medicines that aggravate obesity are narcotics. Narcotics are not only dangerous but sometimes nonproductive. A 2016 article by C Stephan, MD and Fereydoun D Parsa, MD expresses helpful information:

Avoiding Opioids and Their Harmful Side Effects in the Postoperative Patient: Exogenous Opioids, Endogenous Endorphins, Wellness, Mood, and Their Relation to Postoperative Pain.

The primary advantage of eliminating the use of opioids for postoperative pain control appears to be avoidance of the common negative side effects of opioid analgesics. In addition, patients who do not use opioids are often more pleased with their overall postsurgical wellness in our experience. We believe that the profound impact of beta-endorphins are often underscored in the literature. Based on our research, the following guidelines should be implemented to achieve adequate opioid- free postoperative pain control:

1. The patient must be provided adequate preoperative verbal and written education concerning the rationale for eliminating the use of opioids in the perioperative period.

2. The preoperative and intraoperative use of local anesthetic is strongly recommended.

3. Preoperative use of gabapentin and celecoxib (in appropriate-risk patients) is advised.

4. The practitioner should avoid intraoperative use of opioids to preserve the effects of endogenous beta-endorphins.

5. Avoidance of postoperative opioid use is strongly recommended.

(Stephan & Parsa, 2016)

Chapter 6: Healthy vs Unhealthy BMI

"Obesity loads the gun with more bullets when playing Russian roulette"

Obesity increases the risk of arterial and venous diseases. The incidence of coronary artery disease, congestive heart failure, stroke, atrial fibrillation, and deep venous thrombosis increase with increasing BMI. Significant weight loss improves both systolic and diastolic cardiac function, especially in patients with NYHA Class II/III heart failure (Blackburn Course in Obesity Medicine, 2014). Weight loss will improve the risk for initial or recurrent lower extremity DVT, improve claudication symptoms from peripheral arterial disease and reduce the risk for atrial fibrillation by improving obstructive sleep apnea (Blackburn Course in Obesity Medicine, 2014). Hypertension affects nearly one third of the American population with a higher prevalence among individuals with obesity. A patient with refractory rapid atrial fibrillation and obstructive sleep apnea who has failed multiple cardiac ablations could help himself by losing weight therefore decreasing his hypoxia at night and lessen the constant sympathetic discharge associated with hypoxia, hypertension, and arrhythmias. **A 10% weight reduction improves obstructive sleep apnea by 50%. Weight loss promotes so many positive benefits but one aspect that is probably overrated is blood pressure reduction.** The following is an excerpt from an editorial commentary by Lewis H. Kuller in Hypertension.

- Weight loss has been a recommended nonpharmacological therapy for reducing blood pressure levels for many years.
- Weight loss is not a very productive treatment or preventive treatment among most overweight and obese individuals.
- Clinical studies have not been impressive in weight loss reducing BP significantly along with the general unsuccessful nature of maintaining weight loss without regain.
- Eight clinical trials and eight cohort studies tried to evaluate the linear relationship between change in BP and weight change. Overall, there was only a 2.8 kg weight loss which resulted in a 1.9 mm decrease in DBP and 2.9 mm decrease for SBP, neither of which were significant.
- The most puzzling study has been the 8-year follow-up of the Swedish Obese Subjects study. 346 obese participants had gastric surgery to reduce obesity and were matched with 346 obese controls that did not have surgery. Over 8 years, there was no weight loss in the controls and a substantial 20.1 kg weight loss for surgical participants. There was no reduction in either the incidence of hypertension or BP levels over time between the 2 groups.
- The Diabetes Prevention Program showed a 5.6 kg weight loss in the diet arm, 2.1 kg loss in the metformin arm, and 0.1 kg in the placebo group. It showed a small 3.3 mm significant decrease in SBP and 3.1 mm of DBP in the diet arm over a 2.8-year follow-up among prediabetic patients with BMIs averaging 33.

In the **Women on The Move through Activity and Nutrition (WOMAN) Study**, there was a 17-lb weight loss at 18 months in the lifestyle group versus 3-lb in the control group. At 6 months, there was a significant 5-mm decrease in SBP between the 2 groups, but by 18 months this had dissipated and the difference in SBP was no longer significant. Even among a large number of women who lost more than 20-lb over 4 years, there was little evidence of a substantial decrease in SBP or DBP.

Weight loss in overweight and obese individuals to prevent elevated BP has been a nice recommendation that has been

around for 50 years but has had limited successful impact (Kuller, 2009).

Relationship to Cancer

- **The American Institute for Cancer Research reports that only half of all Americans are aware of the link between obesity and cancers. The following percentage of cancers are felt to be related to obesity; 38% breast cancer, 50% colon/rectal cancer, 69% throat cancer, 24% kidney cancers, and 19% pancreatic cancers.**
- As many as 84,000 cancer diagnoses each year are attributed to obesity, and overweight and obesity are implicated in 15 to 20 percent of total cancer-related mortality (Ligibel, et al., 2014).
- Obesity has been associated with greater risks of postmenopausal breast cancer and colon cancer and cancers of the prostate, kidney, pancreas, esophagus, gallbladder, and others.
- **More than 60 diseases and 12 cancers are associated with obesity.** Some of the diseases related to obesity include diabetes, hypertension, hyperlipidemia, obstructive sleep apnea, cancer, fatty liver, reflux, gout, depression, venous insufficiency/stasis, gallbladder disease, accelerated arthritis, asthma, pseudotumor cerebri, and unfortunately the social stigma from family, doctors and the general public.
- **Because of social stigma, many patients avoid routine preventative care and present with later stage diseases with end-organ damage and cancers at advanced non-curable stages. A good example is metastatic cervical cancer, a totally treatable condition if diagnosed before metastases occur.**
- Obese people worry if they will fit in conventional theater seats, airplane seats and even hospital diagnostic equipment. Radiology equipment, toilets, beds, wheelchairs, all have weight limits.
- **In radiology, fluoroscopy is limited to 350 lbs., MRI 350, CT scan 450, open MRI 550. Machines are limited by girth (diameter around the body) and weight.**

BMI and Heart Health

- **Although obesity rates reached epidemic proportions over the last two decades, presently the prevalence has reached a plateau at 35% except for class 3 obesity, (BMI of 40 or higher which translates to about one-hundred pounds' overweight), which has increased.**

- A study of patients with class 3 obesity indicated that this group had a STEMI (ST elevation myocardial infarction) at a younger age, age 55 compared to the typical age of 66 in normal weight patients. Despite this group having less extensive coronary artery disease and better ejection fractions, class 3 obesity (BMI 40 and greater) remained independently associated with higher in-hospital mortality. This study reviewed fifty thousand patients (Blackburn Course in Obesity Medicine, 2014).

- What is even more worrisome is the TEN-FOLD increase in people with BMIs greater than 50. This group has the highest morbidity/mortality and is the fastest growing group. Obesity rates are projected to double over the next 30 years worldwide. Unfortunately, the past projected rates over the last 20 years were accurate in obesity statistics. Will the new projections be just as accurate? Hopefully, we can change this (Das, et al., 2011).

Socioeconomics of BMI

- In the mid-1900s obesity in the United States and Europe was directly associated with income. Individuals with more income were more likely to be overweight or obese (Hruby & Hu, 2015). That relationship no longer holds.

- **Obesity disproportionately affects minorities, and people with low income and limited education. The obesity rates are 47.8% in blacks, 42.5% in Hispanics, 32.6% in whites and 10.8% in Asians. Black women suffer the highest rate at 54% with projections in 2030 of greater than 90% which is hard to believe** (Blackburn Course in Obesity Medicine, 2014).

- One in seven American households experience food insecurity at times during the year. Lack of money and other resources hinder their ability to maintain consistent access to nutritious foods. Food insecurity and obesity

78

continue to be strongly and positively associated in women (Franklin, et al., 2012).

BMI Implications for Children

- **Approximately 90% of children with severe obesity (BMI greater than 40) will become obese adults with a BMI of 35 or higher (Blackburn Course in Obesity Medicine, 2014). Trying to break the "obesity cycle" in families is crucial to prevent future morbidities.**

- In children, severe obesity is also defined as 120% above the age-specific 95th percentile of body-mass index (age-specific percentiles are used for children not BMI due to rapid growth patterns based on age). Obese children exhibit altered gait mechanics compared to healthy-weight children and have an increased prevalence of hip pain and pathology (Lerner & Browning, 2015).

- Obesity prevention in the first 1000 days after birth can lead to reduced incidence and prevalence of obesity (Mameli, Mazzantini, & Zuccotti, 2016). Human subjects that are purposely overfed differ markedly in their response to overfeeding. Despite markedly elevated body fat and elevated leptin levels subsequent food intake was stimulated rather than suppressed showing the inefficient response of in-built appetite control mechanisms in the modern environment when food is plentiful (Jebb, et al., 2006). Some people are compensators (responders) and some are not (non-responders) (Blackburn Course in Obesity Medicine, 2014). Remember, obesity is complicated.

BMI General Information

The diagram below defines weight with BMI. BMI has been endorsed by the National Heart, Lung, and Blood Institute, the World Health Organization, the American Heart Association, American College of Cardiology, and The Obesity Society.

Category ideal Weight	Body Mass Index (kg/m2)	Over
Underweight	less than 18.5	
Normal	18.5-24.9	
Overweight	25.0-29.9	BMI

27 equals 20% Above normal weight

Obesity (class 1)	30-34.9
Obesity (class 2)	35-39.9
Obesity (class 3)	40- higher
Super-Obesity	greater than 50

The body mass index (BMI) is a value derived from the weight and height of an individual. The BMI is the body mass divided by the square of the height, and is universally expressed in units of kg/m^2, with mass in kilograms and height in meters.

The BMI is an attempt to quantify the amount of tissue mass (muscle, fat, and bone) in an individual.

The basis of the BMI was published in 1842 by Adolphe Quetelet, a Belgian astronomer, mathematician, statistician and sociologist. The modern term "body mass index" (BMI) was coined in a paper published in the July 1972 edition of the Journal of Chronic Diseases by Ancel Keys (physiologist). Increasing obesity in prosperous Western societies sparked interest in a measure of body fat.

In Singapore, the BMI cut-off figures were revised in 2005, motivated by studies showing that many Asian populations, including Singaporeans, have higher proportion of body fat and increased risk for cardiovascular diseases and diabetes mellitus, compared with Caucasians at the same BMI. The BMI cut-offs are presented with an emphasis on health risk rather than weight in Singapore.

In 1998, the U.S. National Institutes of Health and the Centers for Disease Control and Prevention brought U.S. definitions in line with World Health Organization guidelines, lowering the normal/overweight cut-off from BMI 27.8 to BMI 25. This had the effect of redefining approximately 29 million Americans, previously healthy, to overweight.

This can partially explain the increase in the overweight diagnosis in the past 20 years, and the increase in sales of weight loss products during the same time.

In France, Israel, Italy and Spain, legislation has been introduced banning usage of fashion show models having a BMI below 18. In Israel, a BMI below 18.5 is banned. This is done in order to fight anorexia among models and people interested in fashion. **BMI generally overestimates adiposity on those with leaner body mass (e.g., athletes) and underestimates excess adiposity on those with less lean body mass (elderly).** BMI is particularly inaccurate for people who are very fit or athletic, as their high muscle mass can classify them in the overweight category by BMI, even though their body fat percentages frequently fall in the 10–15% category, which is below that of a more sedentary person of average build who has a normal BMI number. **It is not clear where on the BMI scale the threshold for overweight and obese should be set. Because of this the standards have varied over the past few decades.** Between 1980 and 2000 the U.S. Dietary Guidelines have defined overweight at a variety of levels ranging from a BMI of 24.9 to 27.1. In 1985 the National Institutes of Health (NIH) consensus conference recommended that overweight BMI be set at a BMI of 27.8 for men and 27.3 for women.

In 1998 a NIH report concluded that a BMI over 25 is overweight and a BMI over 30 is obese. In the 1990s the World Health Organization (WHO) decided that a BMI of 25 to 30 should be considered overweight and a BMI over 30 is obese, the same standards the NIH set. A 2010 study that followed 11,000 subjects for up to eight years concluded that BMI is not a good measure for the risk of heart attack, stroke or death. A better measure was found to be the waist-to-height ratio. A 2011 study that followed 60,000 participants for up to 13 years found that waist–hip ratio was a better predictor of ischemic heart disease mortality.

Waist circumference is a good indicator of visceral fat, which poses more health risks than fat elsewhere. According to the US National Institutes of Health (NIH), waist circumference in excess of 102 centimeters (40 in) for men and 88 centimeters (35 in) for (non-pregnant) women is considered

to infer a high risk for type 2 diabetes, dyslipidemia, hypertension, and CVD. Waist circumference can be a better indicator of obesity-related disease risk than BMI (Body Mass Index, n.d.).

Increased medical risk starts at a BMI above 25 but weight loss programs suggest treatment at a BMI of 27 which corresponds to 20% above desirable weight. **A BMI of 22 probably has the best medical/longevity statistics.** The lowest mortality rates worldwide are those with a BMI of 20-22. **The increased medical risk above a BMI of 25 goes back to 1983 Metropolitan Life Insurance data. Research shows reductions in blood pressure (probably overrated),** glucose control and lipids consistently occur with 5% weight loss making 5% the traditional minimum benchmark for success. Weight loss programs target poor food choices, overeating tendencies, overeating stimuli, increasing physical activity, and promoting a positive support structure. These lifestyle interventions usually achieve a 5-10% reduction. The type of diet needs to be catered to each individual. **Multiple studies comparing diets do not show one diet to be superior than any other. Unfortunately, the usual pattern of weight loss with lifestyle intervention is maximum weight loss at 6 months, followed by plateau and gradual regain over time. 80% of patients will initially lose at least 10% weight but more than 95% of patients will regain all the lost weight or more within the next 2-5 years (Blackburn Course in Obesity Medicine, 2014). Only 10-17% of patients maintain 10% weight loss after one year (Blackburn Course in Obesity Medicine, 2014).**

It is well-recognized that individuals in the same BMI category can have substantial heterogeneity of metabolic features, such as lipid profile, glucose tolerance, blood pressure and waist circumference. Researchers have questioned whether obese individuals with normal metabolic features despite their increased adiposity can be defined as having "benign obesity" or "metabolically healthy obesity." A 2013 study evaluated participants from eight studies looking at all-cause mortality, and/or cardiovascular events and BMI. Metabolically healthy obese individuals had increased risk for events compared with metabolically healthy normal-weight individuals only when studies with 10 or more years of follow-up were considered. All metabolically unhealthy groups had an elevated risk despite having normal weight, being overweight, or obese.

The study concluded that obese people compared with metabolically healthy normal-weight individuals are at increased risk for adverse long-term outcomes even in the absence of metabolic abnormalities, suggesting that there is no healthy pattern of increased weight. Although these clinical outcomes occurred only after long-term follow-up, it should be noted that, regardless of metabolic status, excess weight is associated in the short term with subclinical vascular disease, including impaired vasoreactivity, abnormalities in left ventricular measures, chronic inflammation, and increased carotid artery intima-media thickness and coronary calcification. (Kramer, Zinman, & Retnakaran, 2013). **The typical life-span for an NFL lineman is 55 years-old.**

An exception are overweight people greater than 70 years old with no chronic illnesses. The extra weight in this group is felt to be a sign of good health and they should not lose weight.

Reference Range Body Fat Percentage Chart (American Council on Exercise 2009).

Description	Men	Women
Essential fat	2-5%	10-13%
Athletes	6-13%	14-20%
Fitness	14-17%	21-24%
Average	18-24%	25-31%
Obese	25%+	32%+

Normal body mass index (BMI) can rule out metabolic syndrome: An Israeli cohort study.

- The aim of the study was to assess whether body mass index (BMI) can be used as a simple and reliable survey test for metabolic syndrome.
- The study is an observational cohort study among patients who visited the Rambam Periodic Examinations Institute (RPEI).

- During the study years, 23,993 patients visited the RPEI, and 12.5% of them fulfilled the criteria for metabolic syndrome.
- Women with metabolic syndrome had a higher proportion of obesity, when compared with men (89.9% vs 52.6%; P<.0001).
- Normal BMI had very high NPV (negative predictive value) to rule out metabolic syndrome among men and women (98% and 96%, respectively).
- A BMI of 27 was the ideal value for identification of patients at risk for metabolic syndrome for men and for women.
- BMI below 30 provided NPV of 91.1% to rule out metabolic syndrome.
- The BMI as single survey measurement of obesity offers high NPV for metabolic syndrome and can be used by physician and patients for this purpose. (Ofer, Ronit, Ophir, & Amir, 2019).

Health Effects of Overweight and Obesity in 195 Countries over 25 Years

- We analyzed data from 68.5 million persons to assess the trends in the prevalence of overweight and obesity among children and adults between 1980 and 2015 in 195 countries.
- In 2015, a total of 107.7 million children and 603.7 million adults were obese. Since 1980, the prevalence of obesity has doubled in more than 70 countries. More than two thirds of deaths related to high BMI were due to cardiovascular disease.
- The lowest overall risk of death was observed for a BMI of 20 to 25.
- The overall global prevalence of obesity was 5.0% among children (equal for boys and girls) and 12.0% among adults. Obesity was generally higher among women than among men in all age brackets

BURDEN OF DISEASE RELATED TO HIGH BMI (1990–2015)

- Cardiovascular disease was the leading cause of death and disability-adjusted life-years related to high BMI.
- Diabetes was the second leading cause of BMI-related deaths in 2015. Chronic kidney disease was the second leading cause of BMI-related disability-adjusted life-years in 2015
- Nearly 70% of the deaths that were related to high BMI were due to cardiovascular disease, and more than 60% of those deaths occurred among obese persons. A recent pooled cohort analysis involving 1.8 million participants showed that nearly half the excess risk for ischemic heart disease and more than 75% of the excess risk for stroke that was related to high BMI were mediated through a combination of raised levels of blood pressure, total serum cholesterol, and fasting plasma glucose.
- Recent evidence from a meta-analysis and pooled analysis of prospective observational studies showed a continuous increase in the risk of death associated with a BMI of more than 25.

Our systematic evaluation of prospective observational studies showed sufficient evidence supporting a causal relationship between high BMI and cancers of the esophagus, colon and rectum, liver, gallbladder and biliary tract, pancreas, breast, uterus, ovary, kidney, and thyroid, along with leukemia. (The GBD 2015 Obesity Collaborators, 2017).

A systematic review of the relationship between weight status perceptions and weight loss attempts, strategies, behaviours and outcomes

- It is commonly assumed that a person identifying that they are 'overweight' is an important prerequisite to successful weight management.
- The aim of the present research was to systematically review evidence on the relationship between perceived overweight and (i) weight loss attempts, (ii) weight control strategies (healthy and unhealthy), (iii) weight-related behaviours (physical activity and eating habits), (iv) disordered eating and (v) weight change.

- We synthesized evidence from 78 eligible studies between 1991 and 2017 using PubMed, PsycINFO, Nursing and Allied Health Literature databases.

Results indicated that perceived overweight people;

- Increased likelihood of attempting weight loss with healthy and unhealthy weight control strategies.
- Not reliably associated with physical activity or healthy eating.
- Greater disordered eating in some groups.
- Consistent evidence of weight gain over time.
- There is often a mismatch between the weight status a person believes they have and their objective weight status. Some people with a 'normal' or healthy weight mis-interpret their weight status as 'overweight.' More prevalent, however, is the tendency for individuals with overweight or obesity to underestimate their weight status and fail to identify their weight as being 'overweight'.
- A recent analysis of data from a nationally representative survey of UK adults revealed that approximately one-third of women and one half of men who are overweight failed to identify themselves as such, and similar rates have been reported in adolescents
- Overweight and obesity are widely stigmatized. Perceiving oneself as belonging to a stigmatized group can bring psychological distress and associated negative health consequences. Individuals experience higher levels of body dissatisfaction and may thus have a more extreme desire to lose weight than individuals who do not identify as overweight. It has been associated with extreme weight management strategies such as vomiting and laxative use. Such behaviours can compromise health and lead to disordered eating.
- No evidence to suggest that overweight individuals were actually more likely to enact these behaviours than those who did not identify as overweight. For example, a fear of negative evaluation may make exercising in public unappealing.

- These findings challenge the common assumption that identifying oneself as overweight will be associated with better weight management.
- Despite greater self-reported attempts to lose weight, individuals who may not effectively translate their weight loss intentions into effective weight loss behaviours. This intention–behaviour gap is well-recognized in health psychology. Weight stigma has also been shown to encourage binge eating and overconsumption of unhealthy snack foods.

Some public health approaches are based on the assumption that notifying individuals that they are overweight is necessary to motivate them to adopt healthy behaviours and lose weight, but the evidence reviewed here does not support this proposition. (Haynes, Kersbergen, Sutin, Daly, & Robinson, 2018).

Obesity and the lungs: Not just a crush

- Asthma is not a single simple condition of allergic inflammation driving airway narrowing.
- **Obese asthmatic patients have more symptoms and poorer response to treatment than their non-obese counterparts.**
- Obesity compresses lung volume, thus causing airway narrowing[1] and closure[2] and may be one possible mechanism that explains the high prevalence of wheeze in obese subjects that is not necessarily associated with airway hyper-responsiveness (AHR).
- It is understandable that many obese individuals may be treated for asthma based on wheeze and breathlessness, which are prominent symptoms in obesity, even though they may not have airway hyper-responsiveness (asthma).
- Reduced lung volumes in obesity reduce the forces that distend the airway, which in turn decreases airway caliber and permits airway closure. Hence, there is more airway closure in obese individuals during normal breathing.
- In describing the phenomenon of airway closure over 50 years ago, Milic-Emili *et al.* suggested that repeated

closure of small airways during tidal breathing may cause trauma leading to inflammation and remodeling.

- **Obesity alters the nature of bronchoconstriction, with more expiratory flow limitation, airway closure, hyperinflation and more intense symptoms.**
- Airway closure is an obesity-specific response to bronchoconstriction, which is independent of the presence or absence of asthma and is based on abnormal small airway function (King & Thamrin, 2019).

Daily self-weighing and weight gain prevention: a longitudinal study of college-aged women.

- Daily self-weighing has been suggested as an important factor for weight loss maintenance among samples with obesity. This study examined daily self-weighing in association with weight and body composition outcomes over 2 years among young women with vulnerability for weight gain.
- Women (N = 294) of varying weight status completed self-weighing frequency questionnaires and weight was measured in the clinic at baseline, 6 months, 1, and 2 years.
- Daily self-weighing was associated with significant declines in BMI and body fat percent over time (Rosenbaum, Espel, Butryn, Zhang, & Lowe, 2017).

Addictive Eating and Its Relation to Physical Activity and Sleep Behavior

- Addictive eating, physical activity, and sleep behaviors have all been independently associated with obesity.
- This study aims to investigate the relationship between food addiction with physical activity and sleep behavior.
- Australian adults were invited to complete an online survey.
- The sample comprised 1344 individuals with a mean age of 39.8 ± 13.1 years (range 18–91), of which 75.7% were female.
- Twenty-two percent of the sample met the criteria for a diagnosis of food addiction as per the Yale Food Addiction

Scale (YFAS 2.0) criteria, consisting of 0.7% with a "mild" addiction, 2.6% "moderate", and 18.9% classified as having a "severe" food addiction. Food-addicted individuals had significantly less physical activity (1.8 less occasions walking/week, 32 min less walking/week, 58 min less moderate to vigorous physical activity (MVPA)/week; $p <$ 0.05), reported sitting for longer on weekends (83 min more on weekends/week; $p < 0.001$), and reported significantly more symptoms of poorer-quality sleep (more likely to snore, more likely to have fallen asleep while driving, reported more days of daytime falling asleep; $p <$ 0.05) compared to non-food-addicted individuals.

- These differences were also observed in those with a "severe" food addiction classification.
- The present study suggests frequency and duration of physical activity, time spent sitting and sleep duration are associated with food addiction (Li, Pursey, Duncan, & Burrows, 2018).

Metabolic consequences of overfeeding in humans.
Overfeeding leads to obesity and a plethora of metabolic conditions. The consequences of standardized overfeeding on body weight shows considerable interindividual variability, which suggests different adaptive changes in some individuals.

Recent Findings:
Individuals who gain less body weight during overfeeding are those who experience a greater increase in total energy expenditure. This increase in energy expenditure has been attributed to stimulation of non-exercise physical activity (NEAT- nonexercised activity thermogenesis). Overfeeding also alters the compensatory pathways depending on if the overfeeding is mostly carbohydrate or fat based. The sympathetic nervous system and endocrine system are prime candidates for energy expenditure increase during overfeeding.

Summary:
The mechanisms by which some individuals protect themselves against body weight gain remain poorly understood. Nonvoluntary physical activity may allow one to increase energy expenditure during overfeeding and may therefore

constitute a regulatory factor in body weight control. **This article provides input on how genetics may predispose some people to have better adaptive processes than others with overfeeding** (Tappy, 2004).

Weight Stigma in Men: What, When, and by Whom?

This study assessed the weight stigma experiences of some men.

Methods:

Data from three samples of men were examined (N = 1,513). Sample 1 consisted of men with obesity at elevated risk for weight stigma. Sample 2 comprised a convenience online panel. Sample 3 included men from a national online panel of US adults. Men in all samples completed almost identical questionnaires assessing demographics, anthropometrics, weight stigma, and dieting.

Results:

Approximately 40% of men reported experiencing weight stigma. Weight stigma was associated with increased odds of having a BMI consistent with underweight or obesity relative to normal weight. Verbal mistreatment was the most common form of weight stigma experienced across all life stages for men. The most common sources of weight stigma were peers, family members, and strangers. Men reporting weight stigma were younger and less likely to be married, had higher BMIs, and were more likely to have tried to lose weight in the past year relative to men not reporting weight stigma.

Conclusions:

Understanding differences among men as a function of weight stigma is important for practitioners, as it can identify men who may most benefit from intervention (Himmelstein, Puhl, & Quinn, 2018).

The Risks Associated with Obesity in Pregnancy.

Approximately one-third of all women of childbearing age are overweight or obese. For these women, pregnancy is associated with increased risks for both mother and child.

Methods:

This review is based on PubMed search with special attention to current population-based cohort studies, systematic reviews, meta-analyses, and controlled trials.

Results:

- Obesity in pregnancy is associated with unfavorable clinical outcomes for both mother and child.

- Many of the risks have been found to depend linearly on the body-mass index (BMI). The probability of conception declines linearly, starting from a BMI of 29 kg/m2, by 4% for each additional 1 kg/m2 of BMI.

- A 10% increase of pre-gravid BMI increases the relative risk of gestational diabetes and that of preeclampsia by approximately 10% each.

- An estimated 11% of all neonatal deaths can be attributed to the consequences of maternal overweight and obesity.

Conclusion:

Preventive measures aimed at normalizing body weight before a woman becomes pregnant are, therefore, all the more important (Stubert, Reister, Hartmann, & Janni, 2018).

Body mass index and fatal stroke in young adults: A national study.

- Rates of stroke and obesity have increased in recent years. This study aimed to determine the body mass index (BMI) of fatal stroke cases amongst young adults, their clinical characteristics and the association with BMI with risk factors.

- All cases aged 15-44 years where death was attributed to stroke for whom BMI was available were retrieved from the National Coronial Information System (1/1/2009-31/12/2016).

- 179 cases were identified: haemorrhagic (165), ischaemic (5), thrombotic (6), mycotic (3), embolic (0).

- Proportions in each BMI category were underweight (5.6%), normal weight (37.4%), overweight (27.4%), obese (29.6%).

- There was a significant linear trend in the proportion of subarachnoid haemorrhages as BMI increased (p < 0.05), and between higher BMI and hypertension (p < 0.001).
- Overweight and obese cases were prominent among young fatalities of stroke. Reducing rates of obesity, and associated hypertension, would be expected to reduce the escalating stoke rates among young adult (Darke, Duflou, Kaye, Farrell, & Lappin, 2019).

Interaction of obesity and atrial fibrillation: an overview of pathophysiology and clinical management.

- Obesity, defined as a Body Mass Index (BMI) of ≥30 kg/m2, is the most common chronic metabolic disease worldwide and its prevalence has been strongly increasing.
- Obesity is associated with an increase in atrial fibrillation (AF), the most common arrhythmia in clinical practice. AF is associated with increased cardiovascular morbidity and mortality.
- Obesity, a novel risk factor, is responsible for a 50%-increased incidence of AF.

Expert opinion:
    Cardiac arrhythmias, in particular, AF, are common in patients with obesity. In recent literature, there has been increased interest in the role of epicardial adipose tissue and structural remodeling in obese hearts. (Pouwels, et al., 2019).

Chapter 7: The Roaring Twenties

"There is nothing so tragic on earth as the sight of a fat man eating a potato."

The following article shows tremendous insight and is medically correct despite being written almost a hundred years ago. Of course, the descriptions are politically-incorrect today. A wonderful 1926 editorial in The Canadian Medical Association Journal entitled "THE MENACE OF OBESITY" discusses 2 articles in the British Journal Lancet (September 4, 1926, p. 508). The first is an article on the elements of longevity, "attention is called to the unfavorable experience of thirty-four American life insurance companies regarding the lives of those in whom the circumference of the abdomen exceeds that of the chest, but adds that even here a hereditary tendency to longevity is the ruling factor, for corpulent descendants of long-lived parents have, as a rule, a normal expectancy of life" (genetics vs environment principle). In an issue only one week later (September 11, 1926), it refers to investigations that carried out on an extensive scale in America, which show that "**the optimum weight for men of forty-five years is about twenty pounds less than the accepted average weight for that age; and that the steady decline in physical efficiency, which the carrying of twenty pounds of superfluous matter entails, should in itself be a sufficient check on the dangerous self-complacence with which the middle aged man views an increase in his girth.**"

Obesity: A Clinical Review

In an editorial in 1926 on the subject of obesity it calls attention to Dr. Leonard Williams recent book on "Obesity." This writer states that the infiltration of fat into the subcutaneous tissues frequently results in a raised blood pressure from increased peripheral resistance, and against this high blood pressure a heart embarrassed both on its surface and throughout its musculature has to work with diminished efficiency. Renal disease, it is stated, frequently follows such a condition of affairs, and it is not surprising to learn that the mortality from cardiac and renal diseases among the obese is twice as high as in persons of normal weight. As an additional warning to the obese it is stated that such a diseased heart may give rise to very little in the way of symptoms, and nothing in the way of local physical signs; yet, as Dr. Williams emphasizes, **"the fat man dies the next time he hurries to catch a train."** Obesity does not stop at producing disturbances of the circulatory system.; the respiratory system may also suffer, and not a few asthmatics may be greatly relieved by cutting down their weight. Among other disadvantages, troublesome forms of dyspepsia may result from overweight and an invasion of the liver by fat elements increases such troubles leading probably to the form of diabetes associated with obesity. **"The cure of obesity is largely bound up with the cure of its causation."** Perhaps the most striking advance on the subject within recent times has been the proven complicity in some cases of endocrine insufficiency leading to the broad classification of obesity into that caused by alimentary surfeit (i.e. overindulgence), and that caused by deficient activity of one or more of the endocrine glands.

Nevertheless, **it would appear that most of the obesity commonly seen is due to overfeeding.** "To the scientist," wrote Vance Thompson, **"there is nothing so tragic on earth as the sight of a fat man eating a potato."** The starchy carbohydrate foods rather than the more quickly metabolized fats are responsible for much of the alimentary type of obesity. A more rational diet will go a long way in preventing this troublesome complaint. Muscular exercise, fasting, the use of thyroid extract and special diets such as that associated with the name of William Banting. **It would appear that often the influence of race and heredity have a still more powerful influence. Certain, however, it is that obesity is a serious menace to health, and one which requires the attention of the profession.**

Chapter 7: The Roaring Twenties

The 1926 article does a fine job at discussing genetics as a role player and how obesity or simply being overweight 20 pounds can be detrimental to many organ systems. William Banting was a famous undertaker for the British royalty who followed a diet prescribed to him by Dr William Harvey and wrote a booklet describing his past struggles and failures only to be successful by following a low carbohydrate diet. His 1863 booklet is called "Letter on Corpulence, Addressed to the Public." He is described as "The Father of the Low-Carbohydrate Diet." William Banting was a distant relative of Sir Frederick Banting, the co-discovery of insulin. (Howell, 1926). Genetics or coincidence, you make the call?

Chapter 8: The Soda question? (not completely answered).

Remember the 1975 Pepsi challenge comparing Pepsi versus Coke. This was not very good science since most people generally prefer the sweeter of two beverages based on a single sip, even if they prefer a less sweet beverage over the course of an entire can. The soda question depends on whether you are looking at it as a tool to decrease calories or whether you are looking at it in a more general effect. It reminds me of the Yogi Berra quote "He hits from both sides of the plate. He's amphibious."

The "soda question" goes like this; high fructose corn syrup used in sodas is metabolized in the liver and stimulates a CNS pleasure center and indirectly stimulates starvation pathway signals which leads to increased food consumption. Diet soda using non-nutrient sweeteners promotes weight gain indirectly. Diet drinks increase the risk for diabetes type 2, metabolic syndrome and thus heart disease. They double the risk for going from normal weight to overweight and overweight to obesity. The sweet taste increases appetite despite lack of calories. **Artificial sweeteners do not give a satiety signal to the brain.** The epidemic of obesity has coincided with the introduction of non-caloric sweeteners. **A large study in the journal Circulation followed 9,000 people for several years who drank more than one soda per day, diet or regular. They had an increased risk of metabolic syndrome.** Soda is one of many variables contributing to the obesity epidemic (Dhingra, et al., 2007).

Daily Intake of Sugar-Sweetened Beverages Among US Adults in 9 States, by State and Sociodemographic and Behavioral Characteristics, 2016.

- Examined associations between sugar-sweetened beverage (SSB) intake - a chronic disease risk factor - and characteristics of 75,029 adults ($\geq$18 y) in 9 states by using 2016 Behavioral Risk Factor Surveillance System (BRFSS) data.
- SSB intake were categorized as none (reference), fewer than 1 time per day, and 1 or more times per day, by sociodemographic and behavioral characteristics.
- Overall, 32.1% of respondents drank SSBs 1 or more times per day.
- Found higher odds for 1 or more times per day among younger respondents, men, Hispanic and non-Hispanic black respondents, current smokers, respondents residing in nonmetropolitan counties, employed respondents, and those with less than high school education, obesity, and no physical activity. Findings can inform the targeting of efforts to reduce SSB consumption (Lundeen, Park, Pan & Blanck, 2018)

Association Between Artificially Sweetened Beverage Consumption During Pregnancy and Infant Body Mass Index.

- This cohort study included 3,033 mother-infant pairs from the Canadian Healthy Infant Longitudinal Development (CHILD) Study.
- Women completed dietary assessments during pregnancy, and their infants' BMI was measured at 1 year of age (n = 2686; 89% follow-up).
- Maternal consumption of artificially sweetened beverages and sugar-sweetened beverages during pregnancy were tracked.
- The mean (SD) age was 32.4 years, and their mean (SD) BMI was 24.8.

- Compared with no consumption, daily consumption of artificially sweetened beverages was associated with 2-fold higher risk of infant overweight at 1 year of age.
- These effects were not explained by maternal BMI, diet quality, total energy intake, or other obesity risk factors.
- To our knowledge, we provide the first human evidence that maternal consumption of artificial sweeteners during pregnancy may influence infant BMI (Azad, et al., 2016).

Nonnutritive Sweeteners in Weight Management and Chronic Disease: A Review

- The objective of this review was to critically review findings from recent studies evaluating the effects of nonnutritive sweeteners (NNSs) on metabolism, weight, and obesity-related chronic diseases.
- NNS consumption is associated with higher body weight and metabolic disease in observational studies.
- Randomized controlled trials demonstrate that NNSs may support weight loss, particularly when used alongside behavioral weight loss support.

Introduction

- The 2015 Dietary Guidelines for Americans recommend limiting added sugar to less than 10% of total energy intake, and similar guidance has been put forth by the World Health Organization.
- Considerable pressure has been placed on the food industry to reformulate its products to lower sugar content and provide reduced-calorie alternatives.
- One strategy is to substitute nonnutritive sweeteners (NNSs) for added sugars, as NNSs are highly sweet and palatable but contain no or few calories.
- Until recently, NNSs were found primarily in beverages (e.g., diet sodas) and in sweetener packets (e.g., Equal, Sweet' N Low, Splenda), but they are now widespread in the food supply, including in condiments, reduced-calorie desserts and yogurts, cereals, snack foods, medications, and hygiene products.

- We recently demonstrated that consumption of NNSs increased by approximately 200% among children and adolescents from 1999 to 2000, yet whether NNSs are helpful or harmful for weight management.

Recommendations

- Despite widespread and increasing consumption of NNSs, dietary recommendations for their consumption are inconsistent across different health organizations and are often inconclusive.

- For example, the 2015 Dietary Guidelines Advisory Committee scientific report stated, "added sugars should be reduced in the diet and not replaced with low-calorie [nonnutritive] sweeteners, but rather with healthy options, such as water in place of sugar-sweetened beverages."

- A joint position statement from the American Diabetes Association and American Heart Association also urged caution in the use of NNSs, stating that "at this time, there are insufficient data to determine conclusively whether the use of NNS to displace caloric sweeteners in beverages and foods reduces added sugars or carbohydrate intakes, or benefits appetite, energy balance, body weight, or cardiometabolic risk factors".

Observational Studies

- In 2008, Fowler et al. reported a dose-response relationship between baseline consumption of NNS-containing diet beverages and weight gain 7 to 8 years later. Compared with non-consumers, participants who reported drinking diet beverages were more likely to gain weight over time, even after adjustment for baseline BMI. Interestingly, total daily energy intakes were lower among diet beverage consumers, despite increased weight gain. This phenomenon has been observed in several other studies, suggesting that NNSs may influence body weight via mechanisms independent of increasing energy intake.

- The same group reported that NNS use in the form of diet beverages was associated with greater visceral adiposity after 9 to 10 years of follow-up, independent of baseline BMI and with minimal changes in body weight.

- Results of epidemiologic studies evaluating whether NNS use is associated with a healthier or less healthy overall dietary pattern have been mixed.
- Positive associations between NNS use, type 2 diabetes, metabolic syndrome, cardiovascular disease, and nonalcoholic fatty liver disease have also been observed in longitudinal analyses among adults. O'Connor et al. reported a 22% higher incidence of diabetes among NNS consumers.
- Positive associations between NNSs and other unfavorable health outcomes in longitudinal analyses have been further detailed in recent systematic reviews.
- While well established in adults, limited data on the associations among NNSs, weight, and chronic disease are available in children. However, an emerging body of observational literature suggests that maternal ingestion of diet beverages during pregnancy may increase obesity risk in children. Associations between maternal NNS consumption and infant weight have been recently reported by two independent groups and remained statistically significant after adjustment for confounders, including maternal body weight, calorie intake, diet quality, physical activity, and sociodemographic characteristics. A third group conducted a similar analysis but did not observe differences in child weight at 7 years of age based on maternal NNS consumption.

Proposed Mechanisms Linking NNSs to Weight and Health Outcomes

- Individuals who are already overweight or at risk for diabetes or related diseases may use NNSs to manage their weight or delay disease onset.

Sweet taste receptors

- Sweet tasting compounds, including caloric sugars (e.g., sucrose, fructose), NNSs (e.g., sucralose, aspartame), and sweet proteins (e.g., thaumatin), activate the heterodimeric sweet taste receptor T1R2/T1R3. Although once believed to be present exclusively in the oral cavity, sweet taste receptors have recently been located throughout the body. Whereas sweet taste receptor activation on taste buds triggers the release of neurotransmitters to convey

101

sweetness to the brain, activation of sweet taste receptors extra-orally exerts different downstream effects, only some of which are currently understood.

Disturbance of relationship between sweetness and calories

- Evolutionarily, sweet taste was indicative of calories and nutrients (e.g., fruit), yet this is not the case for NNSs. It has therefore been hypothesized that the sensation of sweetness without the delivery of calories may result in a disturbance of appetite regulation and impaired metabolic signaling.

Alterations in gut microbiota

- NNSs influence the microbial composition of the oral mucosa, and they are viewed positively by the dental community. *In vitro* studies have demonstrated that NNSs, including aspartame, saccharin, and sucralose, have antimicrobial activity against common periodontal pathogens.

- Experimental evidence for NNS-induced alterations in gut microbiota in humans is limited.

Changes in taste preferences

- NNSs are potently sweet at low concentrations, and relative to caloric sugars, they are hundreds or thousands of times sweeter by weight, depending on the specific compound. Aspartame, for example, is 200 times more potent than sucrose, and sucralose is 600 times sweeter, yet advantame, the most recently approved NNS in the United States, is approximately 20,000 times sweeter than sucrose by weight

- Given the innate liking for sweetness, it has been hypothesized that exposure to sweet compounds, particularly early in life, may promote a higher preference for sweet taste. Many highly sweet foods and beverages are also high in calories (e.g., brownies, cookies), and thus, enhanced sweetness preference may promote poor dietary patterns, positive energy balance, and ultimately obesity. However, as previously discussed, cross-sectional findings linking NNSs to dietary patterns have been mixed.

- Analogous results were found in children who were given sugar-sweetened water in infancy. Epidemiologic findings linking NNS consumption to overall dietary patterns in adults are mixed and have not been investigated in children.

Human Intervention Studies

- In contrast to the epidemiologic literature, the majority of human intervention studies suggest neutral or beneficial effects of low-calorie sweetener use for weight management.
- Findings are less conclusive when NNSs are compared with water or unsweetened controls.
- The administration of diet beverages led to both significantly greater weight loss during the intervention as well as to less subsequent weight regain during the maintenance period. Both studies were conducted in the context of behavioral weight loss support, which may not reflect typical NNS use in the general population.
- Maersk et al. compared consumption of aspartame/sweetened beverages with sugar/sweetened beverages, isocaloric milk, and water. Aspartame/sweetened beverages, milk, and water all lowered liver fat, visceral adiposity, triglycerides, fasting glucose, fasting insulin, and the homeostatic model assessment of insulin resistance relative to sugar-sweetened beverages, with similar reductions in the aspartame and water groups.
- Several studies have administered high doses of encapsulated aspartame to individuals with diabetes, with no adverse effects on glycemia. Similar findings were reported in individuals with diabetes after high-dose encapsulated sucralose.

Discussion

- Human randomized controlled trials suggest that NNSs may be a useful, or at least neutral, tool for weight management, particularly when used by individuals cognitively engaged in weight loss and who habitually consume NNSs. Given the discrepancies in the available evidence, the extent to which NNSs are helpful or harmful for weight management and chronic disease prevention warrants further study

- It is also important to determine whether the intense sweetness contributed by adding NNSs to foods and beverages leads to heightened expectations for sweetness throughout the diet.

Conclusion

- Consumption of NNSs is associated with a variety of unfavorable metabolic and health outcomes in observational studies, yet intervention trials demonstrate that NNSs may benefit weight management, specifically when used in the context of calorie restriction and intentional weight loss (Sylvetsky & Rother, 2018).

Low/No calorie sweetened beverage consumption in the National Weight Control Registry.

- The aim of this cross-sectional study was to evaluate prevalence of and strategies behind low/no calorie sweetened beverage (LNCSB) consumption in successful weight loss maintainers.
- An online survey was administered to 434 members of the National Weight Control Registry (NWCR, individuals who have lost ≥13.6 kg and maintained weight loss for > 1 year).

Results:

- While few participants (10%) consume sugar-sweetened beverages on a regular basis, 53% regularly consume LNCSB.
- The top five reasons for choosing LNCSB were for taste (54%), to satisfy thirst (40%), part of routine (27%), to reduce calories (22%) and to go with meals (21%). The majority who consume LNCSB (78%) felt they helped control total calorie intake. Many participants considered changing patterns of beverage consumption to be very important in weight loss (42%) and maintenance (40%). Increasing water was by far the most common strategy, followed by reducing regular calorie beverages.

Conclusions:

Regular consumption of LNCSB is common in successful weight loss maintainers for various reasons including helping individuals to limit total energy intake. Changing beverage consumption patterns was felt to be very important for weight

Chapter 8: The Soda question? (not completely answered).

loss and maintenance by a substantial percentage of successful weight loss maintainers in the NWCR (Catenacci, et al., 2014).

Chapter 9: Diets

"You better cut the pizza in four pieces because I'm not hungry enough to eat six" Yogi Berra

What is the best diet? Every year diet books are routinely on the bestseller list, yet the clear majority of diets are not successful. A systematic review of major commercial weight loss programs in the United States by Adam Gilden Tsai MD, and Thomas Wadden, PhD in the Annals of Internal Medicine in 2005 concluded with the exception of one trial of Weight Watchers, **the evidence to support the use of the major commercial and self-help weight loss programs is suboptimal** (Tsai AG, 2005).

Four popular weight loss diets include Adkins, South Beach, the Zone diet, and Weight Watchers. They produce at best only modest long-term benefits, with few differences across the four. Weight loss at 1 year is modest at 1.7-12 lbs. Longer term data out to 2 years, indicated that some of the lost weight was regained over time. Controlled trials are needed to assess the efficacy and cost-effectiveness of these interventions. **The advertising claims of commercial programs are monitored by the Federal Trade Commission rather than the US Food and Drug Administration**. Programs are not required to submit data on safety or efficacy. Programs can be divided into:

Nonmedical commercial weight loss programs such as Weight Watchers, Jenny Craig and L.A. Weight Loss. Participants in Weight Watchers lost 5.3% of their initial weight at 1 year and maintained a loss of 3.2% at 2 years, compared with 1.5% of their initial weight at 1 year and 0% at 2 years who received self-help intervention. Weight Watchers is $12 per week and Jenny Craig's prepackaged meals ($70 to $100) make it expensive.

Ineffectiveness of commercial weight-loss programs for achieving modest but meaningful weight loss: Systematic review and meta-analysis.

This study collates existing evidence regarding weight loss among overweight but otherwise healthy adults who use commercial weight-loss programs.

- Systematic search of 3 databases identified 11 randomized controlled trials and 14 observational studies of commercial meal-replacement, calorie-counting, or pre-packaged meal programs which met inclusion criteria.
- In meta-analysis using intention-to-treat data, 57 percent of individuals who commenced a commercial weight program lost less than 5 percent of their initial body weight.
- One in two (49%) studies reported attrition ≥30 percent.
- A second meta-analysis found that 37 percent of program completers lost less than 5 percent of initial body weight.
- **We conclude that commercial weight-loss programs frequently fail to produce modest but clinically meaningful weight loss with high rates of attrition suggesting that many consumers find dietary changes required by these programs unsustainable.**

(McEvedy, Sullivan-Mort, McLean, Pascoe & Paxton, 2017)

Levels of adherence needed to achieve significant weight loss.

- Positive associations have been found between adherence and weight loss in behavioral weight-management interventions.
- This study examined the levels of adherence associated with a ≥ 5% - < 10% or ≥ 10% weight loss in Weight Watchers® (WW), which included three modes of access: (1) 24-weekly WW meetings over 6 months, (2) the WW member website, and (3) the WW mobile application.

Methods:

- A total of 292 participants were randomized to a WW (n = 147) or a self-help (SH) (n = 145) condition. To assess the impact of adherence, only participants in the WW condition were included in analyses (n = 147).

Results:

- In a 6-month period, increased likelihood of achieving a weight loss ≥ 5% - < 10% was associated with attending approximately one-third (35.4%) of weekly meetings, use of the member website about 25% of days, and use of the mobile application 16.1% of days.
- Attendance at approximately two-thirds (64.5%) of meetings, use of the member website 41.6% of days, and use of the mobile application 14.7% of days were associated with a clinically significant weight loss of ≥ 10%. Meeting attendance was the strongest predictor of weight loss at 6 months.

Conclusion:

- Although adherence was an important predictor of weight loss, extremely high levels were not needed to achieve clinically significant weight loss. Johnston, et al., 2019). **The study was sponsored by Weight Watchers.**

Randomized Controlled Trial Examining the Ripple Effect of a Nationally Available Weight Management Program on Untreated Spouses.

- Weight within couples is highly interdependent. Spouses often enter marriage at a similar weight status and mirror each other's weight trajectories over time. In a landmark study establishing the spread of obesity in social networks such as friendships and marriages, Christakis and Fowler found that when one spouse develops obesity, the likelihood of the other spouse developing obesity increases by 37%. There is also converging evidence that weight loss can spread within couples, a phenomenon referred to as a ripple effect.
- For married couples, when one spouse participates in weight loss treatment, the untreated spouse can also experience weight loss. This study examined this ripple effect.

Methods

- One hundred thirty couples were randomized to Weight Watchers (WW; $n = 65$) or to a self-guided control group (SG; $n = 65$) and assessed at 0, 3, and 6 months.
- Inclusion criteria were age $\geq$ 25 years, BMI 27 to 40 kg/m^2 ($\geq$ 25 kg/m^2 for untreated spouses), and no weight loss contraindications.
- WW participants received 6 months of free access to in-person meetings and online tools. SG participants received a weight loss handout. Spouses did not receive treatment.

Results

- Untreated spouses lost a small non-significant amount of weight at 3 months and 6 months and did not differ by condition.

Conclusions

- Evidence of a small ripple effect was found in untreated spouses in both formal and self-guided weight management approaches. (Gorin, et al., 2018).
- **This work was supported by Weight Watchers International, Inc.**

Medically Supervised Proprietary Programs such as OPTIFAST, Health Management Resources, and MEDIFAST. Offer a 3-phase meal replacement program consisting of 12-18 weeks of rapid weight loss, a 3-8-week transition phase, and long-term maintenance. Both OPTIFAST and Health Management Resources provide mandatory medical monitoring during the first 2 phases whereas MEDIFAST does not require written documentation of medical monitoring for clients to purchase its meal replacement. OPTIFAST and Health Management Resources are both expensive at $1700 to $2200 for the first 3 months. MEDIFAST is only $840 because of its lack of mandatory medical monitoring (Tsai AG, 2005). **Serious complications, including death, have been reported in obese persons who consumed very-low-calorie diets (800 kcals/day or less) without medical supervision. Medical supervision is critical to the safe use of very-low-calorie diets.**

A few definitions and principles of dieting:

1. 10-400 kcals/day-starvation diet
2. 400-800 kcals VLCD (very low-calorie diet)
3. 800-1500 kcals LCD (low calorie diet)
4. Above 1500 BDD (balanced deficit diet, desire to reduce kcals by 500-1000 kcals per day)
5. **A 500-kcal deficit per day will result in a pound weight loss per week since 3,500 kcals equals one pound.**
6. **Combining LCD (low calorie diet) with exercise produces greater weight loss, 10-15% more than LCD alone. Frequent monitoring of weight, consistent eating patterns, journaling food are very helpful.**
7. NWCR (National Weight Control Registry)-largest prospective observational study of individuals who have maintained a weight loss of at least 30 pounds for at least one year. Currently 10,000 individuals over ten years. Positive behaviors-75% weigh themselves once a week, 62% watch less than 10 hours of TV per week, 90% exercise about 80 minutes per day, 76.6% walk.
8. **People underestimate calories by 33%, overestimate physical activity by 50% (Blackburn Course in Obesity Medicine, 2014).**
9. A ketogenic diet results from varying combinations of calorie and carbohydrate restriction that induce the body to make ketones from fat to feed the brain. Any diet with less than 200 kcals of carbohydrates per day is ketogenic. Dietary protein reduces ketones somewhat. Dietary fat intake has little to no effect on ketones.
10. Dietary fiber is thought to be inversely related to weight gain. Fiber may help to reduce insulin secretion and increase satiety. Carb/fiber ratio, the smaller the better. Avoid 10/1, less than 10/1 good, best if less than 5/1 (Blackburn Course in Obesity Medicine, 2014).

Common Myths About Dieting

1. Small sustained changes in energy intake or expenditure will produce large long-term weight changes. Small changes produce small results plus our bodies adapt to change and we live in a dynamic, not static, system. Essentially you get what you put in. Baby-steps is a great principle but it is just a starting point that needs to be ramped up repeatedly to

succeed. A marathon runner can start training at one mile but needs to increase his training substantially to run 26.2 miles.

2. Setting realistic goals for weight loss is important, otherwise patients get frustrated and will not lose the weight. Empirical data indicates no consistent negative association between ambitious goals and program completion.

3. Large rapid weight loss is associated with poorer long-term weight outcomes than is slow gradual weight loss. It's all about kcals eaten versus burned, that's the deciding factor.

4. Physical education classes play an important role in reducing childhood obesity (Diets are the key). It is true that participation in sports is inversely related to overweight/obesity in children and adolescents.

5. Breast-feeding is protective against obesity (sorry mom).

6. Sexual activity burns 100-300 kcals (sorry only 14 kcals).

A 2007 article in Obesity Reviews by A.J. Hill commented on the concern and influence of the weight-loss industry. **Quick-fix products and diet plans are usually quackery and promise consumers what they want to hear: fast and effortless permanent weight loss. The damage is huge.** Failure to lose weight leads customers to blame themselves rather than the ineffectiveness of the product. A history of failures leads to giving up all together. Unlike pharmaceuticals, diet products do not have to prove their effectiveness. They do not show objective data and rely on personal or celebrity testimony to encourage people to spend their money and ultimately give up hope. For a diet to succeed it must be low in energy (low calories) (Hill, 2007). **Whether the diet is low fat, low carbs, high protein, high carbs has been shown in multiple studies to not be the key component.** There is no necessity for carbohydrates in the human diet because metabolic pathways exist within the body to remove energy from dietary protein and fat. The human body does need fat and protein to survive. **The idea of promising consumers quick fixes and promises is not new. An article April 8, 1911 in the British Medical Journal advertises the results of analyses of medicines for the reduction of obesity that stresses "My treatment allows you to eat what you like and drink what you like, without starvation diet or tiresome exercises."**

A dangerous practice is the "hCG diet." In a 2016 review, Doctors Butler and Cole stated: **"**Trend diets can be commonplace amongst those who are trying to lose weight, but in most cases, there is some shred of evidence to suggest they might be of some benefit. Seldom is there a diet which is such a fad that it is not only completely unfounded but also potential harmful. **The human chorionic gonadotropin or "hCG diet" is such a diet, which after half a century still has no evidence to support its efficacy: in fact, all scientific publications subsequent to the original article counter these claims."** (Butler & Cole, 2016)

The case report by Pektezel et al. **Paradoxical consequences of human chorionic gonadotropin misuse** in 2015 expresses an unfortunate event when a drug is used for unapproved indications. A 29-year-old female with a history of obesity suffered an ischemic stroke. Etiologic workup revealed a large patent foramen ovale and history of recent use of hCG as part of a weight loss regimen. hCG is commonly misused as a weight reducing or performance enhancing agent but is associated with increased risk of thromboembolic events (Pektezel, Bas, Topcuoglu, & Arsava, 2015)

Chapter 10: Carbohydrate Diets

"Without ice cream there would be darkness and chaos"
"There's no such thing as a bad carbohydrate" both quotes are from Don Kardong-1976 Olympic marathoner.

- A few words on low carbohydrate diets (the keto diet is a very low carbohydrate diet- typically about 200 kcals from carbohydrates).
- People consume much more carbohydrates than we need immediately and therefore we store 300-400 grams in muscle glycogen (1200-1600 kcals) and 100 grams in liver (400 kcals).
- Extra sugar is converted to glycogen and lipids (lipogenesis).
- People who do not tolerate carbohydrates due to absolute or relative lack of insulin (i.e. diabetics) convert the extra sugar into lipids. Extra carbohydrates are like kryptonite to people who have diabetes. Kryptonite analogy is an oversimplification to express a point.
- A person with lactose intolerance or gluten sensitivity avoids those particular substances.
- Reduction in carbohydrates provides the cellular trigger to switch fuel from predominately carbohydrates to mainly fat. Low carbohydrate diets (less than 200 kcals/day) will switch burning carbohydrates to burning fat. This takes 2-4

week for our bodies to adapt to. The ketone level is only 0.5mmol/l in a ketone diet whereas ketoacidosis levels are usually greater than 10 mmol/l in diabetic ketoacidosis (DKA).

- **There is really no clinically relevant association between DKA and very low safe dietary ketone levels in ketone diets.** The key point is the large order of magnitude between the two. It is the difference between apples and oranges. Ketones can be used as a source of fuel to the brain.

Do 17 ketogenic diets really suppress appetite? A systematic review and meta-analysis.

- Very-low-energy diets (VLEDs) and ketogenic low-carbohydrate diets (KLCDs) are associated with a suppression of appetite. We conducted a systematic literature search that assessed appetite with visual analogue scales before and during adherence to VLED or KLCD.
- Individuals were less hungry and exhibited greater fullness/satiety while adhering to VLED and KLCD.
- Ketosis appears to provide a plausible explanation for this suppression of appetite (Gibson, et al., 2015)

Effect of A Very Low-Calorie Ketogenic Diet on Food and Alcohol Cravings, Physical and Sexual Activity, Sleep Disturbances, and Quality of Life in Obese Patients.

- Psychological well-being and hunger and food control are two relevant factors involved in the success of weight-loss therapy. This study aims to evaluate food and alcohol cravings, physical and sexual activity, sleep, and life quality (QoL) in obese patients following a very low-calorie ketogenic (VLCK) diet, as well as the role of weight lost and ketosis on these parameters.
- A battery of psychological tests were performed in twenty obese patients (12 females, 47.2 year and BMI of 35.5) through the course of a 4-month VLCK diet on four subsequent visits: baseline, maximum ketosis, reduced ketosis, and endpoint.
- Each subject acted as their own control. The dietary-induced changes in body composition (7.7 units of BMI

lost, 18 kg of fat mass, 1.2 kg of visceral fat mass) were associated with a statistically significant improvement in food craving scores, physical activity, sleepiness, and female sexual function. Overall, these results also translated in a notable enhancement in QoL of the treated obese patients (Castro, et al., 2018).

More sugar? No, thank you! The elusive nature of low carbohydrate diets.

- In the past decades, dietary guidelines focused on reducing saturated fat as the primary strategy for cardiovascular disease prevention, neglecting the harmful effects of sugar.
- A greater intake of soft drinks (sugar-sweetened beverages), for example, is associated with a 44% increased prevalence of metabolic syndrome, a higher risk of obesity, and a 26% increased risk of developing diabetes mellitus.
- Carbohydrates comprise around 55% of the typical western diet, ranging from 200 to 350 g/day (800-1400 kcals) in relation to a person's overall caloric intake.
- For long-term weight gain, food rich in refined grains, starches, and sugar appear to be major culprits. Low-carbohydrate diets restrict daily carbohydrates between 20 and 50 g (80-200 kcals) as in clinical ketogenic diets.
- The results of controlled trials show that people on ketogenic diets (a diet with no more than 50 g carbohydrates/day) tend to lose more weight than people on low-fat diets.
- the consumption of the right carbohydrates (high-fiber, slowly digested, and whole grains), in a moderately lower amount (between 40 and 50% of daily energy content), is compatible with a state of good health and may represent a scientifically-based and palatable choice for people with metabolic disorders (Giugliano, Maiorino, Bellastella, & Esposito, 2018).

Successful treatment of obesity and insulin resistance via ketogenic diet status post Roux-en-Y.

- This is a single case of a 65-year-old American woman who presented with substantial weight gain and insulin resistance (IR) post-Roux-en-Y gastric bypass (RYGB) surgery.
- Before RYGB, she had reached 340 lbs (155 kg) and a body mass index (BMI) of 56.6 kg/m.²
- The surgery resulted in a 70 lbs (32 kg) weight loss, bringing her BMI to 44.9 kg/m². Unfortunately, her BMI would return to 53.6 kg/m².
- Her primary care physician placed her on a ketogenic diet. One year later, she had lost 102 lbs (46.4 kg), resulting in a BMI of 36.6 kg/m.² (Handley, Bentley, Brown, & Annan, 2018)

Metabolic effects, safety, and acceptability of very low-calorie ketogenic dietetic scheme on candidates for bariatric surgery.

- Evaluation of safety, efficacy, and acceptability of a very low-calorie ketogenic diet in patients before bariatric surgery at a University Hospital.
- Patients were given a dedicated Keto Station kit, for use during the first 10 days of the scheme, followed by a hypocaloric scheme for 20 days.
- The study group underwent routine laboratory tests and anthropometric measurements at enrollment (T0), after 10 days (T1), and after 30 days (T2). Ketone body levels were measured in the plasma and urine.
- Results:
- Between January 2015 and September 2015, 119 patients were included in the study.
- Mean body mass index was 41.5 ± 7.6 kg/m².
- Weight, body mass index, and waist circumference at T0 and T1, T0 and T2, and T1 and T2 decreased significantly (P<.05).
- A bioelectrical impedance assay determined a significant reduction in visceral fat after 10 days and 30 days.
- We observed a significant (P<.05) improvement in several clinical parameters, including glycemic and lipid profile parameters. We also observed a mean 30% reduction in liver volume.
- Conclusion:

- Our results confirm the acceptability, safety, and significant advantage of a very low-calorie ketogenic diet for reducing weight and liver volume of patients in preparation for bariatric surgery (Pilone, et al., 2018)

Chapter 11: Keto-Diet and Serious Exercising

There will come a point in the race, when you alone will need to decide. You will need to make a choice. Do you really want it? Rolf Arands (Ironman triathlete).

Metabolism of ketone bodies during exercise and training: physiological basis for exogenous supplementation

- Over the past century, exercise physiologists have appreciated the role of carbohydrate (CHO) and fat in energy provision to exercising skeletal muscle. Much of the work examining the metabolic response to exercise and the impact of exercise on metabolic regulation and adaptive responses to training has focused on the relative contribution of these fuels
- Optimising training and nutrition strategies by manipulating the relative intakes of these macronutrients is central to supporting elite sports performance.
- An alternative fuel source to CHO and fat are ketone bodies (KBs), namely acetoacetate (AcAc), acetone, and β-hydroxybutyrate (βHB), which are produced in the liver during physiological states and nutritional manipulations that result in reduced CHO availability, most commonly during prolonged fasting, starvation, and ketogenic (very low CHO ($\sim$5%), low protein ($\sim$15%), high fat ($\sim$80%)) diets. This relative glucose deprivation and concomitant elevation in circulating free-fatty acids (FFAs) results in the production of KBs to replace glucose as the primary fuel

for peripheral tissues such as the brain, heart and skeletal muscle in these states (Evans, Cogan, & Egan, 2017).

Keto-adaptation enhances exercise performance and body composition responses to training in endurance athletes.

- Low-carbohydrate diets have recently grown in popularity among endurance athletes, yet little is known about the long-term (>4wk) performance implications of consuming a low-carbohydrate high fat ketogenic diet (LCKD) in well-trained athletes.

- Twenty male endurance-trained athletes (age 33±11y, body mass 80±11kg; BMI 24.7±3.1kg/m^2) who habitually consumed a carbohydrate-based diet, self-selected into a high-carbohydrate (HC) group (n=11), or a LCKD group (n=9) for 12-weeks.

- Both groups performed the same training intervention (endurance, strength and high intensity interval training (HIIT)).

- The LCKD group experienced a significantly greater decrease in body mass and percentage body fat percentage.

- Compared to a HC comparison group, a 12-week period of keto-adaptation and exercise training, enhanced body composition, fat oxidation during exercise, and specific measures of performance relevant to competitive endurance athletes (McSwiney, et al., 2018).

A Low-Carbohydrate Ketogenic Diet Reduces Body Mass Without Compromising Performance in Powerlifting and Olympic Weightlifting Athletes.

- The purpose of this study was to determine whether a low-carbohydrate ketogenic diet (LCKD) could be used as a weight reduction strategy for athletes competing in the weight class sports of powerlifting and Olympic weightlifting.

- Fourteen advanced to elite competitive lifting athletes (age 34 ± 10.5, n = 5 female) consumed a usual diet (UD) (>250 g daily intake of carbohydrates) and an ad libitum LCKD (≤50 g or ≤10% daily intake of carbohydrates) in random order, each for 3 months in a **crossover design.**

- Lifting performance, body composition, resting metabolic rate, blood glucose, and blood electrolytes were measured at baseline, 3 months, and 6 months.
- The LCKD phase resulted in significantly lower body mass (-3.26 kg, $p = 0.038$) and lean mass (-2.26 kg, $p = 0.016$) compared with the UD phase. Lean mass losses were not reflected in lifting performances that were not different between dietary phases. No other differences were noted.
- Coaches and athletes should consider using an LCKD to achieve targeted weight reduction goals for weight class sports (Greene, Varley, Hartwig, Chapman, & Rigney, 2018).

Metabolic characteristics of keto-adapted ultra-endurance runners.

- Many successful ultra-endurance athletes have switched from a high-carbohydrate to a low-carbohydrate diet.
- Twenty elite ultra-marathoners and ironman distance triathletes performed a maximal graded exercise test and a 180 min submaximal run at 64% VO2max on a treadmill to determine metabolic responses. One group habitually consumed a traditional high-carbohydrate diet, and the other a low-carbohydrate diet for an average of 20 months (range 9 to 36 months).

Conclusion:

- long-term keto-adaptation results in extraordinarily high rates of fat oxidation, whereas muscle glycogen utilization and repletion patterns during and after a 3-hour run are similar (Volek, et al., 2016).

Chapter 12: Micronutrients, Superfoods and Supplements

**"The concept of superfood is rather ingenious,"
observes Eric Birlouez, a French sociologist and
food historian. "It invokes very positive images of
superheroes and superpowers, rather than health
and medicine.**

**An overview of herb and dietary supplement efficacy,
safety and government regulations in the United States
with suggested improvements.**

- Dietary supplements (DS; includes herbs) exceed over 50,000 in the Office of Dietary Supplement's "Dietary Supplement Label Database.
- The most popular DS were vitamin or mineral supplements (43%) followed by specialty supplements (20%), botanicals (20%; herbs), and sports supplements (16%).
- The 2013 Annual Report of the American Association of Poison Control Centers revealed 1692 fatalities due to drugs, and zero deaths due to DS. Less than 1 percent of Americans experience adverse events related to DS, and the majority was classified as minor, with many of these related to caffeine, yohimbe, or other stimulant ingredients.
- The number one adulterant in DS is drugs, followed by New Dietary Ingredients (NDI) not submitted to the FDA - both are illegal and not DS, but rather "tainted products marketed as dietary supplements."

- The three main categories of DS prone to medical problems are those for sexual enhancement, weight loss, and sports performance/body building.
- **The death rate from supplements is clearly above zero percent due to the contamination of supplements with both legal and illegal substances. This is the risk with taking supplements. The FDA will does not routinely review supplements. It will investigate a product only after multiple public complaints (Brown A. , 2017).**

Effects of superfoods on risk factors of metabolic syndrome: a systematic review of human intervention trials.

- The term "superfoods" was introduced to describe foods with supposedly significant health benefits. This review provides an overview of controlled human intervention studies with foods described as "superfoods." Seventeen superfoods were identified, including a total of 113 intervention trials: blueberries (8 studies), cranberries (8), goji berries (3), strawberries (7), chili peppers (3), garlic (21), ginger (10), chia seed (5), flaxseed (22), quinoa (1), cocoa (16), maca (Peruvian ginseng) (1), spirulina (blue-green algae) (7), wheatgrass (1), acai berries (0), hemp seed (0) and bee pollen (0).
- Overall, only limited evidence was found for the effects of the foods described as superfoods on metabolic syndrome parameters, since results were not consistent or the number of controlled intervention trials was limited (van den Driessche, Plat, & Mensink, 2018).

Micronutrient Gaps in Three Commercial Weight-Loss Diet Plans

- Weight-loss diets restrict intakes of energy and macronutrients but overlook micronutrient profiles. Commercial diet plans may provide insufficient micronutrients.
- We analyzed nutrient profiles of three plans with Dietary Reference Intakes (DRIs) for male U.S. adults.
- hypocaloric vegan (Eat to Live-Vegan, Aggressive Weight Loss; ETL-VAWL)

- high-animal-protein low-carbohydrate (Fast Metabolism Diet; FMD)
- weight maintenance (Eat, Drink and Be Healthy; EDH) diets.
- Seven single-day menus were sampled per diet ($n = 21$ menus, 7 menus/diet) and analyzed for 20 micronutrients with the online nutrient tracker CRON-O-Meter.
- ETL-VAWL diet failed to provide 90% of recommended amounts for B_{12}, B_3, D, E, calcium, selenium and zinc.
- FMD diet was low (<90% DRI) in B_1, D, E, calcium, magnesium and potassium.
- EDH diet met >90% DRIs for all but vitamin D, calcium and potassium.
- Several micronutrients remained inadequate after adjustment to 2000 kcal/day: vitamin B_{12} in ETL-VAWL, calcium in FMD and EDH and vitamin D in all diets.
- **Consistent with previous work, micronutrient deficits are prevalent in weight-loss diet plans** (Engel, Kern, Brenna, & Mitmesser, 2018).

Chapter 13: Diet Counseling

The great Woody Allen went to counseling for years and the only thing he got was 2 Academy Awards.

The following was provided by Kandi D Dawson, RDN, CD, CDE:
<u>**Weight Management Counseling by Kandi D Dawson, RDN, CD, CDE**</u>.

Weight loss and management should be simple, just cut out and control calories, right? It is never that simple.

Patients need customized and specific goals throughout the weight management process.

<u>Assessment:</u>

1. Identifying readiness for change and motivational triggers.
2. Review of pertinent medical history.
3. Review of lifestyle habits such as: work schedule, sleep, food choices, eating schedules, dining out, beverage choices, nutrition knowledge, stress management skills, grocery shopping, and budgeting skills.
4. Psychosocial aspects such as culture, socioeconomics, education level, upbringing, family structure, self-image and history of interpersonal relationships which affect weight.
5. Identifying an initial weight goal. Estimating calorie needs to maintain current weight, support weight loss, and maintain goal weight.
6. Patient beliefs regarding issues that have precipitated weight gain or lead to maintenance of an unhealthy weight.
7. Identifying support persons who can promote positive interactions during the weight loss process

The plan is to "re-frame the brain" or promote a "paradigm shift" for a healthier way of thinking about and managing food intake. Making goals to change behaviors should be paced realistically for the patient. Success comes from the patient committing to reinforce and repeat positive actions daily.

Healthy Nutrition/Healthy Weight

    a. Routine weight monitoring, BMI changes, factors that can influence weekly weights (i.e. constipation, sodium and alcohol intake).

    b. Journaling food, beverage, water, calories and portions to promote avoidance of portion distortion.

    c. Planning: Mealtimes, shopping, food preparation, dining out, special occasions/travel/holidays.

    d. Nutrition awareness of excess calories/fat/sugars (calorie density) and limiting processed foods.

    e. Specific goals for fresh fruit and non-starchy vegetables daily.

    f. Value of increased fiber intake, including sources.

    g. Budget and healthy eating.

    h. Menu and snack ideas.

    i. Food preparation techniques.

    j. **Using the "Two Bite Rule" to avoid deprivation of high calorie treats**.

    k. Assessing and identifying specific unconscious eating habits, brainstorming ideas for specific changes.

    l. Managing the eating cues unrelated to hunger.

    m. Emotional/Boredom/Fatigue/Stress Eating.

    n. Hunger and Fullness Awareness; increase awareness and use your natural "Pause" during a meal to evaluate when it is okay to stop eating.

    o. Promoting self-awareness to identify opportunities to improve mindful food intake.

    p. Influence of other people and identifying toxic food environments.

    q. Holiday, Travel, and Social Situations.

- Healthy Sleep
- Staying hydrated
- Intentional Activity – FITT (frequency, intensity, time, type); individualized and realistic goals; promote getting help to make a safe intentional activity plan.

- Managing appetite with food choices related to timing of meals and snacks.
- Managing depression and stress.
- Managing slips/regression – which is a normal event! Use the motto, "Don't quit."
- Managing plateaus in weight loss.
- Mindful Eating – practicing new ways of viewing and responding to food.

Here is a sample list of "pearls of wisdom" that are sometimes used during the coaching and education process.

- Mindful eating does not include deprivation of "bad" foods. We should learn to pay attention to how much and how often we eat high calorie treats. Teaching the "two-bite rule" moves attention to the physical enjoyment of food without sabotaging a healthy weight.

- Mindful eating requires "practice, practice, practice" creating the habit of listening to what your body is telling you regarding hunger and fullness and learn to respond responsibly.

- Starting out the day with no food usually results in overeating later in the day. **Don't go over 4-5 hours without eating a meal or snack.** A full meal isn't essential at breakfast time, but rather a snack will work.

- **Don't focus on cutting out carbohydrates and/or fats... research points to the fact that calories are key.**

- There is value in eating small portions of protein with meals or snacks, which promote satiety and moderates blood glucose spikes, thus suppressing hunger longer after eating.

- Having a specific plan when traveling, whether for business or pleasure, long or short trips.

- Having a specific plan for holiday or social events.

- Rather than avoid others who have contributed to your past unhealthy food habits, put together a plan for communication. Acknowledge that they care about you, and in turn let them know your decision to change your style of eating. Ask for their support as you seek to improve your health. It doesn't mean you need to exclude them from your life, but rather help them understand why you are making new choices. There should be no implication that you are trying to shame them or change their choices.

- Frequently review your triggers to keep focused on repeating positive changes.

- **Calories are key in losing weight.** Journaling food and calorie content help you understand where calories come from. Choosing healthier items that taste great, provide less calories and are items perhaps you would never have tried if you weren't focusing on attaining a healthier weight.

Follow up visits with the nutrition coach include:

1. Review challenges and successes, including continued progress on prior goals. Assistance in problem solving to manage challenges and providing kudos for successes.
2. Helping to creating a vision for the future such as: managing clothing, using bucket lists, effectively dealing with effect of success on others, and creating a sense of importance to actively use long term goals and strategies to maintain a healthy weight.

If used diligently for at least two years, most patients will maintain their healthier weight for the remainder of their life.

Good Luck,
Kandi. (Kandi Dawson, Personal email, April 27, 2017)

Chapter 14: Medications

For a drug to be approved for weight loss, the FDA requires the drug to be responsible for losing 5% or more body weight in at least 35% of people tested. Also, the weight loss should be double the percentage which occurred in the placebo treated group and should last one year. Medications for obesity treatment must be considered for long-term use when evaluating their safety and efficacy. A lesson from the withdrawal of previous anti-obesity drugs is that serious adverse effects may become apparent only when a drug is used in larger populations or for longer periods of time than in preapproved trials. The Endocrine and Metabolic Drug Advisory Committee has recommended to the FDA that all new medications reviewed for an obesity indication undergo premarket testing to ensure they do not increase cardiac events. The dropout rate in long-term obesity drug trials have historically been high (40-50%). The stronger the ancillary weight loss program (frequent weigh-ins, dietician visits, behavior therapist visits, etc.), the greater the weight loss but the difference between the studied drug and standard of care decreases. Most obesity drug trials minimize the ancillary program to maximize the difference.

Combining medicines has been a successful strategy to treat many diseases for decades and this same strategy is being applied with weight loss medicines. The potential and rationale for combination therapies were confirmed by a recent study that concluded that the transition probability (the chance of a medication studied in phase 1 trials to be approved) of a monotherapy for obesity was 8.5%, jumping to 40% if the pill was a combination therapy (Hussain, Parker, & Sharma, 2015).

I divide medications to lose weight into weight loss meds and diabetic meds with weight loss features. I will describe them briefly followed by more information later. The FDA has approved 5 agents for long-term weight loss- orlistat, lorcaserin (Belviq), phentermine/topiramate (Qysmia), naltrexone/bupropion (Contrave) and high-dose liraglutide (Saxenda). Other weight loss medicines are generic phentermine, generic topiramate, and generic bupropion. Orlistat is approved for weight loss as a fat blocker but realistically is not used much due to side effects of bloating, fatty stools, flatus and other gastrointestinal side effects. It is not very effective at weight loss. Getting the insurance company to pay for the newer meds Qysmia, Belviq and Contrave has been the biggest roadblock despite being approved by the FDA for over 4 years. Getting a Medicare patient the drug is almost always unsuccessful. The same applies to Saxenda which is the higher dose Victoza with a different name. I have yet to have it approved regularly despite being a great drug. Insurance companies are resistant to pay for many expensive medicines. The following article expresses drug coverage.

US health policy and prescription drug coverage of FDA-approved medications for the treatment of obesity

- An alarming 39.8% of men and women in the United States suffer from obesity.
- Lifestyle and behavior modification to lose weight has been an unsuccessful strategy to weight loss for decades. Our body's adaptive biologic responses to weight loss leads to altered physiology that ultimately results in weight regain.
- It is recommended that patients with obesity be treated with adjuncts such as pharmacotherapy and/or bariatric surgery to decrease weight recidivism. Compared to new drugs available for diabetes, these new obesity drugs are 15 times less likely to be dispensed.
- 6 of the 21 states with no coverage for obesity medications are among the states with the highest prevalence of obesity.
- Despite the American Medical Association (AMA) recognizing obesity as a disease in June 2013 and the US government recognizing obesity as a disease in 2004, several factors have improved and several have crippled treating obesity. Some factors are:
  1. Many insurance companies will pay for doctor visits and counseling services for obesity.
  2. Coverage for Bariatric surgery has improved.

3. The stigma of obesity is still widely pervasive.

- Most states do not provide coverage for newer obesity medicines. Among 136 marketplace health insurance plans, 11% had some coverage for the specified drugs in only nine states.
- Medicare policy strictly excludes drug therapy for obesity.
- Few Medicaid programs have drug coverage for obesity (only seven states).
- Ironically, federal government employees, with 2.7 million have health benefit plans that are not allowed to exclude coverage of obesity medications.
- Since cardiovascular disease is the number one leading cause of death in the United States, demonstrating the associated benefit of obesity medication use for cardiovascular disease may ease the concerns of patients and providers and increase the use of these safe medications.

In addition, since more and more patients with obesity are undergoing bariatric surgery, patients still need to manage their obesity, although it may be in remission. For patients who do have weight regain after achieving a healthier body mass index or with inadequate weight loss, pharmacotherapy may be an option for postoperative patients to achieve a healthy weight (Gomez & Stanford, 2018)

Coverage for Obesity Prevention and Treatment Services: Analysis of Medicaid and State Employee Health Insurance Programs.

This study examined changes in coverage for adult obesity treatment services in Medicaid and state employee health insurance programs between 2009 and 2017.

Methods

Administrative materials from Medicaid and state employee health insurance programs in all 50 states and the District of Columbia were reviewed for indications of coverage for adults ($\geq$ 21 years of age) with obesity, including nutritional counseling, pharmacotherapy, and bariatric surgery.

Results

From 2009 to 2017, the proportion of state employee programs indicating coverage increased by 75% for nutritional counseling (from 24 to 42 states), 64% for pharmacotherapy (from 14 to 23 states), and 23% for bariatric surgery (from 35 to 43 states). The proportion of Medicaid programs indicating coverage increased by 133% for nutritional counseling (from 9 to 21 states) and 9% for bariatric surgery (from 45 to 49 states), with no net increase for pharmacotherapy (16 states in both plan years).

Conclusions

Coverage for adult obesity care improved substantially in Medicaid and state employee insurance programs since 2009. However, recommended treatment modalities are still not covered in many states (Jannah, Hild, Gallagher, & Dietz, 2018)

The other group of medicines helpful for weight loss are some diabetic medications. They include metformin, the GLP1 agents - Victoza, Bydureon, Trulicity, Ozempic and the SGLT2 agents- Invokana, Farxiga, Jardiance, and Steglatro.

Metformin helps lower sugars and is weight neutral. It is a great drug but not a game changer. It has been shown to be much safer than past reported and can be given to people with a GFR higher than 30 cc/min. It decreases gluconeogenesis (glycogen to glucose) in the liver and promotes insulin sensitivity.

GLP1(glucagon-like peptide-1) agents decrease glucose and promote weight loss by telling the brain not to be hungry, slowing gastric emptying by promoting a full sensation, decreasing gluconeogenesis/glycogenolysis in the liver and promoting insulin release with hyperglycemia.

SGLT2 (sodium glucose transporter-2) agents cause glucosuria by lowering the renal threshold for glucosuria from about 180 mg% to 90mg%. Any elevated sugar the kidney sees is excreted instead of being absorbed. 90% of the filtered glucose is reabsorbed by the high capacity SGLT2 transporter in the proximal tubule and the remaining 10% of the filtered glucose is reabsorbed by the SGLT1 transporter of the descending proximal tubule. Patients with diabetes have been shown to have an increased renal threshold higher than the normal 180 mg/dl thus promoting more glucose absorption and weight gain.

The FDA's guidance statement to the pharmaceutical industry in 2009 mandated the demonstration of cardiovascular safety for all new glucose-lowering agents (DeFronzo, 2009).

Chapter 15: Phentermine

"A drug must be a pretty good drug if it has its own chapter".

Phentermine has been the main drug I use to help people lose unwanted extra weight. I have prescribed it in very unhealthy people with chronic illnesses without any serious side-effects. I have used it with success in multiple age brackets including 70 to 80 years old. I have become very comfortable with it. It reminds me of metformin regarding the safety and great benefits of it. Metformin has also been around for decades and now is the backbone for type 2 diabetes management.

It is a safe and successful medicine. It has never been removed from the market by the FDA and has been around since 1959. Long-term use is restricted in some states to only 3 months due to low addiction potential. Ohio is one such state. By declaring obesity a disease in 2013 more and more states should be removing the 3-month restriction since chronic diseases usually require medicines for more than 3 months. It is not an amphetamine but has some amphetamine-like characteristics. Many doctors think it is an amphetamine which is not correct. Because of this misinformation, many patients and doctors hesitate to take it or prescribe it. Amphetamines and narcotics are schedule 2 drugs due to addiction potential and phentermine is a schedule 4 drug. Schedule 4 drugs have much lower abuse potential and include benzodiazepines, Ambien, tramadol, Belviq (weight loss med), and phentermine. A physician can write refills up to a 6-month supply with phentermine, whereas narcotics and amphetamines cannot be given refills.

Phentermine has a half- life of 4-19 hours and is excreted by the kidney. **It releases norepinephrine granules in the lateral hypothalamus with stimulation of beta-2 adrenergic receptors.** Most doctors have used it for long-term weight loss for years and it is by far the most popular and successful medicine for this for decades. From 2008-2011, 25.3 million scripts were written for an estimated 6.2 million people (Hampp, Kang, & Borders-Hemphill, 2019) **In Europe, weight loss medicines don't exist due to the belief that obesity is more a lifestyle than a disease. Phentermine, Belviq, Qysmia and Contrave are not approved in Europe.** Phentermine was withdrawn in 2000 in Europe due to perceived unfavorable risk to benefit ratio. Orlistat is the only agent approved in the European Union for weight loss. It is not used much in the United States due to oily, foul smelling stools and other unpleasant GI side-effects. I guess medieval times still exist in Europe. Even members of Monty Python would pass on taking orlistat due to uncivilized GI side effects. To keep the article well-balanced and give Great Britain the respect it deserves, I must state that the idea that British people have poor dentition is really not true.

Studies up to eight years suggest long-term phentermine therapy is a safe and useful treatment for weight loss and weight maintenance. There are no published reports that orally administered phentermine has been associated with abuse or psychological dependence as defined by DSM-IV. Common side-effects include insomnia 1.1%, increased blood pressure 0.8%, nervous/shakiness 1%, palpitations 0.4% and the risk of abuse is 0.4 per 100,000. The risk of abuse with narcotics is 92.5 per 100,000 and 32.7 per 100,000 for anti-depressants. Abrupt cessation of phentermine after 90-day use or longer has resulted in no withdrawal symptoms or cravings. **Intermittent usage or drug holidays is a viable and clinically effective use since the addictive potential is so low.** By comparison, as many as 97% of amphetamine-dependent users will experience a withdrawal syndrome within 24 hours of stopping an amphetamine. Telephone surveys in 2010-2011 of 23 rehab centers in Kentucky with an experience of treating 24,000 patients have never admitted or treated phentermine abuse or addiction. A telephone survey of medical directors of 50 drug treatment centers and 50 major hospital emergency centers in each of 50 states has documented that no physician could recall ever having diagnosed or treated phentermine abuse, addiction or withdrawal (Hendricks, et al., 2014).

The 2014 study in the International Journal of Obesity by Dr. Hendricks et al. entitled **Addiction potential of phentermine prescribed during long-term treatment of obesity** looked at 269 obese, or overweight subjects treated with phentermine from 1.1 years to 21.1 years at doses from 18.75 to 112.5 mg/day or short-term use of 4-22 days at 15-93.75 mg/day were interviewed and underwent several dependence and addiction questionnaire scales showing no abuse, dependence, or cravings. It did show a return of appetite and hunger when phentermine was stopped. **The doses ranged from 18.75 to 112.5 mg/day. This study provides evidence of the long duration and high dose of phentermine that some patients have received without trouble.** The most common dose I prescribe is 37.5 mg/day which is probably over 80% in my practice. Most people take 18.75 to 60.0 mg/day with 30-37.5 mg/day the most common doses which is similar to other prescribers. I faxed the above 2014 study to one pharmacist who questioned the dose and safety of phentermine (Hendricks, et al., 2014).

There has been one case report in 2005 in Anesthesia Intensive Care where a woman had two perioperative hypertensive crises felt to be due to phentermine. Even though the half-life would indicate that phentermine is completely metabolized in a few days, the conservative recommendation based on this one case report is to hold phentermine one week before surgery. (Stephens & Katz, 2005).

Phentermine: A Systematic Review for Plastic and Reconstructive Surgeons.

Phentermine is the most prescribed anti-obesity drug in America, with 2.43 million prescriptions written in 2011. There are no published guidelines for the perioperative management of phentermine use in the plastic surgery literature. A systematic review was undertaken using the search engines PubMed/MEDLINE, EMBASE, and Scopus.

Results:

A total of 251 citations were reviewed, yielding 4 articles that discussed perioperative phentermine use and complications with anesthesia. One was a review article, 2 were case reports, and 1 was a letter. Complications included hypotension, hypertension, hypoglycemia, hyperthermia, bradycardia, cardiac depression, and acute pulmonary edema.

Conclusion:

The relationship between phentermine and anesthesia, if any, is unclear. Hypotension on induction of general anesthesia is the most reported complication of perioperative phentermine use. Specifically, phentermine-induced hypotension may be unresponsive to vasopressors that rely on catecholamine release, such as ephedrine. Therefore, the decision to perform surgery, especially elective surgery, in a patient taking phentermine should be made with caution. **Because of the half-life of phentermine, we recommend discontinuing phentermine for at least 4 days prior to surgery.** This differs from the classic 2-week discontinuation period recommended for "fen-phen." The patient should be made aware of the increased risk of surgery, and a skilled anesthesiologist should monitor intraoperative blood pressure and body temperature for signs of autonomic derailment (Lim, et al., 2018).

Phentermine will cause a urine drug screen to be false positive for amphetamine with a confirmation test identifying phentermine. Pilots and truckers need to look at the list of medicines prohibited in their respective professions. If a false positive occurs with a patient of mine, I would write a letter stating the above false positive result. This has never happened in my practice so far. Amphetamines are 10-fold as potent as phentermine in maintaining self-administration behavior in baboons, and phentermine has been demonstrated to decrease self-administration behavior in baboons (Hendricks & Greenway, 2011). Baboons were chosen over politicians in these studies due to less innate erratic behavior. **Phentermine is considered a performance enhancing medicine by the Olympic Committee since it is a beta-agonist and therefore not allowed in the**

Olympics. Beta-blockers are also not allowed but only in archery and shooting to lessen any tremor.

Very common side effects are dry mouth, constipation and insomnia. No data is present in peer-reviewed medical literature to support that phentermine increases blood pressure or heart rate at a sustained elevated level. I added the words "sustained" to emphasize the difference between acute and chronic. The occurrence of hypertension is rare rather than common. I would qualify that chronic hypertension is rare but short-term elevated blood pressure is very common. I see an elevation in blood pressure mostly in medication naïve patients. I usually observe it and wait several visits with the person usually not needing an anti-hypertensive. Short-term elevation of blood pressure does not defer me from using phentermine daily. I would rather be conservative and comment on the short-term elevated blood pressure than have a physician start prescribing it and stop using it since he or she sees some initial elevated blood pressure that clinically is not significant. The general idea is the weight loss offsets the potential elevated blood pressure. I do believe that hypertension is mostly genetic since ideal weight patients can have blood pressure that is as difficult to treat as an obese individual. I definitely decrease or stop more blood pressure medicines than start them in phentermine treated patients. My mindset is phentermine is a beta-agonist similar to breathing medication with its potential warning of heart disease. I have several hundred patients on phentermine and over 90% tolerate it well. The ones that stop are usually non-responders meaning that they did not show a 12-lb. weight loss over 12 weeks or chose to go off for other reasons such as constipation, insomnia, anxiety, cost or a desire to lose weight on their own. By using the"12-week rule," **(12 pounds in 12 weeks)** we limit exposure to weight loss drugs and hopefully select out the subpopulation that has the best chance at long-term success. **Most studies have shown that initial weight loss response at 12 weeks predicts later weight loss at 1 year and afterwards** (Colman, et al., 2012) (Rissenen, Lean, Rossner, Segal, & Sjostrom, 2003) (Finer, Ryan, Renz, & Hewkin, 2005).

Genetics plays an important factor in selecting out responders and non-responders. Based on my experience, phentermine works well. It is generic and costs about 20 dollars per month. **The** contraindications are unstable heart disease, untreated hyperthyroidism, unstable accelerated hypertension, drug addiction, pregnancy and unstable psychiatric illness. It is well tolerated dating back as early as 1968 and was even given to children. A 2016 study in the International Journal of Obesity compared 25 adolescents on phentermine matched to a comparison group of 274 with standard of care. Phentermine use was associated with a greater change in BMI at 1 month (minus 1.6%), 3 months (minus 2.9%), and 6 months (minus 4.1%). No differences in systolic or diastolic blood pressure occurred between groups but heart rate was higher at all time-points in the phentermine group (Ryder, et al., 2016). **The 12-week rule is very important since it limits exposure to medicines in non-responders.**

The concern for phentermine abuse and potential cardiovascular risk is overestimated based on literature. Long-term studies as long as eight years suggest long-term phentermine therapy may be a safe and useful treatment for weight maintenance. The 2011 article by Hendricks et al in Obesity is reassuring:

> **Blood Pressure and Heart Rate Effects, Weight Loss and Maintenance During Long-term Phentermine Pharmacotherapy for Obesity.** There were no significant differences in SBP, DBP, or HR comparing patient cohorts at the five dose levels of 0, 18.75 mg, 30-37.5, 48.75-56.25, and 60-75 mg phentermine per day (Hendricks, Greenway, Westman, & Gupta, 2011).

The most obvious effect was appetite and hunger suppression. The second effect was more subtle and variously described as improved or stronger control of eating, diminution or absence of food cravings or improved ability to follow their eating plan. The occurrence of hypertension with phentermine is rare rather than common. Aside from a few anecdotal reports, there is no data in the peer-reviewed medical literature to support the perception that phentermine increases blood pressure or heart rate. Phentermine was part of the combination medicine fenfluramine/phentermine (fen-phen). It was taken off the market in 1997 due to cardiac fibrosis and valvular heart disease (mild aortic regurgitation) due to

Chapter 15: Phentermine

fenfluramine. Fenfluramine activates 5-HT2b receptors on cardiac valves causing mitogenesis leading to cardiac hyperplasia, pulmonary hypertension and in some cases cardiac fibrosis. It was found that phentermine was not responsible for the harm. **There have been no cases of valvular heart disease described with phentermine monotherapy use in over half a century** (Connolly HM, 1997) (Roth, 2007) (Meltzer & Roth, 2013).

An exaggerated concern is the idea that phentermine causes pulmonary hypertension. Pulmonary hypertension is defined as a mean pulmonary artery pressure of greater or equal to 25 mmHg at rest with a normal pressure defined as less than 20 mmHg. Pulmonary arterial hypertension (PAH) is a proliferative vasculopathy promoting remodeling of pulmonary circulation by vasoconstriction, cell proliferation, fibrosis and thrombosis. A low-pressure system becomes a high-pressure system causing right ventricular overload and cor pulmonale. PAH is caused mostly by left heart disease, lung disease, thromboembolic disease, and some chronic systemic/metabolic disorders. A very small percentage is due to drug and toxin exposure. The supposed mechanism for drug exposure is an increase in serotonin which acts as a growth factor for pulmonary artery smooth muscle cells. Pulmonary hypertension has been associated with appetite suppressants such as aminorex, fenfluramine, dexfenfluramine and benfluorex. These drugs have been confirmed to cause PAH and were removed from the market decades ago. Fenfluramine and its derivatives were banned from commercial use in 1997. Fenfluramine-induced PAH patients share clinical, functional, hemodynamic and genetic features with idiopathic PAH patients, as well as similar overall survival rates.

In an analysis by Rich et al., phentermine was not retained as a potential risk factor for PAH. **Simply stated phentermine does not cause pulmonary hypertension. We will catch a whole bunch of people with pulmonary hypertension by thinking of obstructive sleep apnea** (Rich, Rubin, Walker, Schneeweiss, & Abenhaim, 2000).

Safety and Effectiveness of Longer-Term Phentermine Use: Clinical Outcomes from an Electronic Health Record Cohort

- Lifestyle interventions remain the cornerstone of treatment for patients with obesity, typically yielding a peak weight loss of 5% to 10% after 6 months.
- Up to one-third of patients do not respond to such programs and weight regain is common.
- Pharmacotherapy can increase the proportion of individuals who respond to lifestyle interventions as well as the duration and magnitude of response.
- The most commonly used weight-loss medication in the United States is phentermine, a sympathomimetic amine that acts by inhibiting appetite and that was originally approved for weight loss in 1959.
- Longer-term use of phentermine in the United States indeed appears to be a pervasive practice.
- 30% of our cohort was made up of individuals with at least one phentermine episode lasting > 12 weeks.

Study

- The aim of this work was to study weight loss and risk of cardiovascular disease (CVD) or death associated with longer-term phentermine use

Methods

- Using electronic health record data, 13,972 adults were identified with a first phentermine fill in 2010 to 2015. Percent weight loss at 6, 12, and 24 months and risk of composite CVD or death, up to 3 years after starting phentermine were measured.

Results

- The cohort was 84% female and 45% white, with a mean (SD) baseline age 43.5 years and BMI of 37.8 kg/m^2.
- Longer-term users of phentermine experienced more weight loss; patients using continuously for > 12 months lost 7.4% more than the reference group at 24 months ($P < 0.001$). Discontinuation of phentermine consistently resulted in weight regain.

- The composite CVD or death outcome was rare (0.3%, 41 events), with no significant difference in hazard ratios between groups.

Conclusions

- **Greater weight loss without increased risk of incident CVD or death was observed in patients using phentermine monotherapy for longer than 3 months.**

- **Recommendations to limit phentermine use to less than 3 months do not align with current concepts of pharmacological treatment for patients with obesity** (Lewis, et al., 2019).

Combination of venlafaxine and phentermine/topiramate induced psychosis: A case report.

- Venlafaxine, a first-line medication for depression, inhibits the reuptake of both serotonin and norepinephrine and weakly inhibits the reuptake of dopamine. Phentermine/topiramate (Qsymia®), specifically the phentermine component, functions by blocking the dopamine and norepinephrine transporter, similar to amphetamine. Various publications have noted increases in dopamine, specifically in the mesolimbic region of the brain, to have a direct correlation to psychotic-like symptoms.

CASE REPORT:

A 40-year-old Hispanic woman was admitted to the inpatient mental health unit based on reports of delusional thinking and several attempts of self-harm. Past medical history was significant for major depressive disorder, posttraumatic stress disorder, anxiety, irritable bowel syndrome, and migraines. The patient was started on venlafaxine (75 mg extended-release by mouth once daily) for depression approximately 1 month prior to admission. Furthermore, the patient was restarted on a previously prescribed medication, oral phentermine/topiramate for weight loss, in combination with venlafaxine, approximately 1 week prior to the bizarre behavior. The patient denied any psychosis or changes in behavior when medications were taken individually prior to the combination. The patient was treated with lurasidone (anti-psychotic/40 mg by mouth daily) with resolution of psychosis.

DISCUSSION:
A PubMed search revealed no current literature or case reports on psychosis induced by the combination of venlafaxine and phentermine/topiramate. Individual case reports of psychosis in patients on venlafaxine alone and the phentermine component of phentermine/topiramate alone have been reported (Homola & Hieber, 2018).

The FDA recently approved **Lomaira** in September 2016. It is an 8-mg tablet formulation of phentermine that can be taken up to three times per day before meals. I do not have any personal experience with it but suspect it may be helpful in people who cannot tolerate 30 mg, 37.5 mg or ½ tab of 37.5 mg. The low dose allows for flexibility and may be a good choice for maintenance weight management. One price comparison revealed the wholesale price for phentermine is $10.50, and for Lomaira, $43.50.

Chapter 16: Prediabetes

Prediabetes is important to look for and treat. It is not benign. Most topics with "pre-" before them mean something significant. Just think of the words pretrial, premature, prenuptial, precancer, pre-op, preeclampsia and prehistoric. Enough said.

Prediabetes: Why Should We Care?

- The 2017 National Diabetes Statistics Report estimates that 33.9% of the adult U.S. population has prediabetes. The prevalence is higher in those aged 65 years and older, at 48.3%. Not surprisingly, only 11.6% of U.S. adults know they have prediabetes.

- Diagnosis of prediabetes is based on the presence of impaired fasting glucose, impaired glucose tolerance, and/or elevated HbA1c levels between 5.7% and 6.4%. Impaired glucose tolerance is defined as blood glucose levels of 140 to 199 mg/dL during a 75-gram oral glucose tolerance test (normal < 140 mg/dL), and impaired fasting glucose is defined as blood glucose levels of 100 to 125 mg/dL.

- In multiple studies, prediabetes is shown to have a cause-effect relationship to cardiovascular disease and all-cause mortality. In a cohort meta-analysis by Huang et al., prediabetes was associated with an increased risk of coronary heart disease, stroke, and all-cause mortality.

- The prediabetes state is not only a noteworthy risk factor for type 2 diabetes but is also a significant risk factor for macrovascular disease. A meta-analysis of 38 prospective studies in which cardiovascular disease (CVD) or mortality was the end point concluded that increasing glucose levels displayed a linear relationship with CVD risk.

- Strong evidence suggests that patients with prediabetes have an increase in fibrinogen and high-sensitivity C-reactive protein (hs-CRP)—both proatherogenic factors—compared with normoglycemic patients.

- Sen et al. conducted a study on 62 acute coronary syndrome patients who were admitted to a tertiary facility in India to identify the proportion that had prediabetes; they discovered that 48.4% of this patient population had prediabetes and 25% had diabetes.

- In a study by the American Diabetes Association (ADA) 67 patients with established coronary artery disease (CAD) underwent catheterization. Per ADA guidelines, 16 of the patients were classified as nondiabetic, 28 were considered prediabetic, and 23 were diabetic. The number and grade of yellow plaques were higher in the prediabetic patients than in nondiabetics but similar in both prediabetic and diabetic patients.

- In a larger study done by Scicali et al., the impact of prediabetes on coronary artery calcium (CAC) scores and mean common carotid media thickness (IMT) was compared in prediabetic patients and nondiabetic patients. Of the 272 patients enrolled, both the CAC scores and mean IMT were significantly higher in the prediabetes group.

- Di Pino et al. studied the effects of prediabetes on diastolic function in 167 patients with HbA1c between 5.7% and 6.4%. In patients with prediabetes, they found significant early signs of diastolic dysfunction.

- Diet and exercise can halt the progression towards type 2 diabetes in patients with prediabetes. Among the first studies to prove this was the Finnish Diabetes Prevention Study (DPS), a controlled randomized trial including 522 overweight subjects with impaired glucose tolerance who were randomized to either an intensive lifestyle intervention group or a standard-of-care control group. Weight reduction, lipid and glycemic parameters showed more improvement in the intervention group. A 58% reduction in the risk of developing diabetes was noted. During the total 7-year follow-up period, the study showed a 36% reduction in relative risk in developing type 2 diabetes.

- Another large study that reproduced similar results was from the Diabetes Prevention Program (DPP), which was similar to the Finnish study in its design but included a group treated with metformin for comparison. A total of 3,234 high-risk adults were recruited; 1,079 participants underwent intensive lifestyle intervention, 924 were treated with metformin, and 932 were treated with a placebo. The lifestyle group achieved two important goals: loss of 7% of their initial body weight and a minimum of 150 min of physical activity per week. Diabetes incidence was reduced by 58% in the lifestyle group and by 31% with metformin compared to placebo. Analysis was by intention-to-treat, with one case of diabetes prevented for every 6.9 people. After a 10-year follow-up, the study concluded that the effects of lifestyle modification on diabetes prevention were maintained.

- De la Cruz-Muñoz and colleagues performed a retrospective analysis of 1,602 adults who underwent bariatric surgery; they were categorized into those with diagnosed type 2 diabetes, those with prediabetes, those with high fasting plasma glucose (FPG), and those with normal FPG. At 1- and 3-year follow-up post bariatric surgery, all four groups had normal FPG, but the prediabetes group had more significant weight loss (47 kg) than the diabetes population.

- 4,032 participants from the Swedish Obese Subjects study, half of whom had bariatric surgery and the other half received usual care. After 15 years of follow-up, bariatric patients in the diabetes, prediabetes, and normoglycemic groups had a reduced incidence of macrovascular complications. Interestingly, the largest risk reduction for macrovascular complications was seen in the prediabetes group.

- The first step in managing patients with prediabetes is to encourage strict lifestyle modifications consisting of ≥ 180 min of physical activity per week and a calorie intake of

1,200 to 1,800 kcal per day. In addition to lifestyle
management, anti-obesity agents should be considered for
obese patients with prediabetes.

- Complications of prediabetes include macrovascular effects
such as myocardial infraction, stroke, and peripheral
vascular disease as well as microvascular changes such as
retinopathy, neuropathy, and nephropathy. (Zand,
Ibrahim, & Patham, 2018),

DYSGLYCEMIA-BASED CHRONIC DISEASE: AN AMERICAN ASSOCIATION OF CLINICAL ENDOCRINOLOGISTS POSITION STATEMENT

- This document represents the official position of the
American Association of Clinical Endocrinologists and the
American College of Endocrinology.

- The American Association of Clinical Endocrinologists
(AACE) has created a dysglycemia-based chronic disease
(DBCD) multimorbidity care model consisting of four
distinct stages that are actionable in a preventive care
paradigm to reduce the potential impact of T2D,
cardiometabolic risk, and cardiovascular events.

Dysglycemia-Based Chronic Disease (DBCD)
- stage 1 represents "insulin resistance"

- stage 2 "prediabetes"

- stage 3 "type 2 diabetes"

- stage 4 "vascular complications"

- This model encourages earliest intervention focusing on
structured lifestyle change. Further scientific research may
eventually reclassify stage 2 DBCD prediabetes from a pre-
disease to a true disease state.

- The most recent 2017 National Diabetes Statistics Report;

- 30.3 million U.S. residents of all ages (9.4% of the
population) with diabetes

Chapter 16: Prediabetes

- 84.1 million age 18 and over (33.9% of the population) with prediabetes.

- According to a recent analysis using data from the U.S. National Health and Nutrition Examination Surveys (NHANES; 1988-2014), patients with prediabetes have increased prevalence rates of hypertension, dyslipidemia, chronic kidney disease, and cardiovascular disease (CVD) risk.

- What is particularly alarming is that in 2015, 23.8% of patients with diabetes (7.2 million) and 88.4% of patients with prediabetes (74.3 million) did not even know they had the condition.

- The critical question is whether making the diagnosis of "prediabetes" can improve health?

- Prediabetes was first described in 1956 in the perspective of gestational diabetes but now identifies people at higher risk for T2D, hypertension, and CVD than the general population.

- Prediabetes is diagnosed based on fasting plasma glucose (FPG), standardized 2-hour post-challenge glucose testing, or A1C levels, though diagnostic cutoffs may vary. The concept of prediabetes hinges on a preventive care approach to chronic disease. Hence, those with overweight are at higher risk for obesity, prehypertension for hypertension, metabolic syndrome (MetS) for CVD, and so forth. In the 15-year follow-up of the Diabetes Prevention Program Outcomes Study, those patients with prediabetes randomized to lifestyle intervention had significant reduction in T2D development. Moreover, among all patients in the study, there was a 28% lower prevalence of microvascular complications in those not developing T2D.

- The current paradigm of diabetes care is plagued by patient adherence problems, inertia among health care professionals adopting contemporary clinical practice guidelines, and a lack of reverent, consistent, and universal insurance coverage for diagnostics, lifestyle medicine, and pharmaceuticals, all prompting the need for a new approach involving patient-centered and preventive care.

- With respect to obesity, AACE has recently proposed a new Adiposity Based Chronic Disease (ABCD) diagnostic term and a complications-centric obesity care model. AACE takes the firm stance that patients with prediabetes fall within the progressive spectrum of DBCD (insulin resistance-prediabetes-T2D) and are well-suited for structured lifestyle and/or pharmaco-therapeutic preventive measures.

- The essential component of DBCD is insulin resistance. Since up to 70% of patients with prediabetes have a lifetime risk of converting to T2D (74% of individuals at age 45), primary prevention of T2D is paramount. Also, since those with prediabetes have significant CVD risk factors (36.6% with hypertension, 51.2% dyslipidemia, 24.3% tobacco use, and 5 to 7% 10-year cardiovascular event risk), secondary prevention is paramount. There are three aspects to reducing the impact of prediabetes using primary and secondary prevention strategies.

- The first aspect is to prevent T2D. Progression to T2D can be prevented with interventions that improve insulin sensitivity, such as weight loss, healthy eating patterns, regular and sustained physical activity, and/or the use of diabetes medications (e.g., metformin, thiazolidinediones, and incretin-based therapies). Left unchecked, prediabetes will progress to T2D in a majority of patients.

- The second aspect is to prevent CVD. Prediabetes represents a state of clustered CVD risk factors, accelerated atherosclerosis, and increased risk for CVD events. Epidemiologically, elevated postprandial plasma glucose levels are more associated with increased CVD risk than FPG levels, particularly in women.

- The third aspect is to prevent T2D-related complications. The degree of dysglycemia in prediabetes is sufficient to cause microvascular complications of diabetes in some patients, as demonstrated in the Diabetes Prevention Program, where up to 10% of patients developed background retinopathy or neuropathy. Insulin resistance in association with overweight/ obesity gives rise to Metabolic Syndrome, which may or may not be accompanied by prediabetes. In these patients, there is an infiltration of inflammatory macrophages in adipose tissue; dysregulated secretion of adipokines; impaired lipid storage leading to redistribution of lipid to the intra-abdominal compartment, liver, and muscle cells; and an exacerbation of insulin resistance. Hence, in those patients who develop prediabetes, ABCD (Adiposity Based Chronic Disease) is essentially indistinguishable from DBCD. However, not all patients with ABCD have DBCD.

Dysglycemia is loosely defined as any abnormality in glycemic status that is associated with disease, or the potential for disease, with the earliest citation in PubMed in 1951. Furthermore, reciprocal effects of b-cell function can reduce the number of a-cells, the relative a-cell/b-cell distribution, and a-cell function. Specifically, in a meta-analysis of prospective cohort studies, Huang et al found that for those patients with prediabetes (defined by various impaired fasting glucose and impaired glucose tolerance criteria), the range of relative risks for composite CVD was 1.13 to 1.30, coronary heart disease 1.10 to 1.20, stroke 1.06 to 1.20, and all-cause mortality 1.13 to 1.32 (Mechanick, Garber, Grunberger, Handelsman, & Garvey, 2018).

Chapter 17: Diabetes Mellitus Type 2

Clinical features similar to diabetes mellitus were described 3000 years ago by the ancient Egyptians. The term "diabetes" was first coined by Araetus of Cappodocia (81-133AD). Later, the word mellitus (honey sweet) was added by Thomas Willis (Britain) in 1675 after rediscovering the sweetness of urine and blood of patients (first noticed by the ancient Indians) (Ahmed, 2002).

By understanding the metabolic defects with the diabetic state, it makes it easier to approach treatment. As individuals progress from normal to impaired fasting glucose (prediabetes), there is a 50% decline in beta-cell volume, suggesting a significant loss of beta-cell mass long before the onset of type 2 diabetes. By the time the diagnosis of diabetes is made, many patients have lost over 80% of his/her beta-cell function. Peripheral neuropathy also is a common finding in prediabetes occurring in as many as 5-10% (DeFronzo, 2009).

One of the most difficult issues with improving management of diabetes is called clinical inertia. Clinical inertia is defined as lack of treatment intensification in a patient without good clinical reason. Recent work suggests that clinical inertia related to the management of diabetes, hypertension, and lipid disorders may contribute to up to 80% of heart attacks and strokes. Clinical inertia is, therefore, a leading cause of potentially preventable adverse events, disability, and death (O'Connor, Sperl-Hillen, Johnson, & Rush, 2005).

A good example of treatment intensification is in an article by Vos and colleagues entitled **"Insulin monotherapy compared with**

the addition of oral glucose-lowering agents to insulin for people with type 2 diabetes already on insulin therapy and inadequate glycemic control." This article points out a very simple idea. It looked at 37 trials comparing 40 different treatment plans involving 3,227 patients. It compared multiple different insulin schedules compared with insulin in combination with adding an oral agent. The oral agents included several different sulfonylureas, metformin, pioglitazone, alpha-glucosidase inhibitors, dipeptidyl peptidase-4 inhibitors (DDP-4 inhibitors), and combination metformin/glimepiride. The conclusion was that the addition of all glucose-lowering agents in people with type 2 diabetes and inadequate glycemic control had positive effects on glycemic control and insulin requirements. It also showed the addition of sulfonylurea agents results in more hypoglycemic events. (Vos, et al., 2016)

In my opinion, the article brings out a few ideas. Simply stated, doing something to a patient with inadequate glycemic control is better than not doing anything. I would argue adding a sulfonylurea to insulin is almost always a bad idea since it usually does not help since beta-cell function is usually exhausted by the time insulin is used and if it is not exhausted then the risk of hypoglycemia is too high considering the much better, safer alternative agents available to us presently. A good physician needs to know his comfort level and either educate himself on the new agents available or relinquish this task to someone more qualified. Generally speaking, an endocrinologist usually does diabetes care better than an internist and an internist usually does better than a family physician.

Another great article for further reading is **"Clinical inertia with regard to intensifying therapy in people with type 2 diabetes treated with basal insulin."** Khunti and colleagues completed a retrospective cohort study of 11,696 patients looking at treatment intensification between 2004 and 2011 in the United Kingdom in patients who were already taking basal insulin. A HbA1c level equal to or greater than 7.5% was the threshold level used for intensification. Among all patients, 36.5% had therapy intensification with 50% bolus insulin, 42.5% with premix insulin and 7.4% with a GLP-1 agent (glucagon-like peptide-1 receptor agonist). **The median time from initiation of basal insulin to treatment intensification was 4.3 years. Using a threshold HbA1c equal to or greater than 8.0% showed a median time to intensification of 3.2 years.** Among patients with HbA1c levels equal or greater than 7.5%, 32.1 % stopped basal insulin therapy. This delay in treatment intensification was more pronounced among older people and those with a longer duration of diabetes (Khunti, et al., 2016).

Some basic concepts for diabetes.

1. Who's at risk for diabetes: overweight or obese individuals, minorities, family history of diabetes, elderly, females more often than males, delivery of baby greater than 9 lbs., gestational diabetes, and abnormal lipid profile with elevated triglyceride level and low HDL cholesterol.
2. The use of insulin by itself does not classify the type of diabetes a person has. 90-95% of diabetics have type 2 diabetes and only 5-10% have type 1 diabetes. This straight-forward principle is poorly appreciated by both doctors and nurses many times. People with type 2 diabetes usually need about one unit of insulin per kilogram. (70 kg man needs about 70 units per day). A person with type 1 may need only ½ unit or less per kg.
3. Our pancreas releases insulin and adjusts on a minute-by-minute basis to treat glucose from our meals. It should not be a surprise that our attempts at glucose control with 1-4 shots per day cannot even compare to the sophisticated control that our pancreas and other hormones engage in. An insulin pump with a continuous glucose sensor provides the best technology presently and mostly is a tool for people with type 1 diabetes but the number of people with type 2 diabetes using this technology is increasing yearly. Insurance approval and patient preference are the two key questions. It is absolutely necessary that a person with type 1 diabetes uses a pump or does multiple daily injections (MDI). Remember, a person with type 1 diabetes does not make insulin and needs exogenous insulin to survive. Children in the past with type 1 diabetes before insulin was discovered essentially starved themselves until they died before adulthood. Type 1 diabetics need a basal insulin and

mealtime insulin to try to primitively mimic the normal pancreas. It is very hard to tell a healthy child that from now on you need to prink your finger 6 times a day and stick a needle in your belly 4 times a day while your friends do not understand this or accept this. Growing up with a chronic illness can devastate a child and family. Hypoglycemia is frightening to everyone especially children.

One can assume the "state of the art" approach to a person with type 2 diabetes would be an insulin pump or multi-daily injections if we are only looking at insulin and not taking into consideration medications like metformin, SGLT-2, GLP-1 agents. The problem is compliance. People do not want to take multiple injections, do glucoscans regularly, or upset the doctor so multiple daily injections ends up being one shot of Lantus and one shot of short-acting insulin many times. A very common scenario I see routinely in the hospital is a patient taking a basal insulin like Lantus or Levemir and supposedly also taking short-acting insulin for meals. They usually have a HgbA1c level above 8% and I am seeing them after they are admitted for acute coronary syndrome and or are scheduled for CABG. I will typically change them to a premix 70/30 or 75/25 insulin and do two shots per day. This is not as physiologic as basal/bolus administration but decreases the number of shots and improves compliance and HgbA1c levels.

A study by Giugliano D et al., in March 2016, looked at thirteen randomized-controlled trials lasting 16-60 weeks and involving 5,255 patients comparing intensification of insulin therapy with either basal-bolus or premixed insulin regimens. There was no statistical significance for hypoglycemic rate, weight change, and total daily insulin dose. The likelihood for reaching the HbA1c less than 7% was 8% higher with basal-bolus compared with pre-mix (Giugliano, Chiodini, Maiorino, Bellastella, & Esposito, 2016).

Compromise is the most realistic option with certain patients. Sometimes, an HbA1c of 7-8% rather than a non-compliant HbA1c of 9 or 10% is the best one can do. Remember the complication rate curve stays pretty flat till about 8% before it starts to climb. Always think of thyroid disease, iron deficiency anemia, obstructive sleep apnea and hypogonadism (in men) when seeing a person with diabetes. It's like fishing in a stocked pond, you are going to catch something. There are multiple studies showing many different ways to improve HBA1c levels using various combinations of differing insulins, so this is just one approach that sometimes is helpful.

Understanding the onset, duration and peak of different insulins is essential to appropriately dose insulin.
For example:

- Morning sugar reflects intermediate insulin (NPH) at dinnertime or bedtime.
- Noontime sugar reflect short-acting insulin at breakfast.
- Dinnertime sugar reflects intermediate insulin at breakfast or short-acting insulin at lunch.
- Bedtime sugar reflect short-acting insulin at dinnertime.

4. Counterregulatory hormones- hormones such as cortisol, epinephrine, growth hormone, glucagon are increased in times of stress. These can aggravate hyperglycemia and promote an inflammatory state. Hormones like Ghrelin, NPY, agRP are other examples. Combatting counterregulatory hormones is why using several drugs with different mechanisms of action are important and effective in treating certain common disease processes.

5. An FBS of 100 or greater indicates inadequate glucose handling and glucose pathology and needs to be followed and not ignored.

6. **Physicians use insulin as a last resort for poor control rather than the logical next step in diabetes management. We need to emphasize insulin from the very first visit, not as a threat, but the realization that most patients with type 2 diabetes will eventually need insulin. Hopefully this will motivate them to improve diet and exercise.** Many physicians exhibit inertia (a tendency to do nothing or to remain unchanged) when the time comes to starting insulin. Insulin is not the enemy; diabetes is the issue. The discovery of insulin was one of the greatest discoveries in medicine and has saved millions of lives. People afflicted with type 1 diabetes went from

slow starvation and death to having children and having long productive lives. Insulin is an anabolic hormone, not a catabolic hormone. I strongly recommend reading the 1982 book by Michael Bliss "The Discovery of Insulin." It's the definitive story of how insulin was discovered and became clinical.

7. **Diabetic patients with no previous cardiovascular disease have the same long-term morbidity and mortality as nondiabetic patients with established cardiovascular disease. The 2000 OASIS study provided evidence for this foundation principle** (Malmberg, et al., 2000).

8. If the HgbA1c is 10% (average sugar 247), it's a guarantee that the fasting glucose level is elevated. If you bring down the fasting glucose you are likely to get to a HgbA1c down to 7.5-8.0%, but to get lower you have to control the postprandial glucose levels. Postprandial sugars more closely correlate with CV events than do fasting sugars. This makes sense since we are most of the time in a postprandial state.

9. By converting the HgbA1c to an average sugar it makes it easier for patients to understand where their sugar control is. **HgbA1c x 33.3 − 86 = average sugar.** Glycosylated hemoglobin (hgbA1c) measures glucose on red blood cells and red blood cells live for 120 days therefore it measures the average sugar over the last 4 months. A transfusion dependent person will not have an accurate hgbA1c since he is always receiving new red blood cells from someone else.

10. A good example of the importance of postprandial control involves gestational diabetes. Most pregnant woman will have a normal HgbA1c or mildly elevated HgbA1c level but significant insulin resistance. By controlling and making insulin adjustments based on postprandial sugars, lower complication rate, lower C-section rate, and lower neonatal ICU admissions have been noted.

11. The main predictors of weight gain are the initial glucose level and its response to treatment. The patient with poor glucose control, and large kcal losses per day due to glucosuria, is at greater risk for weight gain once a good

treatment response occurs. **A rough but accurate estimate is a 5-lb. weight gain for every 1% decrease in HgbA1c level.** This is a very important clinical concept to always keep in mind and is one of the reasons I became interested in obesity medicine. For example, **most diabetic medicines will decrease HgbA1c by about a point except for insulin.** If I have a person with a HgbA1c level of 10% I know that it will take several medicines to bring his sugars under control. I can start him on insulin and he will gain a lot of weight, or I can try metformin and an SGLT-2 agent while working on diet and exercise.

12. **Secondary failure. Decline in drug effectiveness due to disease progression.** For example, a person goes from HgbA1c level of 6.4 to 8.0 over 2 years on Amaryl only. It is not a surprise that this happens because diabetes is a progressive beta-cell failure disease which will require more medicines to counteract decreasing beta-cell function. This is just one of many reasons why patients with diabetes need to be seen every 3-4 months. Also, metformin is the standard first-line drug in type 2 diabetes and not Amaryl.

13. 1500 rule-tool used to assess how much one unit of insulin will decrease a person's sugar. For example, a person takes 50 units of insulin per day. 1500 divided by 50 equals 30. One unit of insulin will decrease the person's sugar by 30 mg/dl.

14. **Despite a revolution of new diabetic medicines and new insulins over the last 2 decades, the majority of people with type 2 diabetes do not achieve the goals outlined by the American Diabetes Association, the American Association of Clinical Endocrinologists and the American College of Endocrinology.**

15. For every 1% reduction in HgbA1c level, there is about a 14% reduction in coronary events. Elevated HbA1c is a strong predictor of mortality and morbidity irrespective of previous diabetic status. In particular, the mortality risk for CABG is quadrupled at HbA1c levels >8.6%. In elective situations, it has been proposed that these patients should be delayed for surgery until adequate glycemic control is achieved (Tennyson, Lee, & Attia, 2013).

A 2008 study examined 3,089 diabetic and non-diabetic patients. HbA1c proved to be a powerful predictor of in-hospital mortality and morbidity postoperatively. Significant increases in mortality (P = 0.019) and deep sternal wound infection (DSWI) (P = 0.014) were identified per unit increase in HbA1c. **Elevated HbA1c ≥8.6% caused a four-fold increase in mortality. Postoperative complications such as renal failure (RF), cerebrovascular accident (CVA), and DSWI (deep sternal wound infection) occurred more frequently at HbA1c ≥ 8.6%.** Complication rates were significantly higher in poor control HbA1c ≥7% vs good control <7% (Halkos, et al., 2008).

1. Cardiovascular risk doubles for each 20 mm. Hg systolic/10 mm. diastolic rise in blood pressure.
2. **Greater than 2/3 of patients with hypertension require more than one drug to reach goal.**
3. The standard of care is to offer diabetes education to every patient with newly diagnosed diabetes. A person cannot be labeled noncompliant if he is never informed.
4. **Remember the ABC's of diabetes care- A1c level, Blood pressure, Cholesterol.**
5. "RULE OF 6"-each doubling of the statin dose produces an average additional decrease in LDL of about 5-6%. I typically do not see this when I increase from 40 mg to 80 mg atorvastatin.
6. **The main reason to start a statin is really to promote cholesterol plaque stability. By using this principle, one does not have to debate about whether to start a statin drug on a person with diabetes who has a very favorable lipid profile. The answer will always be yes unless statin intolerance is present.**
7. Insulin stacking- accumulation of insulin following repetitive doses of short-acting insulin given too early to correct hyperglycemia. Many times, this leads to hypoglycemia. For example, a Nursing home nurse has a patient with a sugar of 340 mg/dl and gives insulin based on a sliding scale every hour instead of 4-6 hours and leads to a sugar of 70 mg/dl three hours later. The

subsequent insulin doses add up since the first dose has not had adequate time to work.

8. Freestyle Personal Libre – a continuous glucose monitor (CGM) designed to provide multiple glucose levels throughout a period of time up to 14 days. It requires no finger sticks to calibrate the system. It is a water-resistant plastic sensor placed on the body(arm) as a patch the size of a one-dollar coin. It provides real-time information. Was approved October 2016. Glucose sensors have shown that hypoglycemia is more common than appreciated. The majority of episodes occur without symptoms and/or while the patient is asleep. The Freestyle Personal Libre \ is very easy to use and is cost-effective.

9. Lipodystrophy- area of skin that may have diminished or unpredictable absorption from repeatedly injecting at the same site. Solution is to always rotate sites for injections or for pump insertion site.

10. **It is well known that too much sugar causes tooth decay, but it seems hard to convince patients that too much sugar causes the same decay in many important organs we have.**

We Know More Than We Can Tell About Diabetes and Vascular Disease: The 2016 Edwin Bierman Award Lecture

Progress in Vascular Complications

- Authentic progress has been made to decrease the incidence of diabetes-related complications involving both macrovascular and microvascular disease.
- Relative risks for acute myocardial infarction, stroke, amputations, and end-stage renal disease associated with diabetes decreased between 1990 and 2010.
- How this happened is probably multifactorial, including the use of statins and inhibitors of the renin-angiotensin system, more options for glucose lowering, and less tobacco use.

- Despite this progress in relative risk, the overall burden of vascular complications continues to increase for at least two reasons;
  (1) people with diabetes remain much more likely than those without diabetes to have heart attacks, strokes, limb loss, and renal failure.
  (2) the incidence of both type 1 and type 2 diabetes has increased.

Relationships between vascular diseases in diabetes

- Tacit knowledge (knowledge from life's experience) implies that some of the distinctions between macrovascular (larger vessel disease leading to heart attacks, strokes, and limb loss) and microvascular (smaller vessel disease leading to retinopathy, nephropathy, and neuropathy) disease are artifactual. Recent studies support this concept.

- In a very large (more than 49,000 subjects) population-based cohort of people with type 2 diabetes, the cumulative burden of microvascular disease was associated with major adverse cardiovascular events (MACE). This study also reported a dose-response relationship between the number of microvascular disease states and MACE hazard ratio as well as death from cardiovascular disease.

- In a discovery cohort as well as a replication cohort of individuals with type 2 diabetes representing a broad spectrum of ethnicity, subtle decrements in renal function over time were associated with a greater risk of MACE. These findings suggest that changes in the renal vasculature mirror progression of macrovascular disease.

- There is also evidence that specific vascular complications in diabetes may be interactive, i.e., the pathophysiology of one complication may modulate progression of another.

Conundrums in diabetic vascular disease

- These conundrums are in part the product of studying clinical end points from the perspective of circulating biomarkers. Biomarkers may be associated with vascular disease as in the case of HDL particles, which are strongly inversely related to disease in multiple populations. But this association does not ensure a direct role in disease.

- Fenofibrate appears to decrease the risk of both cardiovascular events (in selected subgroups) and retinopathy in diabetes.
- The Action to Control Cardiovascular Risk in Diabetes (ACCORD) Lipid trial did not demonstrate cardiovascular benefit for the addition of fenofibrate to a statin, but long-term follow-up suggests that fenofibrate is beneficial in a subgroup of people with diabetes, triglycerides >204 mg/dL, and HDL cholesterol <34 mg/dL.
- The Fenofibrate Intervention and Event Lowering in Diabetes (FIELD) study, another fibrate trial, showed that fenofibrate did not reduce the coronary event primary outcome but did demonstrate decreased need for laser treatment of diabetic retinopathy, an effect independent of circulating lipids.

A practical approach to vascular disease in diabetes

- many patients are not deriving maximal benefit from currently available therapies.
- In more than 2,000 adults with diabetes but no cardiovascular disease followed for 11 years, achieving blood pressure, LDL cholesterol, and HbA_{1c} goals was associated with substantially lower risk of heart disease.
- **only about 7% of patients reached these relatively modest targets for blood pressure (130/80 mmHg), LDL cholesterol (100 mg/dL), and HbA_{1c} (7% [53 mmol/mol]).**

One approach to decrease vascular risk in type 2 diabetes

- **Improve glycemic control, with metformin and SGLT2 inhibitor or GLP-1 receptor agonist**
- **Exercise, diet, and smoking cessation counseling**
- **Blood pressure control, often with more than one agent**
- **High-intensity statin, as tolerated**
- **Fenofibrate, especially in males with elevated triglycerides and low HDL cholesterol**
- **Consideration of PCSK9 inhibition based on clinical circumstance**

(Semenkovich, 2017)

Myocardial cell death in human diabetes.

This is a very nice description of why ace-inhibitors are essential in treating patients with diabetes. The dynamic duo of diabetes and hypertension can do some dynamic damage to our hearts. ACE (angiotensin converting enzyme) inhibitors block angiotensin I conversion to the potent vasoconstrictor angiotensin II of the renin-angiotensin system. The renin-angiotensin system is upregulated with diabetes, and this may contribute to the development of a dilated myopathy. Angiotensin II (Ang II) locally may lead to oxidative damage, activating cardiac cell death. Moreover, diabetes and hypertension could synergistically impair myocardial structure and function by apoptosis and necrosis. Damage can be ascertained in ventricular myocardial biopsies obtained from diabetic and diabetic-hypertensive patients by measuring the accumulation of a marker of oxidative stress, nitrotyrosine, and labeling Angiotensin II. The diabetic heart showed cardiac hypertrophy, cavitary dilation, and depressed ventricular performance. These alterations were more severe with diabetes and hypertension.

Diabetics was characterized by an

- 85-fold apoptosis of myocytes
- 61-fold apoptosis of endothelial cells
- 26-fold increase in apoptosis of fibroblasts
- necrosis by 4-fold in myocytes, 9-fold in endothelial cells, 6-fold in fibroblasts
- Diabetes and hypertension increased necrosis by 7-fold in myocytes and 18-fold in endothelial cells.

Similarly, Ang II labeling in myocytes and endothelial cells increased more with diabetes and hypertension than with diabetes alone. In conclusion, local increases in Ang II with diabetes and with diabetes and hypertension may enhance oxidative damage, activating cardiac cell apoptosis and necrosis (Frustaci, et al., 2000).

The pathogenesis of myocardial fibrosis in the setting of diabetic cardiomyopathy.

Chapter 17: Diabetes Mellitus Type 2

The increasing incidence of diabetes in young individuals is particularly worrisome given that the disease is likely to evolve over a period of years. In 1972, the existence of a diabetic cardiomyopathy was proposed based on the experience with four adult diabetic patients who suffered from congestive heart failure in the absence of discernible coronary artery disease, valvular or congenital heart disease, hypertension, or alcoholism.

An important component is the accumulation of extracellular matrix (ECM) proteins, in particular collagens. The excess deposition of ECM in the heart mirrors what occurs in other organs such as the kidney and peritoneum of diabetics. Mechanisms responsible for these alterations may include the excess production, reduced degradation, and/or chemical modification of ECM proteins. These effects may be the result of direct or indirect actions of high glucose concentrations (Asbun & Villareal, 2006).

The "Ominous Octet": Multiple Pathophysiological Abnormalities in Type 2 Diabetes (Dr. Ralph DeFronzo)

1. Beta-cell decline/failure (reduced insulin secretion by pancreas).
2. Insulin resistance in muscle. Decreased glucose uptake in muscle. More insulin needed to move glucose into muscle to do work. Lipid infiltration (lipotoxicity) into muscle impairs muscle function and worsens insulin resistance.
3. Insulin resistance in liver. Takes more insulin to suppress liver gluconeogenesis. Lipid infiltration into liver (fatty liver/non-alcoholic steatohepatitis)
4. Increased activity of alpha cells in pancreas releasing more glucagon to liver to promote gluconeogenesis. Glucagonemia promotes elevated hepatic glucose production (gluconeogenesis).
5. Increased glucose reabsorption in kidney. The renal threshold increases before glucosuria occurs. Instead of losing glucose in urine at a level of 180 mg/dl, it may be 240 mg/dl, causing increased calories kept in circulation promoting weight gain and glucotoxicity.

6. Loss of incretin function from gut (decreased GLP-1). Both GLP-1 and GIP (Gastric Inhibitory Peptide, or Glucose-dependent insulinotropic peptide) are called incretin hormones. Incretin hormones are released from the GI tract when we eat. The existence of them explains why a greater sugar lowering response occurs when we eat compared to receiving the same calories intravenously. GLP-1 is released from the ileum of small bowel and also the colon. It does the following:

1. Decreases appetite.
2. Promotes insulin release by pancreas when glucose is present.
3. Decreases liver gluconeogenesis by inhibiting glucagon.
4. Decrease gastric emptying.

GIP is released from duodenum of small bowel and stimulates pancreas to release insulin when glucose is present. GIP plays a minor role.

Incretins have been shown to improve beta-cell function and maintain durability of glycemic control.

7. Increased lipids cause increased fatty acids in bloodstream which aggravates insulin resistance (lipotoxicity). Excessive calorie intake leads to elevated free fatty acids which creates a pro-inflammatory and insulin resistant environment. A simple observation notes that a lipid infusion markedly impairs both the first and second phases of C-peptide release and reduce insulin secretory rate. Weight loss and Actos (TZD) that mobilize fat out of the beta-cell would be expected to reverse lipotoxicity and preserve beta-cell function. Beta-cell function has first and second phase insulin release. The first phase consists of a brief spike lasting 10 minutes followed by the second phase, which reaches a plateau at 2-3 hours. It is widely thought that diminution of first-phase insulin release is the earliest detectable defect of beta-cell function in individuals destined to develop type 2 diabetes and that this defect largely represents beta-cell exhaustion after years of compensation for antecedent insulin resistance.

8. Insulin resistance in brain (higher insulin required to suppress appetite).

(DeFronzo, 2009)

Chapter 17: Diabetes Mellitus Type 2

When I see a person that has diabetes, I try to get them off insulin by using metformin, GLP1, SGLT2 agents along with phentermine if appropriate. **Try to use drugs with "triple bottom line" or "triple threat"- good glycemic control, low risk of hypoglycemia, and weight loss**. Encouraging physical activity is a must. Many insurance companies require a person to be on metformin or intolerant of it before paying for additional higher priced drugs. Losing weight is clearly the best treatment in many individuals. If someone has a BMI of 27 or higher, I will offer phentermine.

Chapter 18: Diabetes Mellitus Type 2 Medications

The number of medications to help treat diabetes has escalated over the last 25 years, especially the last 15 years. Medications have been developed coinciding with the basic science behind understanding how diabetes interacts with many organ systems.

The European Medicines Agency's approval of new medicines for type 2 diabetes.

Since 2005, more than 40 new medicines for the treatment of type 2 diabetes have been introduced on the market.
These consist of 15 new active substances establishing three new classes of non-insulin products, and several new or modified insulin products and combinations.
For the majority of these new medicines approved since 2005, cardiovascular outcome trials have now been completed, and have invariably supported the cardiovascular safety of these products. In some of these trials additional important benefits have been observed, for instance, a reduction in major adverse cardiovascular events and improvement of renal outcome (Blind, Janssen, Dunder, & de Graeff, 2018).

Classes of Diabetic Medications

1. Sulfonylureas- the first sulfonylurea, tolbutamide, was in 1956 in Germany. In 1984, glyburide and glipizide, became available in the United States.
Popular ones are glyburide, glipizide, glimepiride- stimulate additional insulin release. Downside-hypoglycemia and only

effective in first few years of diabetes. Generic and inexpensive. Higher doses no more effective than lower doses. Promotes weight gain. Along with the obvious dangers in elderly, hypoglycemia induces prothrombotic changes while increasing subclinical inflammation markers. **Oral hypoglycemic agents and warfarin account for nearly half of adverse drug events leading to the emergent hospitalization of elderly** (Budnitz & Richards, 2011).

If a practice uses sulfonylurea medicines frequently or the patients have been on them for several years, then the practice needs to be re-educated or the patients need to be referred to someone else.

2. Insulin secretogogues- repaglinide (Prandin), nateglinide (Starlix). Shorter acting than sulfonylureas, therefore lower hypoglycemia risk. Downside-take with meals several times per day. Causes weight gain.

3. Glucose suppressors- **metformin- gold standard as initial medicine. First line treatment for DM2, prevention of DM2, pre-DM2, gestational DM and weight loss.** Decreases hepatic glucose production. Much safer than initially thought. Cannot give if GFR less than 30 cc/min. I have never seen lactic acid with metformin (most dangerous side-effect). Diarrhea most common side effect. Less diarrhea with extended release form. Helps lose weight. Free at some pharmacies. Not a game changer for weight loss. Although decreasing hepatic glucose production is main focus it does a lot more. It increases insulin-mediated glucose utilization. Decreases intestinal glucose absorption, triggers GLP-1 secretion, increases fatty acid oxidation, decreases appetite by decreasing hormones NPY (neuropeptide Y), agRP (agouti-related peptide), and increases expression of appetite-lowering POMC (pro-opiomelanocortin). It is approved for treatment of DM2 in children greater than 10 years old. A great drug. Need to hold 48 hours before and after radiology contrast or surgery to lessen any potential acute kidney injury. **Metformin has been associated with 39% relative risk reduction for MI and 36% reduction in all-cause mortality. Reduced the progression of diabetes by 31% over 4- year period.**

Metformin has also been used to prevent or ameliorate weight gain with atypical anti-psychotic agents and mood stabilizers (Hasnain, Vieweg, & Fredrickson, 2010)

4. Insulin sensitizers- pioglitazone (Actos) -improves insulin sensitivity. Causes fluid retention and should not be used if CHF is a possibility. Weight gain and edema are dose-dependent. Has been shown to maintain glucose stability for at least four years. Increases the size and buoyancy of LDL particles to less atherogenic form. Lipid benefits are not simply explained by its effects on glycemic control. I still use it and find very helpful. I am cognizant of potential edema/CHF. Takes about a month to show full effect. Generic. May improve fatty liver and preserve beta-cell function.

5. SGLT-2 inhibitors-(Sodium glucose transporter 2 agents) Blocks reabsorption of glucose in renal tubules. Lowers renal threshold from 180 mg/dl or higher to 90 mg/dl. (Renal threshold is level where glucosuria occurs). Promotes renal glucosuria. Great class of medicine. Very helpful for weight loss and preventing weight regain. 15% develop yeast genital infection (mostly women). Can cause dehydration but clinically do not see as often as expected. Many times, I will decrease diuretic dose or stop diuretic when SGLT-2 started. Effects of drug is insulin-independent. Efficacy dependent on GFR. Expensive. Very effective class. I prescribe it almost daily. Used off-label in some type1 diabetics understanding that it can increase risk of DKA.

- **Invokana (canaglifozin)** 100 mg dose, can increase to 300 mg dose. Not to be used if GFR 30 cc/min of less. I have found that the 300 mg dose seems to cause much more diuresis with patient's not tolerating as well as the 100 mg dose.
- **Jardiance (empagliflozin)** 10 mg/day starting dose. 25 mg is given for a little better effect. Use 10 mg if GFR less/equal to 60 and stop if GFR less/equal to 45. Recent literature supports cardioprotective benefit.
- **Farxiga (dapagliflozin)** 5 mg starting dose and 10 mg for a little more additional benefit. Results in spilling of about

280 kcals/day of glucose in urine. Not effective if GFR less than 60. Side effects same as others.

- **Steglatro (ertugliflozin)** 5 mg/day starting dose with 15 mg/day for a little more additional benefit. Not recommended if GFR less than 60 cc/min. Newest SGLT-2.

Recent clinical studies have shown significant benefits in this class of medicine.

EMPA-REG OUTCOME: The Endocrinologist's Point of View.

- For many years, it was widely accepted that control of plasma lipids and blood pressure could lower macrovascular risk in patients with type 2 diabetes mellitus (T2DM), whereas the benefits of lowering plasma glucose were largely limited to improvements in microvascular complications. The Empagliflozin Cardiovascular Outcome Event Trial in Type 2 Diabetes Mellitus Patients-Removing Excess Glucose (EMPA-REG OUTCOME) study demonstrated for the first time that a glucose-lowering agent, the sodium glucose cotransporter 2 (SGLT2) inhibitor empagliflozin (Jardiance) could reduce major adverse cardiovascular events, cardiovascular mortality, hospitalization for heart failure, and overall mortality when given in addition to standard care in patients with T2DM at high cardiovascular risk. These results were entirely unexpected and have led to much speculation regarding the potential mechanisms underlying cardiovascular benefits (Perreault, 2017).

EMPA-REG OUTCOME: The Cardiologist's Point of View.

- Cardiologists could view empagliflozin (Jardiance) as a cardiovascular drug that also has a beneficial effect on reducing hyperglycemia in patients with type 2 diabetes mellitus (T2DM). The effects of empagliflozin in lowering the risk of cardiovascular death and hospitalization for heart failure in T2DM patients with high cardiovascular risk during the recent Empagliflozin Cardiovascular Outcome Event Trial in Type 2 Diabetes Mellitus Patients-Removing Excess Glucose (EMPA-REG OUTCOME) trial may be explained principally in terms of changes to cardiovascular physiology; namely, by the potential ability of empagliflozin to reduce cardiac workload and myocardial oxygen consumption by lowering blood pressure, improving aortic compliance, and improving ventricular arterial coupling (Pham & Chilton, 2017).

EMPA-REG OUTCOME: The Nephrologist's Point of View.

- There is increasing evidence that sodium glucose cotransporter 2 (SGLT2) inhibitors have renoprotective effects, as demonstrated by the renal analyses from clinical trials including Empagliflozin Cardiovascular Outcome Event Trial in Type 2 Diabetes Mellitus PatientsRemoving Excess Glucose (EMPA-REGOUTCOME), CANagliflozin Treatment And Trial Analysis versus SUlphonylurea (CANTATA-SU), and the dapagliflozin renal study. The potential mechanisms responsible are likely multifactorial, and direct renovascular and hemodynamic effects are postulated to play a central role (Wanner, 2017).

6. DPP-4 Inhibitors (Dipeptidyl peptidase 4 inhibitor)-

sitagliptin (Januvia), saxagliptin (Onglyza), linagliptin (Tradjenta). Slows the inactivation of incretin hormones. Inhibits enzyme that breaks down incretins. Allows incretins to last longer which promotes better glucose control. Nausea, diarrhea side effects. Usually tolerated very well. Easy medicine to add on to care. Weight neutral. Expensive.

- **Januvia (sitagliptin)** Usual dose is 100 mg /day. 50 mg/day if GFR less than 30. 25 mg/day if on dialysis.
- **Tradjenta (linagliptin)** 5 mg /day. No dose adjustment for renal or hepatic issues.
- **Onglyza (saxagliptin)** 5 mg/day. Decrease to 2.5 mg if GFR less than 50.

7. GLP-1 Agonists (Glucagon-like peptide-1)- injectable

agent in pen. Victoza-once/day, while Bydureon, Tanzeum,

Trulicity and Ozempic (once/week). Decreases appetite, and gastric emptying. Promotes insulin release by pancreas when glucose is present, and decreases liver gluconeogenesis by inhibiting glucagon. Helps weight loss. Expensive.

- **Victoza (liraglutide)**-once per day pen injection. Dose is started at 0.6 mg SQ followed by 1.2 mg SQ a week later and then 1.8 mg SQ daily. Most common side effects are nausea, headache. Weight loss beneficial side effect.
- **Trulicity (dulaglutide)**-once per week injection. Doses are 0.75 mg and 1.5 mg pens. Most common side effects are nausea, vomiting, diarrhea. Easiest pen to use. No mixing required.
- **Tanzeum (albiglutide)**-discontinued August 2017.
- **Bydureon (exenatide)**-once per week injection. Single dose. Needs reconstitution.
- **Ozempic (semaglutide)**- once weekly starting at 0.25 mg SQ for 4 weeks, then 0.5 mg SQ weekly. Can increase to 1 mg SQ weekly if needed.

Effects of Liraglutide on Weight Loss, Fat Distribution, and β-Cell Function in Obese Subjects with Prediabetes or Early Type 2 Diabetes.

It has been shown that obese adult visceral adipose tissue (VAT) and insulin resistance are independently associated with incident prediabetes and type 2 diabetes, but this is not the case for general adiposity or subcutaneous adipose tissue (SAT)

- Liraglutide, a glucagon-like peptide 1 analog, is associated with weight loss, improved glycemic control, and reduced cardiovascular risk.
- We determined whether an equal degree of weight loss by liraglutide or lifestyle changes has a different impact on subcutaneous adipose tissue (SAT) and visceral adipose tissue (VAT) in obese subjects with prediabetes or early type 2 diabetes. We chose the loss of 7% of initial body weight as the target weight loss based on previous reports where such a weight loss was associated with improved metabolic outcomes.

Conclusions

- We observed significantly enhanced abdominal visceral fat loss and improved β-cell function with liraglutide (Victoza). The liraglutide effects on visceral obesity and β-cell function might provide a rationale for its use in obese subjects in an early phase of the natural history of glucose dysregulation (Santilli, et al., 2017).

Pharmacologic therapy to induce weight loss in women who have obesity/overweight with polycystic ovary syndrome: a systematic review and network meta-analysis.

Compare the effectiveness of metformin, inositol, liraglutide and orlistat to induce weight loss in women with PCOS and overweight/obesity.

Methods:

A search was conducted using the MEDLINE, EMBASE, PubMed and CENTRAL databases.

Results:

Twenty-three trials reporting on 941 women were included in the meta-analysis. The amount of weight lost differed significantly among the drugs (in descending order): liraglutide, orlistat and metformin. Liraglutide alone, liraglutide/metformin and metformin alone significantly reduced waist circumference, but no change was found with orlistat.

Conclusion:

Liraglutide (Victoza) appears superior to the other drugs (orlistat, metformin) in reducing weight and waist circumference in women with PCOS. (Wang, et al., 2018).

8. Amylin mimetic- pramlintide (Symlin) - injectable approved March 2005. Symlin is a synthetic analog of amylin, a naturally occurring neuroendocrine hormone synthesized by pancreatic beta-cells that contribute to glucose control during the postprandial period. Amylin is co-located with insulin in secretory granules and co-secreted with insulin in response to food intake. Amylin and insulin show similar fasting and postprandial patterns in healthy individuals. Amylin slows gastric emptying, suppresses glucagon secretion, and regulates food intake due to centrally-mediated modulation of appetite. In patients with diabetes, glucagon concentrations are abnormally elevated during the postprandial period, contributing to hyperglycemia. Symlin has been shown to decrease postprandial glucagon concentrations in insulin-using patients. Symlin is administered prior to a meal and has been shown to reduce total caloric intake.   Several benefits but requires couple shots per day. Nausea is main side effect. Decreases insulin requirements along with promoting weight loss. Expensive. Used mostly by some endocrinologists with type 1 diabetics. A difficult drug to use and not popular.

9. Bile acid sequestrant- colesevelam (Welchol) - improves glucose control and lowers LDL cholesterol. Downside-6 big tablets per day, can interfere with thyroid medicine absorption. GI side effects. Probably good choice with person with post-GB diarrhea or someone who wants more natural remedy. Moderate price.

10. Alpha-Glucosidase inhibitors- acarbose (Precose). Delays absorption of carbohydrates in intestines thus decreasing glucose levels. Lowers postprandial hyperglycemia. Does not cause hypoglycemia. Downside-gas, diarrhea. Not used much in United States.

11. Dopamine agonists- dopamine receptor agonist. Trade name "Cycloset." 1st approved May 2009. Centrally-acting but exact mechanism unknown. Works by increasing insulin sensitivity. Is an add-on medicine at best. Nausea occurs in 26%. Starting dose is 0.8 mg in morning with food and is increased weekly as tolerated up to 6 tablets per day. HgbA1c improvement only 0.6 or less. I have no experience and suspect I will never use it. Expensive. I find it interesting that neurotransmitters are so often intricately involved in diabetes, weight gain and weight-loss.

12. Insulin - see chapter on insulin.

Combination Medicines

Chapter 18: Diabetes Mellitus Type 2 Medications

Very helpful drugs but confusing. Many are metformin combinations that emphasize the fundamental role of metformin in type 2 diabetes care. Understanding each component helps clarify using them. It is very hard to keep up with all the new drugs and insulins on the market now. If a practice does not focus and purposely attracts patients with diabetes, I would suggest having those patients see a diabetes practice for their management.

1. **Glyambi** (SGLT-2-Jardiance and DPP4-Tradjenta). Doses are 10 mg/5 mg and 25 mg/5 mg.
2. **Syngardy** (Jardiance and metformin). Doses are 5 mg/500 mg, 5 mg/1000 mg, 12.5 mg/500 mg, 12.5 mg/1000 mg.
3. **Synjardy XR** (Jardiance and extended release metformin). Doses are 10 mg /1000 mg, 12.5 mg /1000 mg, 25 mg /1000 mg.
4. **Xigduo** (SGLT-2 Farxiga and metformin XR). Doses are 5 mg /500 mg, 5 mg /1000 mg, 10 mg /500 mg, 10 mg /1000 mg.
5. **Qtern** (SGLT-2 Farxiga and DPP-4Onglyza). Dose is 10 mg /5 mg.
6. **Invokamet** (Invokana and metformin). Doses are 50 mg /500 mg, 50 mg /1000 mg, 150 mg/500 mg, 150 mg/1000 mg.
7. **Kombiglyze** (DPP4 Onglyza and metformin). Doses are 5 mg /500 mg, 5 mg /1000 mg, and 2.5 mg /1000 mg.
8. **Oseni** (DPP4 Alogliptin and TZD Actos). Doses are 12.5 mg /15 mg, 12.5 mg /30 mg, 12.5 mg /45 mg, and 25 mg/15 mg, 25 mg/30 mg, 25 mg/45 mg.
9. **Glucovance** (glyburide, metformin). Doses are 1.25 mg/250 mg, 2.5 mg /500 mg, 5 mg /500 mg.
10. **Actoplus Met** (Actos, metformin). Doses are 15 mg/500 mg, 15 mg/850 mg.
11. **Duetact** (Actos, Amaryl). Doses are 30 mg/2 mg, 30 mg/4 mg.
12. **Janumet** (Januvia, metformin). Doses are 50 mg /500 mg, 50 mg/1000 mg.
13. **Jentadueto** (Tradjenta, metformin). Doses are 2.5 mg/500 mg, 2.5 mg /850 mg, 2.5 mg/1000 mg.

14. **Prandimet** (prandin, metformin). Doses are 1 mg /500 mg, 2 mg/500 mg.
15. **Kazano** (metformin, alogliptin). 500 mg /12.5 mg.

Insulin resistance improvement by cinnamon powder in polycystic ovary syndrome: A randomized double-blind placebo controlled clinical trial.

- Assess the effect of cinnamon powder capsules on insulin resistance in women with polycystic ovarian syndrome (PCOS).
- 66 were enrolled in this randomized double-blind placebo-controlled clinical trial.
- The women in the first group were treated with cinnamon powder capsules 1.5 g/day in 3 divided doses for 12 weeks and the second group by similar placebo capsules.
- **The present results suggest that complementary supplementation of cinnamon significantly reduced fasting insulin and insulin resistance in women with PCOS.** (Hajimonfarednejad, et al., 2018).

Curcumin, the golden nutraceutical: multitargeting for multiple chronic diseases

Among the numerous natural remedies, turmeric has gained considerable attention due to its profound medicinal values. This agent possesses antioxidant, anti-inflammatory, anticancer, antigrowth, antiarthritic, antiatherosclerotic, antidepressant, antiaging, antidiabetic, antimicrobial, wound healing and memory-enhancing activities. Moreover, it exerts chemopreventive, chemosensitization and radiosensitization effects as well.

Conclusions

There is an abundance of preclinical and clinical evidence indicating that curcumin has potential as a therapy for a wide variety of chronic diseases. Unlike most pharmaceutical drugs, curcumin modulates multiple targets that affect different diseases. Safety, efficacy and affordability are some of the added advantages exhibited by this compound.

It seems that curcumin has potential but does not have FDA approval for any disease process and therefore use is off label. It does seem to be very safe. Curcumin is just one of many compounds found in the bright yellow Indian spice Turmeric that belongs to the ginger plant family. It is the main spice used in curry (Kunnumakkara, et al., 2017).

Chapter 19: C-peptide

"An unappreciated tool"

A Practical Review of C-Peptide Testing in Diabetes

- C-peptide is the part of proinsulin which is cleaved prior to co-secretion with insulin from pancreatic beta cells and is produced in equimolar amounts to endogenous insulin.

What is C-Peptide and Why Might it be Useful in Clinical Practice?

- C-peptide is a useful and widely used method of assessing pancreatic beta cell function.

So why is C-Peptide testing preferable to insulin as a guide to beta cell function?

- The degradation rate of c-peptide in the body is slower than that of insulin (half-life of 20–30 min, compared with the half-life of insulin of just 3–5 min). In healthy individuals the plasma concentration of c-peptide in the fasting state is 0.9-1.8 ng/ml, with a postprandial increase of 3-9 ng/ml. In insulin-treated patients with diabetes, measurement of c-peptide also avoids the pitfall between exogenous and endogenous insulin.

What are the Potential Problems with C-Peptide Measurement?

- The majority of c-peptide is metabolized by the kidneys with 5–10% then excreted unchanged in the urine. This can make c-peptide measurement in individuals with chronic kidney disease inaccurate.
- The presence of large numbers of anti-insulin antibodies that bind both proinsulin and c-peptide can give a falsely high c-peptide reading.

The various practical applications of C-Peptide measurement

Diagnostic
- Criteria for acceptance for CSII (continuous subcutaneous insulin infusion-pump)
- To determine whether T1DM or T2DM
- Diagnostic test for MODY (maturity-onset diabetes of the young), LADA (latent autoimmune diabetes of adults)

Prognostic
- Marker of duration of diabetes
- Lower levels are associated with microvascular complication risk in T1DM
- Associated with glycemic variability/HbA1C level
- Lower levels are associated with greater hypoglycemia risk

Therapeutic response
- Lower baseline levels associated with increased need for insulin
- Higher levels present in patients who respond to metformin, thiazolidinediones
- Correlates with reduction in HbA1C following initiation of GLP-1 agonist therapy

Prediction of Response to Non-Insulin Therapies in T2DM
- High fasting C-peptide is associated with response to the thiazolidinediones, pioglitazone, which is in keeping with their action of reducing insulin resistance. Higher c-peptide levels do seem to predict response to GLP-1 agonists.
- In patients taking SGLT-2 inhibitors, c-peptide may be able to identify those patients who are at risk of diabetic ketoacidosis. Unfortunately, low C-peptide is not a consistent finding in patients on SGLT-2 inhibitors who have ketoacidosis.

Can C-Peptide Predict Diabetes Complications?
- Lower c-peptide values have been associated with poorer glycemic control and hence increased HbA1c values.
- Lower levels of C-peptide and decreased beta cell function have been linked to greater levels of glucose variability. As

glucose variability is known to be associated with increased complications and mortality in patients with diabetes it is possible that c-peptide may be a predictor of future outcomes independent of HbA1c levels (Leighton, Sainsbury, & Jones, 2017).

Association of C-peptide with diabetic vascular complications in type 2 diabetes.

- Fasting serum C-peptide is a biomarker of insulin production and insulin resistance. This study aimed to investigate whether C-peptide is associated with cardiovascular disease (CVD) and diabetic retinopathy (DR).

- A total of 4793 diabetic patients were enrolled from seven communities in Shanghai, China, in 2018.

RESULTS:

- Prevalence of CVD increased with increasing C-peptide levels (Q1, Q2, Q3 and Q4: 33%, 34%, 37% and 44%, respectively; $P_{for\ trend} < 0.001$), whereas diabetic retinopathy prevalence decreased with increasing C-peptide quartiles (Q1, Q2, Q3 and Q4: 21%, 19%, 15% and 12%, respectively; $P_{for\ trend} < 0.001$).

- C-peptide levels were significantly associated with CVD prevalence (1.27, $P < 0.001$) and C-peptide quartiles (Q1: reference; Q2: 1.31, Q3: 1.53, Q4: 1.76, $P_{for\ trend} < 0.001$).

- **C-peptide was positively associated with CVD, but inversely associated with diabetic retinopathy progression** (Wang, et al., 2019).

Random non-fasting C-peptide testing can identify patients with insulin-treated type 2 diabetes at high risk of hypoglycaemia.

The aim of this study was to determine whether random non-fasting C-peptide (rCP) measurement can be used to assess hypoglycaemia risk in insulin-treated type 2 diabetes.

In a population-based cohort with insulin-treated type 2 diabetes, self-reported hypoglycaemia was twice as frequent in those with rCP < 0.6 ng/ml (OR 2.0, p < 0.001) and the rate of episodes resulting in loss of consciousness or seizure was five times higher.

Low rCP< 0.6 ng/ml is associated with increased glucose variability and hypoglycaemia in patients with insulin-treated type 2 diabetes and represents a practical, stable and inexpensive biomarker for assessment of hypoglycaemia risk (Hope, et al., 2018).

Type 1 diabetes defined by severe insulin deficiency occurs after 30 years of age and is commonly treated as type 2 diabetes.

Late-onset type 1 diabetes can be difficult to identify. Measurement of endogenous insulin secretion using C-peptide provides a gold standard classification of diabetes type in longstanding diabetes that closely relates to treatment requirements.

Clinicians should be aware that patients progressing to insulin within 3 years of diagnosis have a high likelihood of type 1 diabetes, regardless of initial diagnosis (Thomas, et al., 2018).

Dynamics in insulin requirements and treatment safety.

- The majority of insulin users have elevated HbA1c levels There is growing recognition that insulin requirements are dynamic and not static. Thus, frequent dosage adjustments are needed. In practice, adjustments occur sporadically due to limited provider availability.

- insulin dosage is seldom adjusted and thus transient periods of decrease in insulin requirements and overtreatment are usually overlooked.

- **Simply put, glucose control can be improved if patients call sugars into a doctor's office for insulin adjustments on a regular basis instead of every 3-4 months office visit.**

Two-thirds of patients on insulin fail to achieve the American Diabetes Association's (ADA) target HbA1c level of below 7.0%. Yet a clinical trial showed that if insulin doses were adjusted every 1–4 weeks, 88% of patients reached that goal (R, et al., 2016).

Chapter 19: C-peptide

Weight change and mortality and cardiovascular outcomes in patients with new-onset diabetes mellitus: a nationwide cohort study.

- We aimed to investigate whether changes in weight early after type 2 DM diagnosis influence the incidence of CVD and all-cause mortality in patients.
- 173,246 subjects with new-onset DM who underwent health examinations during 2007-2012 were included.
- Weight was measured at the time of diabetes diagnosis and 2 years later. Weight change over 2 years was divided into five categories of 5% weight change, from weight loss $\geq$ -10% to weight gain $\geq$ 10%.
- There were 3113 deaths (1.8%), 2060 cases of stroke (1.2%), and 1767 myocardial infarctions (MIs) (1.0%) during a median follow-up of 5.5 years.
- Subjects with weight gain $\geq$ 10% had a significantly higher risk of stroke (hazard ratio [HR] 1.51) compared with the group with stable weight.
- Weight changes of more than 10% after diabetes diagnosis were associated with higher mortality and over 10% weight gain was associated with increased risk of stroke. I suspect the larger weight variations reflect higher HgbA1c levels (Kim, et al., 2019).

Chapter 20: Insulin. We cannot live without it.

The discovery of insulin was one of medicine's greatest achievements. Without the manufacture of insulin millions of people would die every year, many of them teenagers and young adults. People afflicted with type 1 diabetes cannot survive without exogenous insulin since they do not make any insulin themselves. The vast majority of people with diabetes, 90%, have type 2 diabetes meaning they do not have an adequate supply of insulin to keep normal levels of glucose in their bloodstream. One of the most profound misconceptions with patients is believing that insulin is the "bad guy". The typical scenario is someone stating that they do not want to take insulin because their grandmother had her leg amputated and died two months after starting insulin. The problem with that idea is the fact that grandmother waited too long before starting insulin and essentially the game was already over before insulin was started. I cannot think of any other drug that takes so long to get started on someone that has proven benefits. The blame is not only on the patient, but many doctors too. Doctors are notorious for clinical inertia with insulin. Insulin is an anabolic hormone. It works in everyone but promotes weight gain.

Insulin is the only drug that has long-term sustainability. Its effective longevity over several years of use is not debated like the majority of diabetic medicines. The price of insulin has substantially increased over the last decade. The price of insulin is now several hundred dollars per month.

- An interesting sidebar shows the percent increase in insulin prices from 2005 to 2015:
- Humalog insulin increased 264%
- Novolog increased 389%
- Lantus increased 348%
- NPH increased 364%
- U-500 insulin increased 508%.
- The cost of one vial of Lantus in different countries are: USA $386, Spain $81, Argentina $286, and Germany $102.
- **North America accounts for 7% of diabetes in the world and pays 52% of the cost of insulin in the world.** Cynically, the US is truly exceptional.
- As stated earlier, insulin was one of the great discoveries in medicine and is a necessity for survival not only in humans but in many organisms. **Insulin** (from the Latin, **insula** meaning island) is a peptide hormone promoting the absorption of glucose from the blood into fat, liver and skeletal muscle cells. The secretion of insulin and glucagon into the blood in response to the blood glucose concentration is the primary mechanism responsible for keeping the glucose levels in the extracellular fluids within very narrow limits at rest, after meals, and during exercise and starvation (Koeslag, Saunders, & Terblanche, 2003). Insulin may have originated more than a billion years ago (Souza & López, 2004). The molecular origins of insulin go at least as far back as the simplest unicellular eukaryotes.

  Within vertebrates, the amino acid sequence of insulin is strongly conserved. Even insulin from some species of fish are similar enough to human insulin to be clinically effective in humans.

  Insulin is produced and stored in the body as a hexamer (a unit of six insulin molecules), while the active form is the monomer. The hexamer is an inactive form with long-term stability, which serves as a way to keep the highly reactive insulin protected, yet readily available. The hexamer-monomer conversion is one of the central aspects of insulin formulations for injection (Dunn, 2005).

Chapter 20: Insulin. We cannot live without it.

One million to three million islets of Langerhans (pancreatic islets) form the endocrine part of the pancreas, which is primarily an exocrine gland. The endocrine portion accounts for only 2% of the total mass of the pancreas. Within the islets of Langerhans, beta cells constitute 65–80% of all the cells.

Beta cells in the islets of Langerhans release insulin in two phases. The first phase consists of a brief spike lasting 10 minutes followed by the second phase, which reaches a plateau at 2-3 hours. It is widely thought that diminution of first-phase insulin release is the earliest detectable defect of beta-cell function in individuals destined to develop type 2 diabetes and that this defect largely represents beta-cell exhaustion after years of compensation for antecedent insulin resistance (Gerich, 2002). Even during digestion, in general, one or two hours following a meal, insulin release from the pancreas is not continuous, but oscillates with a period of 3–6 minutes, changing from generating a blood insulin concentration more than about 800 pmol/l to less than 100 pmol/l. This oscillation avoids downregulation of insulin receptors in target cells, and to assist the liver in extracting insulin from the blood (Hellman, Gylfe, Grapengiesser, Dansk, & Salehi, 2007). This oscillation is important to consider when administering insulin-stimulating medication, since it is the oscillating blood concentration of insulin release, which should, ideally, be achieved, not a constant high concentration.

The body's blood sugar range is carefully controlled in a healthy individual, which will usually measure 80 mg/dl in the blood. So, how much actual sugar (or glucose) is in the body? This amounts to 4 grams of sugar (16 kcals) in the blood, which is less than a teaspoon of sugar! The American Diabetes Association draws the line between a healthy individual and someone being pre-diabetic at 100 mg/dl. This 100 mg/dl is about 1 teaspoon. For someone to be diagnosed as diabetic, her fasting blood sugar is over 126 mg/dl. or about 1 ¼ teaspoons. The difference between being healthy and being diagnosed as diabetic is a quarter of a teaspoon of sugar. If one eats something with 400 kcals and 50% are carbohydrates (200 kcals or 50 grams of glucose), then your body is exposing itself to greater than 10x the amount of sugar in your bloodstream at that time.

The actions of insulin on metabolism include:

- Increase of glucose in muscle and adipose tissue (about two-thirds of body cells).
- Increase of DNA replication and protein synthesis via control of amino acid uptake.
- Modification of the activity of numerous enzymes.
- Increase glycogen synthesis – insulin forces storage of glucose in liver (and muscle) cells into glycogen; lowered levels of insulin cause liver cells to convert glycogen to glucose and excrete it into the blood.
- Increase potassium uptake
- Decrease gluconeogenesis and glycogenolysis – decreases production of glucose from non-carbohydrate substrates, primarily in the liver. (the vast majority of endogenous insulin arriving at the liver never leaves the liver); decrease of insulin causes glucose production by the liver from assorted substrates.
- Increase lipid synthesis – insulin forces fat cells to convert glucose into triglycerides; decrease of insulin causes the reverse.
- Increase esterification of fatty acids – forces adipose tissue to make triglycerides from fatty acids; decrease of insulin causes the reverse.
- Decrease lipolysis – forces reduction in conversion of fat cell lipid stores into fatty acids and glycerol; decrease of insulin causes the reverse.
- Decrease proteolysis – decreasing the breakdown of protein.
- Decrease autophagy - decreased level of degradation of damaged organelles. Postprandial levels inhibit autophagy completely.
- Increase amino acid uptake – forces cells to absorb circulating amino acids; decrease of insulin inhibits absorption (Dimitiriadus, Mitrou, Lambadiari, Maratou, & Raptis, 2011).

Chapter 20: Insulin. We cannot live without it.

A brief history of insulin, from Wikipedia's Insulin page:

- 1869-Paul Langerhans, a medical student in Berlin, identified previously unnoticed tissue clumps scattered throughout the bulk of the pancreas. The function of the "little heaps of cells," later known as the islets of Langerhans.

- 1889- physician Oskar Minkowski, in collaboration with Joseph von Mering, removed the pancreas from a healthy dog to test its assumed role in digestion. Several days after the removal of the dog's pancreas, Minkowski's animal-keeper noticed a swarm of flies feeding on the dog's urine. On testing the urine, they found sugar, establishing for the first time a relationship between the pancreas and diabetes.

- 1901-Eugene Lindsay Opie established the link between the islets of Langerhans and diabetes: "Diabetes mellitus ... is caused by destruction of the islets of Langerhans and occurs only when these bodies are in part or wholly destroyed.

- 1916- Nicolae Paulescu, a Romanian professor of physiology developed an aqueous pancreatic extract which, when injected into a diabetic dog, had a normalizing effect on blood sugar levels.

- October 1920-Canadian Frederick Banting concluded that it was the very digestive secretions that Minkowski had originally studied that were breaking down the islet secretion(s), thereby making it impossible to extract successfully. He jotted a note to himself: "Ligate pancreatic ducts of the dog. Keep dogs alive till acini degenerate leaving islets. Try to isolate internal secretion of these and relieve glycosurea."

- The idea was the pancreas's internal secretion regulates sugar in the bloodstream, might hold the key to the treatment of diabetes. A surgeon by training, Banting knew certain arteries could be tied off that would lead to atrophy of most of the pancreas, while leaving the islets of Langerhans intact. He theorized a relatively pure extract could be made from the islets once most of the rest of the pancreas was gone.

- Banting's method was to tie a ligature around the pancreatic duct; when examined several weeks later, the pancreatic digestive cells had died and been absorbed by the immune system, leaving islets. They then isolated an extract from these islets, producing what they called "isletin" (what we now know as insulin).

- January 11, 1922, Leonard Thompson, a 14-year-old diabetic who lay dying at the Toronto General Hospital, was given the first injection of insulin.

- The drug firm Eli Lilly and Company had offered assistance not long after the first publications in 1921. Lilly was able to produce large quantities of highly refined insulin. Insulin was offered for sale shortly thereafter.

- The Nobel Prize committee in 1923 credited the practical extraction of insulin to a team at the University of Toronto and awarded the Nobel Prize to two men: Frederick Banting and J.J.R. Macleod. They were awarded the Nobel Prize in Physiology/Medicine in 1923 for the discovery of insulin. Banting, insulted that Charles Best was not mentioned, shared his prize with him, and Macleod immediately shared his with James Collip. The patent for insulin was sold to the University of Toronto for one half-dollar.

- The primary structure of insulin was determined by British molecular biologist Frederick Sanger. It was the first protein to have its sequence be determined. He was awarded the 1958 Nobel Prize in Chemistry for this work.

- Rosalyn Sussman Yalow received the 1977 Nobel Prize in Medicine for the development of the radioimmunoassay for insulin.

- The work published by Banting, Best, Collip and Macleod represented the preparation of purified insulin extract suitable for use on human patients. Paulescu already succeeded in extracting the antidiabetic hormone of the pancreas and proving its efficacy in reducing the hyperglycaemia in diabetic dogs but his saline extract could not be used on humans. In a private communication, Professor Tiselius, former head of the Nobel Institute, expressed his personal opinion that Paulescu was equally worthy of the award in 1923 (Insulin, n.d.).

Chapter 20: Insulin. We cannot live without it.

Insulin resistance is a two-sided mechanism acting under opposite catabolic and anabolic conditions.

The regulation of glucose is controlled by opposing signaling pathways where anabolic processes are activated by insulin and catabolic action is activated by glucagon or stress hormones (catecholamines and cortisol). Insulin increases glucose uptake in muscles and fat, and inhibits hepatic glucose production, thus serving as the primary regulator of the blood glucose concentration. Insulin also stimulates cell growth, and promotes the storage of energetic reserve in fat, liver, and muscles by stimulating lipogenesis, glycogen, and protein synthesis and inhibiting lipolysis and protein breakdown. Catabolic stress hormones and glucagon act in opposite via activation of lipolysis, producing non-esterified fatty acids (NEFAs) which reduce the cellular sensitivity to insulin action (Schwartzburd, 2016).

Sometimes reading another description of how the body regulates glucose catalyzes a lasting reaction in our understanding.

Association between insulin-induced weight change and CVD mortality: Evidence from a historic cohort study of 18,814 patients in UK primary care.

- This study explores the association of insulin-induced weight (wt) gain on cardiovascular outcomes and mortality among patients with type 2 diabetes (T2D) following 1-year insulin initiation using real-world data.
- A historical cohort study was performed in 18,814 adults with insulin-treated T2D.

Patients were grouped into 5 categories (>5 kg wt loss; 1.0-5.0 kg wt loss; no wt change; 1.0-5.0 kg wt gain; >5.0 kg wt gain) and followed-up for 5 years. The median age was 62.8 years, HbA$_{1c}$: 8.6% and mean BMI 31.8.

Results:

- **Insulin-induced weight gain did not translate to adverse cardiovascular outcomes and mortality in patients with T2D. These data provide reassurance on the cardiovascular safety of insulin patients with T2D**

(Anyanwagu, Mamza, Donnelly, & Idris, 2018)

New insulins
Insulin pens were first introduced in 1985

Basal Insulin (long-acting insulin that provides slow release with essentially no peak) Concentrated insulins - key point is one unit equals one unit when dialing pens. The pens deliver different volumes.

TOUJEO (U-300 Lantus/glargine)- approved 2/25/2015. it is Lantus insulin concentrated 3x.
Basal insulin (last 18-24 hours). 450 units/pen. One box is 3 pens (1350 units). Expensive.

TRESIBA (insulin degludec)-approved 9/25/2015 - 42-hour insulin. Stable basal insulin injection once per day. After 3-4 days, a stable continuous insulin dose is administered. No insulin stacking occurs (doses do not accumulate).
Comes in 2 varieties- normal concentration and double concentration.
A single injection of 80 units or 160 units is top single injection dose depending on single or double concentration.
Pens are either 300 units/pen or 600 units/pen. 5 pens/box. Expensive.

BASAGLAR KwikPen (glargine)- same as Lantus. Final approval 12/16/2015. Comes only in 3ml pens with total 300 units glargine per pen.

Not every good idea works out clinically. The following article expresses this:

How Can a Good Idea Fail? Basal Insulin Peglispro [LY2605541] for the Treatment of Type 2 Diabetes.
Lack of control in diabetic patients has stimulated the development of new insulin analogues. One of these was basal insulin peglispro (BIL) or LY2605541; it had a flat pharmacokinetic profile, half-life of 2-3 days and acted preferably in the liver.
Results:
Unfortunately, it caused higher transaminase and triglyceride levels in data from the IMAGINE trials. This led the company to

discontinue development. (Muñoz-Garach, Molina-Vega, & Tinahones, 2017).

Short-Acting Meal insulin (prandial insulin).
1. Humalog 200u/ml KwikPen: Approved May 22, 2015. Short-acting insulin. Same as U-100 insulin but U-200 means double concentrated. Remember 1 unit is still 1 unit but pen causes only half the volume to be administered.

Afrezza (inhaled insulin): Approved June 22, 2014. Insulin is dry powder stored in small packages that are punctured by inhalation device. The doses are cartridges of 4, 8 and 12 units of insulin. A person inhales it with each meal. Very simple easy device to use. Cough, decrease in pulmonary function, and lack of coverage by insurance companies has crippled the drug. Essentially the second inhaled insulin that has failed in the diabetes market. The future of the drug is very speculative.

A brief review:
Place of technosphere inhaled insulin in treatment of diabetes.
Technosphere insulin (TI), Afrezza, is a powder form of short-acting regular insulin taken by oral inhalation with meals. Action of TI peaks after approximately 40-60 min and lasts for 2-3 hours. TI is slightly less effective than subcutaneous insulin aspartate, with mean hemoglobin A1c (HbA1c) reduction of 0.21% and 0.4%, respectively. Apart from hypoglycemia, cough is the most common adverse effect of TI reported by 24%-33% of patients vs 2% with insulin aspartate. TI is contraindicated in patients with asthma and chronic obstructive pulmonary disease. While TI is an attractive option of prandial insulin, its use is limited by frequent occurrence of cough, need for periodic monitoring of pulmonary function, and lack of long-term safety data. Candidates for use of TI are patients having frequent hypoglycemia while using short-acting subcutaneous insulin, particularly late post-prandial hypoglycemia, patients with needle phobia, and those who cannot tolerate subcutaneous insulin due to skin reactions.

Chapter 20: Insulin. We cannot live without it.

Cannot be used with COPD, asthma, lung disease, and the person has to abstain from smoking for at least 6 months. Patients need spirometry before starting, repeated at 6 months and annually to evaluate FEV1. (forced breath out in one second).
Cartridges consist of 4 units and 8 units of insulin.
The inhaler needs to be replaced every 15 days (Mikhail, 2016).

Combination insulin products

Soliqua (insulin glargine (lantus)/lixisenatide)-Combination basal insulin/GLP-1-approved November 21, 2016. One unit of Soliqua contains 1 unit of Lantus and 0.33 mcg of lixisenatide. Dose ranges from 15 to 60 units SQ once daily. Top dose is 60 units lantus and 20 mcg lixisenatide. Each pen has 300 units of lantus or 5-day supply of highest dose.

Xultophy 100/3.6 (insulin degludec 100 units/ml and liraglutide 3.6 ml injection) – Combination basal insulin/GLP-1-approved November 21, 2016. Recommended starting dose is 16 units (16 units of insulin degludec and 0.58 mg of liraglutide). It is essentially combination pen of Victoza and Tresiba. Maximum dose is 50 units (50 units of Tresiba and 1.8 mg Victoza). As with Victoza this carries a blackbox warning regarding potential risk of medullary thyroid tumors and contraindicated in patients with Multiple Endocrine Neoplasia syndrome type 2 (MEN2).

Insulin therapy, weight gain and prognosis.
- Insulin treatment is needed when people with type 2 diabetes have failed other therapies and have become insulin-deficient.
- Almost all those with type 2 diabetes who start insulin therapy gain weight, which may potentially diminish the prognostic advantage of improved glycaemia.
- To date, all available guidelines emphasize both the attainment of glycated haemoglobin (HbA1c) goals

and weight control, without directing the clinician as to which element is of a higher priority.

- The following review attempts to clarify the issue using the available literature.

- **The body of evidence indicates that glycaemic management with exogenous insulin replacement is of a much higher priority than weight gain.**

Lower weight or weight loss do not show prognostic benefit in advanced stages of diabetes; therefore, weight gain should not discourage providers from achieving and maintaining HbA1c goals with insulin therapy, regardless of insulin dosage or other medications (Hodish, 2018).

Outcomes and treatment patterns of adding a third agent to 2 OADs in patients with type 2 diabetes.

- The transition to insulin has been shown to be delayed in current practice, potentially through clinical inertia--the failure of health care providers to initiate or advance therapy when indicated.

- Patients and physicians may be resistant to insulin therapy because of beliefs about side effects and limitations to patients' lifestyle, while patients may consider that starting injectable therapy signifies a considerable worsening of their disease and may feel they have "failed" to manage it effectively.

- To describe current treatment patterns and outcomes among adult patients with T2DM in the United States who were treated with 2 OADs (oral antidiabetic drugs) and added a third antidiabetic drug.

- This retrospective study followed patients with T2DM who added a third OAD (the "3OAD" cohort), insulin ("+Insulin"), or a GLP-1 ("+GLP-1") between July 2000 and March 2009. Patients were followed for up to 2 years.

Results:

- A total of 51,771 patients adding a third agent to their 2OAD regimen were included in this study.

- Most patients added a third OAD (n = 41,052) over insulin (n = 6,904) or GLP-1 (n = 3,815).

Chapter 20: Insulin. We cannot live without it.

- At baseline, +Insulin patients were older, with higher comorbidity burden and higher HbA1c.
- During follow-up, 3OAD patients were more likely to be persistent with their treatment than +Insulin or +GLP-1 patients, but +Insulin patients had the greatest HbA1c reduction from baseline.
- Among 3OAD patients, most of those who switched a third agent started insulin, and those who switched early during the follow-up period had greater HbA1c reduction than those who continued with the 3OAD treatment regimen. Average annual health care costs declined in +Insulin patients but increased among 3OAD and +GLP-1 patients.
- Treatment persistence and HbA1c reduction in +GLP-1 patients were low.

Conclusions:

- This study found that in current practice, physicians seem to be reluctant to prescribe injectable agents for patients with uncontrolled T2DM despite combination OAD therapy.
- Despite higher treatment persistence among patients adding a third OAD, this persistence did not translate into better glycemic control and may not necessarily be a long-term cost-saving solution (Levin, Wei, Zhou, Xie, & Baser, 2014).

Chapter 21: Metformin and Geroprotection (anti-aging)

The fountain of youth will not be found in a mythical place like "Shangri-La" but probably in a research lab looking at gene manipulation and mitochondria.

The effects of metformin on simple obesity: a meta-analysis.

To evaluate the efficacy of metformin versus a placebo in the treatment of patients with simple obesity without obesity related diseases.

A search was done on Pub-Med, EMBASE, Cochrane, and Science Citation Index Expanded databases.

- There was no significant difference in the reduction of waist circumference between the metformin group and the control group.
- The fasting blood glucose levels and body weight were significantly lower in the metformin group than in the control group.
- no hypoglycemia was noted in the metformin group or the control group.

Conclusion:

Metformin is effective in reducing body weight of simple obesity patients, and metformin does not induce hypoglycemia as a side effect (Ning, et al., 2018).

Homer Simpson stated "Donuts, what can't they do!" My quote is "Metformin, what can't it do!"

Metformin reduces all-cause mortality and diseases of ageing independent of its effect on diabetes control: A systematic review and meta-analysis.

This systematic review investigated whether the insulin sensitizer metformin has a geroprotective effect in humans. Overall, 260 full-texts were reviewed, 53 met the inclusion criteria for a combined population of 417,316.

- Diabetics taking metformin had significantly lower all-cause mortality than non-diabetics.
- Diabetics taking metformin had significantly lower all-cause mortality compared to diabetics receiving non-metformin therapies, insulin or sulfonylureas.
- Metformin users also had reduced cancer compared to non-diabetics.
- Metformin users had reduced cardiovascular disease (CVD) compared to diabetics receiving non-metformin therapies or insulin.
- **The apparent reductions in all-cause mortality and diseases of ageing associated with metformin use suggest that metformin could be extending life and health spans by acting as a geroprotective agent** (Campbell, Bellman, Stephenson, & Lisy, 2017).

Geroprotection: A promising future

- Geroprotection is to improve the quality of life and lifespan of the concerned individual.
- One intervention, which has been shown to prolong lifespan by 30-50% in species ranging from roundworms to primates, is calorie restriction. Metformin acts as a CRM (calorie restriction mimetic), it tries to conserve energy by reducing hepatic gluconeogenesis, while promoting uptake in peripheral tissues and fatty acid oxidation. Metformin has seemed to reduce the incidence of cancer.
- Reservatrol – nutraceutical found in red wine. The term "red-wine endocrinology" has been coined to describe the various hormonal and metabolic effects of this nutraceutical.
- Rapamycin reduces progression of atherosclerosis but causes hyperlipidemia (Magon, Chopra, & Kumar, 2012).

Chapter 21: Metformin and Geroprotection (anti-aging)

Geroprotectors as a novel therapeutic strategy for COPD, an accelerating aging disease.

Aging is defined as the progressive decline of homeostasis that occurs after the reproductive phase of life is complete, leading to an increasing risk of disease or death due to impaired DNA repair after damage by oxidative stress or telomere shortening as a result of repeated cell division.

Geroprotectors are therapeutics that affect the root cause of aging and age-related disease, and thus prolong the life-span of animals. Geroprotectors such as melatonin, metformin, rapamycin and resveratrol are anti-oxidant or anti-aging molecule regulators. The average lifespan at the beginning of the 20th century was 46 years compared to 68 years in 2005-2010.Underlying the aging process is a lifelong, bottom-up accumulation of molecular damage and progressive chronic inflammatory state.

Sirtuins are well documented anti-aging molecules. Seven molecules have been identified in the human sirtuin family (SIRT1-SIRT7) and they are known to be NAD+ dependent histone/protein deacetylases which are involved in gene expression, cell cycle regulation, apoptosis, metabolism, DNA repair and senescence.

Geroprotectors

- Metformin can slow down the rate of aging, and decrease glucose, insulin and IGF-1 level.
- Melatonin is involved in the circadian rhythms (the sleep-wake cycle). It has powerful antioxidant activity.
- Resveratrol found in grapes, berries and peanuts, red wines. It has anti-oxidant and activates SIRT-1.
- Rapamycin (Sirolimus) is an immunosuppressive agent used to prevent rejection in transplantation.
- Sirtuins are anti-aging molecules and control oxidative stress resistance, DNA repair and inflammation (Ito, Colley, & Mercado, 2012).

Chapter 22: Laurel & Hardy (Leptin & Ghrelin)

This chapter and the next chapter are difficult to comprehend. Obesity is very complicated.

Ghrelin

- Leptin and Ghrelin are 2 important hormones that started a tremendous interest in obesity research in the 1990s. They are like salt and pepper, heads and tails on a coin, Muhammad Ali and Joe Frazier, Laurel and Hardy (famous slapstick comedy duo in 1920-1940s). I use these terms as a simple analogy to 2 very different hormones; while they are very different, they function at their best when together. They both act on the same cells in the brain to help regulate hunger and appetite.

- Ghrelin was initially reported in 1999. The name indicates that it is a growth hormone releasing peptide; the root **ghre-** means *to grow*. Ghrelin is like Hardy, a large, stout man. **Ghrelin is called the hunger hormone, and is a neuropeptide produced in the GI tract.** The stomach produces ghrelin when it is empty, and secretion stops when the stomach is full. It signals an increase in hunger to the hypothalamus and stimulates gastric acid secretion and gastrointestinal motility for food intake. Ghrelin crosses the blood-brain-barrier and triggers receptors in the arcuate nucleus that include the orexigenic neuropeptide Y (NPY) and the agouti-related protein (agRP) neurons. Ghrelin reduces the mechanosensitivity of gastric vagal afferents, so they are less sensitive to gastric distension. Ghrelin induces appetite and is associated with feeding behaviors and acts as a body weight regulator. If you were to test for the hormone, you would find ghrelin levels at their highest right before a meal and the lowest right after. Studies indicate ghrelin levels decrease with weight gain. Ghrelin levels increase during weight loss, which promote increased food consumption and weight gain. Remember, **our body thinks we are still in the stone-age and that dieting is not a voluntary act, but a threat to our survival.**

- Ghrelin can be related to many other systems in the body as well.

- Ghrelin suppresses gastrointestinal pro-inflammatory mechanisms and augments anti-inflammatory mechanisms, leading to a potential for treatment of inflammatory diseases of the GI tract. Ghrelin can promote gastrointestinal and pancreatic malignancy. Ghrelin also inhibits glucose-stimulated insulin secretion.

- Ghrelin has a marked relationship with sleep cycles as well. Sleep deprivation results in high levels of ghrelin, which can lead to obesity. As individuals get more sleep, ghrelin levels trend lower and the chance of obesity is reduced. Lack of sleep increases ghrelin, and decreases leptin, both effects producing increased hunger and obesity (Yildiz, Suchard, Wong, McCann, & Licinio, 2014). The strong association between sleep disorders, obesity and diabetes is not a coincidence.

- **Gastric bypass surgery has been shown to dramatically lower ghrelin levels while voluntary weight loss has to compete with increasing ghrelin. Bariatric surgeries involving vertical sleeve gastrectomy reduce plasma ghrelin levels close to 60% over time. Ghrelin plasma concentration increases as people age, which may contribute to the tendency for people to gain weight as they get older** (Cummings, et al., 2001).

In a 2016 Romanian study entitled **Effects of ghrelin in energy balance and body weight homeostasis,** researchers stated:

Ghrelin is a gut peptide composed of 28 amino acids mostly secreted in the gastric fundus mucosa. In humans, there is a pre-prandial rise and a postprandial fall in plasma ghrelin levels, which strongly suggest that the peptide plays a physiological role in meal initiation and may be employed in determining the amount and quality of ingested food. Besides the stimulation of food intake, ghrelin determines a decrease in energy expenditure and promotes the storage of fatty acids in adipocytes. Thus, in the human body ghrelin induces a positive energy balance, an increased adiposity gain, as well as an increase in caloric storage, seen as an adaptive mechanism to caloric restriction conditions. In the current world context, when we are witnessing an increasing availability of food and a reduction of energy expenditure to a minimum level, these mechanisms have become pathogenic (Mihalache, et al., 2016).

Another 2016 study, **Ghrelin and the Cardiovascular System,** presented information about the stated relationship:

Ghrelin is a small peptide released primarily from the stomach. It is a potent stimulator of growth hormone secretion from the pituitary gland and is well known for its regulation of metabolism and appetite. There is a strong relationship between ghrelin and the cardiovascular system. Ghrelin receptors are present throughout the heart and vasculature and have been linked with molecular pathways, including, but not limited to, the regulation of intracellular calcium concentration, inhibition of pro-apoptotic cascades, and protection against oxidative damage. Ghrelin shows robust cardioprotective effects including enhancing endothelial and vascular function, preventing atherosclerosis, inhibiting sympathetic drive, and decreasing blood pressure. After myocardial infarction, exogenous administration of ghrelin preserves cardiac function, reduces the incidence of fatal arrhythmias, and attenuates apoptosis and ventricular remodeling, leading to improvements in heart failure. It ameliorates cachexia in end-stage congestive heart failure patients and has shown clinical benefit in pulmonary hypertension. Nonetheless, since ghrelin's discovery is relatively recent, there remains a substantial amount of research needed to fully understand its clinical significance in cardiovascular disease (Lilleness & Frishman, 2016).

Leptin

- **"Leptin is called the satiety hormone and the word "leptin" originates from the Greek root "leptos," which means "thin,"** and cited by the medical community in 1994"
- Leptin is like Laurel who also has an L in the name. Laurel was the thin man in the comedy duo. He purposely exhibited a resistance to understanding causing great frustration to the obese Hardy. The resistance of Laurel (i.e. leptin) aggravated the obese Hardy.
- The following is a collection of highlights from a 2014 study published in Physiology and Behavior by researchers Pan, Guo, and Su about the issue of leptin resistance and how it relates to obesity.
- Various factors influence leptin secretion and expression. The most important factors are the distribution of subcutaneous fat and the status of its energy stores because leptin is mainly expressed in the adipose tissue, and circulating leptin concentrations in the fed state are highly correlated with the degree of adiposity.
- Glucocorticoids directly induce hyperleptinemia and stimulate leptin synthesis in cultured adipocytes, for example, leptin expression increases in response to the chronic elevation of cortisol in humans.
- Unfortunately, treatment with leptin alone in obese individuals fails to counteract common obesity. Leptin is not the cure for obesity.
- A large number of studies demonstrated that most individuals with diet-induced obesity (DIO) manifest leptin resistance characterized by increased leptin levels in the blood and decreased leptin sensitivity, which is in proportion to the individual's adipose mass and BMI.
- **Leptin levels are high in obesity due to leptin resistance.**

- A growing number of biologists have reached extensive consensus on the idea that leptin resistance is a hallmark of obesity, especially DIO (diet induced obesity), indicating that drugs aimed at ameliorating leptin resistance might prevent the development of DIO. Consequently, understanding the mechanisms that may underlie "leptin resistance" is crucial for both determining the causes of obesity and identifying the potential mechanisms that may be targeted for therapy. Leptin resistance resulting in the failure of elevated leptin levels to control or reverse obesity enhances the susceptibility to obesity, and obesity can also aggravate leptin resistance, which further sustains obesity, leading to a vicious cycle of escalating metabolic derangement.

- The results of a large number of studies displayed that obese individuals exhibit high peripheral leptin levels but relatively lower cerebrospinal fluid (CSF) concentrations, suggesting that defective leptin transport into the central nervous system (CNS) across the BBB (blood brain barrier) conduces to leptin resistance (Pan, Guo, & Su, 2014).

Adaptations of leptin, ghrelin or insulin during weight loss as predictors of weight regain: a review of current literature

- **Sixty-eight percent of men and women in the United States are classified as overweight (body mass index ≥25) or obese (body mass index ≥30)**

-

- **Clinically significant weight losses of ~5–10% have been shown to reduce disease risk.**

- Weight regain is common.

- Caloric restriction and weight loss induce significant increases in the concentration of ghrelin, a potent orexigenic hormone.

- Elevations in ghrelin concentration, are associated with feelings of hunger and increased food intake.

Discussion:

- **Despite the important roles that leptin, ghrelin and insulin seem to exert in energy homeostasis, their**

<u>changes during weight loss, taken alone, are not
sufficient predictors of weight regain in humans</u>
(Strohacker, McCaffery, MacLean, & Wing, 2014)<u>.</u>

Chapter 23: Smorgasbord of hormones

- <u>Other hormones involved in weight control;</u> our body does not like change and will do everything to prevent this.
- The physiological control of appetite regulation involves circulating hormones with orexigenic (appetite-stimulating) and anorexigenic (appetite-inhibiting) properties that induce alterations in energy intake via perceptions of hunger and satiety. **Orexigenic and anorexigenic neuropeptides are constantly orchestrating are responses to food and attempts at dieting** (Hazell, Islam, Townsend, Schmale, & Copeland, 2016).
- By understanding how certain hormones react with other hormones and neurons, it is easier to understand how things work.

- <u>**Orexigenic-stimulates appetite (parasympathetic**</u>)- ghrelin, NPY (neuropeptide Y), AgRP (agouti-Related Peptide), MCH (melanin concentrating hormone), Orexin A, Orexin B, Cannabinoid-1 receptor.

- <u>**Anorexigenic-decreases appetite (sympathetic**</u>)- amylin, POMC (proopiomelanocortin), CART (cocaine and amphetamine regulated transcript), leptin, serotonin,

BDNF (brain-derived neurotrophic factor), alpha-MSH (melanocortin-stimulating hormone), obestatin, PYY, GLP-1, GIP, cholecystokinin.

The following abstract from a 2015 article by Jong-Woo Sohn, entitled "**Network of hypothalamic neurons that control appetite**" supports these ideas:

- The central nervous system (CNS) controls food intake and energy expenditure via tight coordination between multiple neuronal populations. Specifically, two distinct neuronal populations exist in the arcuate nucleus of hypothalamus (ARH): the anorexigenic (appetite-suppressing) pro-opiomelanocortin (POMC) neurons and the orexigenic (appetite-increasing) neuropeptide Y (NPY)/agouti-related peptide (AgRP) neurons. The coordinated regulation of neuronal circuit involving these neurons is essential in properly maintaining energy balance, and any disturbance therein may result in hyperphagia/obesity or hypophagia/starvation. Thus, adequate knowledge of the POMC and NPY/AgRP neuron physiology is mandatory to understand the pathophysiology of obesity and related metabolic diseases (Sohn, 2015).

Effects of exercise intensity on plasma concentrations of appetite-regulating hormones: Potential mechanisms.

- The physiological control of appetite regulation involves circulating hormones with orexigenic (appetite-stimulating) and anorexigenic (appetite-inhibiting) properties that induce alterations in energy intake via perceptions of hunger and satiety. As the effectiveness of exercise to induce weight loss is a controversial topic, there is considerable interest in the effect of exercise on the appetite-regulating hormones such as acylated ghrelin, peptide YY (PYY), glucagon-like peptide-1 (GLP-1), and pancreatic polypeptide (PP). Research to date suggests short-term appetite regulation following a single exercise session is likely affected by decreases in acylated ghrelin and increases in PYY, GLP-1, and PP. In an effort to guide future research, it is important to consider how exercise alters the circulating concentrations of these appetite-regulating hormones. Potential mechanisms include blood redistribution, sympathetic nervous system activity, gastrointestinal motility, cytokine release, free fatty acid concentrations, lactate production, and changes in plasma glucose and insulin concentrations. This review of relevant research suggests blood redistribution during exercise may be important for suppressing ghrelin, while other mechanisms involving cytokine release, changes in plasma glucose and insulin concentrations, SNS activity, and muscle metabolism likely mediate changes in the anorexigenic signals PYY and GLP-1. Overall, changes in appetite-regulating hormones following acute exercise appear to be intensity-dependent, with increasing intensity leading to a greater suppression of orexigenic signals and greater stimulation of anorexigenic signals. A better understanding of how exercise intensity and workload affect appetite across the sexes and life stages will be a powerful tool in developing more successful strategies for managing weight (Hazell, Islam, Townsend, Schmale, & Copeland, 2016).

Acute exercise and hormones related to appetite regulation: a meta-analysis

- Understanding the impact of an acute bout of exercise on hormones involved in appetite regulation may provide insight into some of the mechanisms that regulate energy balance. In resting conditions, acylated ghrelin is known to stimulate food intake, while hormones such as peptide YY (PYY), pancreatic polypeptide (PP) and glucagon-like peptide 1 (GLP-1) are known to suppress food intake.
- The results of the meta-analyses indicated that exercise had small to moderate effects on appetite hormone levels, suppressing acylated ghrelin (median decrease 16.5 %) and increasing PYY (median increase 8.9 %), GLP-1 (median increase 13 %), and PP (median increase 15 %).

Conclusions:

- An acute bout of exercise may influence appetite by suppressing levels of acylated ghrelin while simultaneously increasing levels of PYY, GLP-1 and PP, which may contribute to alterations in food and drink intake after acute exercise. (Schubert, Sabapathy, Leveritt, & Desbrow, 2014).

Chapter 24: Rainbow Pills.

Sometimes ideas get out of hand. A lot of the baggage and negative opinions regarding weight loss medicines and the doctor's that prescribe them stem from rainbow pills. This is the perfect chapter for the Yogi Berra quote "Even Napoleon had his Watergate"

The Return of Rainbow Diet Pills

The US Food and Drug Administration (FDA) has recently warned consumers about the risks of weight loss supplements adulterated with multiple pharmaceutical agents. Some of these supplements combine potent anorectics, such as amphetamines derivatives, with benzodiazepines, beta-blockers, and other medications to suppress the anorectics' adverse effects. These weight loss supplements represent the most recent generation of rainbow diet pills, named for their bright and varied colors, which date back more than 70 years. Beginning in the 1940s, several US pharmaceutical firms aggressively promoted rainbow pills to physicians and patients. By the 1960s the pills had caused dozens of deaths before the FDA began removing them from the US market. We used a variety of original resources to trace these deadly pills from their origins in the United States to their popularity in Spain and Brazil to their reintroduction to the United States as weight loss dietary supplements.

Physicians have prescribed a wide range of combination weight loss regimens for more than a century. Some regimens combine multiple anorectics, and others have included additional classes of pharmaceuticals to mask the anorectics' unpleasant side effects. The modern use of weight loss regimens with opposing pharmaceutical actions can be traced to the 1890s, when clinicians combined desiccated thyroid with strychnine and other drugs to ameliorate the thyroid's cardiac effects.

By the 1940s, the newly discovered anorectic effects of amphetamine generated tremendous interest in combination weight loss regimens. These brightly colored capsules and tablets, commonly referred to as rainbow diet pills, combined amphetamines, diuretics, laxatives, and thyroid hormones to maximize weight loss with digitalis, benzodiazepines, barbiturates, potassium, corticosteroids, and antidepressants to suppress the insomnia, palpitations, anxiety, and other common side effects. As deaths and injuries linked to these pills accumulated over the years, the US Food and Drug Administration (FDA) eventually removed the rainbow pills from the US market in the late 1960s. Rainbow pills have once again returned to the United States, now in the guise of weight loss dietary supplements.

A Brief History

A cultural shift in body image of the late 19th and early 20th centuries by the advertising industry and Hollywood helped to cultivate the ideal image of the slender woman and athletically trim man.

Thyroid preparations emerged in the 1890s with some physicians prescribing strychnine or digitalis leaf to prevent thyroid's adverse effects on the heart.

The next major players were amphetamines with their anorectic effects. Rainbow pills emerged in the 1940s with their bright colors and the marketing strategy suggesting personalized attention.

The rainbow pill firms sold their products directly to physicians. Physicians specializing in rainbow pill practices could see an impressive number of patients. "On a slow day" one physician was able to see more than 100 patients.

By promoting an all-out endogenous etiology of obesity, the firms justified a wide range of pharmaceutical ingredients.

By contrast, standard medical texts emphasized proper diet and exercise. The theoretical foundation of the rainbow pill practice distinctly opposed what physicians were taught in training. By 1967, 5000 MDs and DOs devoted a majority of their practices to weight loss. Of these, 2000 practices focused exclusively on weight reduction.

Chapter 24: Rainbow Pills.

A rainbow pill clinic could be both profitable and relatively easy to operate, even if it flew in the face of professional standards and ethics. The AMA characterized these drugs as having "no rational therapeutic use, and therefore [their] administration for treatment of obesity must be regarded as misuse."

Adverse events, including deaths, began to be reported to the FDA as early as the 1940s and 1950s.

Two important events outside of the FDA changed the regulatory landscape in 1968. A slim investigative reporter, Susanna McBee, for *Life* magazine reported on her experiences posing as a patient at 10 obesity clinics where she was prescribed more than 1500 pills. That same month, the US Senate, identified at least 60 deaths launched hearings into the rainbow diet pill industry.

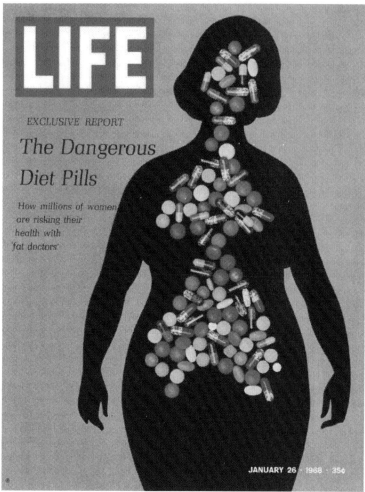

The FDA began to respond aggressively by January 1968. Within two months the agency seized 43 million tablets from a dozen manufacturers.

The federal government also moved to tighten control of amphetamine abuse. The Comprehensive Drug Abuse Prevention and Control Act of 1970 established different schedules for certain drugs based on their medical abuse potential. Amphetamines was relegated to Schedule II. In the 1970s, the FDA ruled that amphetamines were effective but only safe for short-term use.

Small, local compounding pharmacies, often with close financial relationships to the prescribing physicians, specialized in rainbow pills. In the early 1990s, the number of pharmacies specializing in rainbow diet pills increased five-fold. [62] Eighty-six percent of patients experienced side effects and in one study almost 4% of pill users required hospitalization from adverse effects of the pills. Compounding rainbow pills was subsequently banned in 2007.

Throughout the 2000s, with increasingly restrictive laws governing their prescribing, rainbow pills became more frequently marketed as herbal weight loss products.

The Dietary Supplement Health and Education Act of 1994 allowed rainbow pills and other potentially dangerous medicines to escape FDA initial scrutiny.

The 1994 Dietary Supplement Act does not require that dietary supplements prove to be safe or effective before they are marketed. The FDA does not scrutinize a dietary supplement before it enters the marketplace (Cohen, Goday, & Swann, 2012).

Chapter 25: Weight Loss Medications and Past Bad Players

"We made too many wrong mistakes" Yogi Berra

Several medicines are available to assist in weight loss. Over the years several medicines have been given for weight loss only to be removed from the market due to safety concerns. It is important to look at history to give perspective and avoid repeating the same mistakes. In 1947, the FDA approved methamphetamine. In 1959 phentermine was approved. In 1973 with the country struggling with a long-running epidemic of amphetamine abuse and Rainbow pill abuse (not phentermine abuse-big difference), the FDA limited the indication of all obesity drugs to short-term use , hence, the 3 month restriction on phentermine use in some states. The discovery in the early 1990s of leptin prompted more obesity research. Phentermine and other obesity drugs suffered under the "negative amphetamine halo."

Bad Players

Weight loss medications that have failed and have been removed are:

1. **Aminorex**-amphetamine like appetite suppressant. Removed due to pulmonary hypertension.
2. **Fenfluramine/phentermine (Fen-Phen).** Removed 1997 due to valvulopathy (mild aortic regurgitation) from fenfluramine
3. **Phenylpropanolamin**e- sympathomimetic similar to pseudoephedrine. Removed due to hemorrhagic strokes in women. Removed 2000.

4. **Ephedrine**-sympathomimetic. Ephedrine was combined with caffeine and/or acetylsalicylic acid (ASA). Ephedrine increases thermogenesis and caffeine and ASA reduce ephedrine breakdown, thus potentiating its action. The best way to promote thermogenesis is exercise not medicines. Ephedrine is used by anesthesiologists routinely to increase blood pressure intraoperatively. It is also the ingredient in Primatene mist to help asthma. Unfortunately, a 2009 survey found that 1.4% of specialist physicians in the United States still employed ephedrine with caffeine in the treatment of obesity (Hendricks, Rothman, & Greenway, 2009). Ephedra alkaloids were banned in the United States in 2004.

5. **Romonabant**- CB1 cannabinoid receptor antagonist. Never approved in US but approved in 38 other countries. Concern for suicidal ideation/behavior.

6. **Sibutramine (Meridia**)- serotonin norepinephrine reuptake inhibitor. Removed 2000 due to myocardial infarction/stroke.

7. **Thyroid preparations**- used off label in past. Danger – arrhythmias.

Post-marketing withdrawal of anti-obesity medicinal products because of adverse drug reactions: a systematic review

- We searched for anti-obesity medications that had been withdrawn between 1950 and December 2015.
- 25 anti-obesity medications were withdrawn between 1964 and 2009, 23 of which had centrally acting mechanisms via monoamine neurotransmitters (dopamine, epinephrine, norepinephrine and serotonin)
- Cardiovascular and psychiatric adverse drug reactions and drug abuse and dependence together accounted for 83% of the withdrawals.
- In 28% of cases, deaths were attributed to the products.
- Among the centrally acting agents, re-uptake inhibitors were more likely to be withdrawn because of cardiotoxicity, while the neurotransmitter releasers were more likely to be withdrawn because of drug abuse and dependence.

Profile of centrally acting anti-obesity products withdrawn because of associated deaths over the last 50 years

Aminorex

- First introduced in 1962
- Became available within 3 years of introduction as an over-the-counter weight loss pill
- Between 1965 and 1972, there was an alarming increase in the incidence of primary pulmonary hypertension.
- The pulmonary hypertension epidemic ended in 1972 following withdrawal.

Benfluorex

- Approved in 1976 as an add-on treatment in obese patients with diabetes mellitus
- Cases of valvulopathy began to appear from 2003
- Withdrawn in 2009 following an epidemic of valvulopathy.
- Several deaths reported
- To date, more than 3000 hospitalizations and at least 1300 deaths attributed to its use in France alone

Fenfluramine

- First approved in 1973
- Reports of pulmonary hypertension first appeared in 1981
- Epidemiological studies showed an association between fenfluramine and pulmonary hypertension
- Withdrawn worldwide in 1997

Methamphetamine (desoxyephedrine)

- First introduced in 1944
- Within 10 years of its introduction, cases of its misuse had been reported
- By the early 1970s, reports of its abuse as an anorectic were reported
- Was withdrawn in the USA and other countries in 1973
- Several cases of cardiac abnormalities related to its abuse have subsequently been reported

Phentermine

- First approved in 1959
- Several cases of lung phospholipidosis in animals and humans reported thereafter
- Reports of death began to appear in 1974
- Withdrawn from most countries where it was marketed in 1981

- Still available for short-term management of obesity in the USA

Rimonabant

- Approved in Europe in 2006 for obesity treatment
- Within 1 year of approval, concerns about the risk of depression and suicide
- Five deaths attributed to its use in the UK
- Withdrawn in 2007

Sibutramine

- Approved in 1997 in the USA and Europe in 2001
- Within a year of its European approval, serious cardiovascular adverse reactions were reported, resulting in temporary withdrawal in Italy
- Several cases of severe cardiovascular adverse reactions, including deaths, were subsequently reported
- Withdrawn in Europe and USA in 2010

Several medicinal products with similar mechanisms of action to the withdrawn psychotropic anti-obesity medications have been successfully used for treating other medical conditions, and they have not been withdrawn from the market. This may be because in those conditions their mechanisms of action are specifically targeted against abnormal pathways. For example, several analogues of amphetamine are available for treating attention deficit hyperactivity disorder (ADHD) and narcolepsy.

There were no new approvals of anti-obesity medications during the 20 years from 1976 to 1995. No new drugs that cause neurotransmitter release have been marketed since 1974. Drug developers have largely abandoned the use of chemical entities that inhibit re-uptake in favour of releasing agents.

Conclusions

Psychiatric disturbances, cardiotoxicity, or drug abuse and dependence accounted for more than 80% of withdrawals. Centrally acting products that caused release of monoamines were significantly more likely to be withdrawn because of adverse cardiovascular reactions, while monoamine re-uptake inhibitors were more likely to be withdrawn because of drug abuse and dependence (Onakpova, Heneghan, & Aronson, 2016).

Good Players

Five medications have been approved for the management of obesity. **Remember, for a drug to be approved for weight loss, the FDA requires the drug be responsible for losing 5% or more body weight in at least 35% of people tested. The lost weight should be double the percentage which occurred in the placebo treated group and should last one year.** The following articles look at them.

Association of Pharmacological Treatments for Obesity with Weight Loss and Adverse Events. A Systematic Review and Meta-analysis.

Twenty-eight randomized clinical trials with 29,018 patients (median age 46 years old, 74% women, median BMI 36.1). **All active agents were associated with significant excess weight loss compared with placebo at 1-year.**

1. Qysmia (phentermine/topiramate) – 8.8 kg
2. Saxenda (liraglutide) – 5.3 kg
3. Contrave (naltrexone/buproprion – 5.0 kg
4. Belviq (lorcaserin) – 3.2 kg
5. Orlistat – 2.6 kg

Compared with placebo, liraglutide and naltrexone/bupropion were associated with the highest odds of adverse event-related treatment discontinuation. High attrition rates (30%-45% in all trails) were associated with lower confidence in estimates. High attrition rates are the norm in obesity trials (Khera, et al., 2016).

A Comparison of New Pharmacological Agents for the Treatment of Obesity

- No head-to-head trials have been identified between the four agents. The approved agents are lorcaserin (Belviq), phentermine/topiramate (Qysmia) in 2012 and naltrexone/bupropion (Contrave), liraglutide (Saxenda) in 2014.
- The American Heart Association/American College of Cardiology/The Obesity Society and the Endocrine Society recommend that medications be considered as an adjunct

to lifestyle or behavioral interventions in patients with a BMI of 30 or higher or patients with a BMI of 27 or greater plus one or more associated comorbid medical conditions.

- All four agents have a pregnancy category of X, contraindicating use.
- **No clear first line agent has emerged, so treatment should be based on patient-specific factors.**
- Ranking of overall weight loss in studies (remember no direct head-to-head trials) looking at percentages achieving both great/equal 5% and 10% weight loss.
    1. Phentermine/topiramate (Qysmia).
    2. Naltrexone/bupropion (Contrave).
    3. Liraglutide (Saxenda).
    4. Lorcaserin (Belviq).

Completion rates in studies (tolerability).
1. Phentermine/topiramate
2. Liraglutide
3. Lorcaserin and Naltrexone/bupropion tied.
(Nuffer, Trujillo, & Megyeri, 2016)

Pricing using Good Rx coupon 6/23/19
1. Qysmia (Phentermine/topiramate) $193 per month   2. Contrave (Naltrexone/bupropion) $272 per month 3. Belviq (Lorcaserin) $305 per month
4. Saxenda (Liraglutide) $1243 per month

Personally, the cost of the above agents are a daily issue with individuals with private insurance and even more difficult with Medicare patients. More than 90% of the time, my patients cannot afford them. Saxenda has been clinically not obtainable in my practice due to lack of coverage from insurance providers. It has outpriced itself for over 4 years.

Good Players

1. Saxenda
- Approved **12/23/2014**.

- The dose is titrated to 3.0 mg SQ daily whereas the dose of Victoza is 1.8 mg/day. The dose is titrated weekly from 0.6 mg/day to 1.2 to 1.8 to 2.4 to 3.0 mg/day SQ.
- **Patient has to lose 4% body weight by week 16 or medicine is discontinued.** Not paid for by Medicare, Medicaid and most insurances.
- Great drug. Essentially not obtainable since insurance companies rarely approve it.

Effects of liraglutide plus phentermine in adults with obesity following 1 year of treatment by liraglutide alone: A randomized placebo-controlled pilot trial.

This pilot study evaluated whether adding phentermine to liraglutide would induce further weight loss in participants who had previously lost weight with liraglutide alone.

Subjects/Methods:
Participants were 45 adults with obesity (75.6% female, 55.6% white, BMI 34.3 who had lost an average of 12.6% of initial weight during a prior 1-year randomized trial with liraglutide and intensive behavioral treatment.
Participants were re-randomized, in a double-blinded fashion, to liraglutide 3.0 mg (Saxenda) plus phentermine 15.0 mg (liraglutide-phentermine) or liraglutide plus placebo (liraglutide-placebo).

Results:
At week 12, the liraglutide-phentermine and liraglutide-placebo groups lost a mean (±SEM) of 1.6% and 0.1% of re-randomization weight, respectively (p = 0.073).

Conclusions:
The combination of liraglutide and phentermine appeared to be well-tolerated but did not produce additional meaningful weight loss in individuals who had already lost 12.6% of initial weight with liraglutide alone (Tronieri, et al., 2019).

A criticism of the study is the low dose of phentermine used. My experience is the starting dose of phentermine is 30 mg daily followed by increasing the dose to 37.5 mg daily if needed.

2. Phentermine
- beta-2- receptor agonist. See chapter 15 for more information.

3. Qysmia
- Approved **2012**-schedule IV drug- low dose phentermine/extended release topiramate.
- Not approved in 2010 owing to concerns over possible birth defects (Fortress study using retrospective data showed the prevalence of orofacial cleft in pregnant women on topiramate was 0.29% compared to 0.16% off it.
- Doses are 3.75 mg phentermine/23 mg topiramate starting dose, 7.5/46 mg titration dose, 11.25/69 mg titration dose, 15/92 mg top dose. Dose is titrated every 14 days as desired.
- Qsymia was approved with a post-marketing trial to assess long-term cardiovascular safety.
- The rationale for the combination, besides more effective weight loss, is phentermine is a stimulant, and topiramate has a more sedative effect and potential negative cognitive effect. Thus, it was hypothesized that one drug could counteract the side-effect profile of the other (Halpern, Faria, & Halpern, 2013).
- The EQUIP trial (1,267 patients). Had 40% withdrawal rate. One-year mean weight loss was 10.9% for top dose versus 1.6% for placebo.
- A later trial, CONQUER trial- 2,487 patients with BMI 27-45 plus 2 obesity related co-morbid conditions. 31% withdraw rate. One-year weight loss was 7.8% with 7.5/46 mg dose and 9.8% with 15/92 mg dose versus 1.2% with placebo. Many CV risk factors improved with top dose.
- 78% of the CONQUER trial patients who completed 56 weeks continued for total 108 weeks (2 years) in The SEQUEL study. Of these participants 84% completed the second year with sustained weight loss of 9.3% at 7.5/46 mg and 10.5% at 15/92 mg dose versus 1.8% for placebo (Yanovski & Yanovski, 2014).
- Topiramate (other component) is used routinely for seizures and migraine prophylaxis. Shown to promote weight loss incidentally. Side effects are memory issues,

paresthesias (tingling, numbness in arms, fingers), dysgeusia (bad taste in mouth), and metabolic acidosis. Paresthesia side effect due to being weak carbonic anhydrase inhibitor along with slightly increased risk of renal stones. Because topiramate can cause cleft palate, birth control needs to be documented.

Low dose generic topiramate at 25-100 mg qhs or 25-50 mg BID sometimes helps phentermine when patient is at a weight loss standstill. An extended release topiramate called Trokendi is available also but is expensive.

4. Belviq

- lorcaserin- approved **2012**-schedule IV drug-selective serotonin 2C receptor agonist.
- Rejected in 2010 owing to concerns about tumor growth in preclinical trials. Indirectly decreases satiety (stimulates alpha MSH causing activation of MC4R which decreases satiety).
- Serotonin has three receptors 2A, 2B, 2C. Lorcaserin preferentially activates 2C receptor 61-fold greater than 2B receptor which is found in heart muscle. At the recommended dose lorcaserin is not expected to activate the 2B receptor in heart muscle. Although neither incidence of valvulopathy nor hypertension was significantly greater with lorcaserin than placebo treatment, both were numerically more prevalent and the FDA has requested that a post-approval trial be done to assess the long-term cardiovascular effects of lorcaserin (Colman, et al., 2012). On the basis of echocardiographic data from more than 5,200 patients who received lorcaserin for up to one year, the relative risk of FDA-defined valvulopathy was 1.16%. Well-tolerated drug. Expensive.

A One -Year Randomized Trial of Lorcaserin for Weight Loss in Obese and Overweight Adults: The BLOSSOM Trail

- Randomized, placebo-controlled, double-blind, parallel arm trial at 97 U.S. research centers. 4,008 patients, aged 16-65 years old, with a BMI 30-45 or between 27-29.9 with an obesity-related comorbid condition.

- Patients were randomized in a 2:1:2 ratio to receive lorcaserin 10 mg twice daily (BID), lorcaserin 10 mg once daily (QD), or placebo.

- All patients received diet and exercise counseling. 47.2% treated with 10 mg BID, 40.2% treated with 10 mg QD, and 25.0% with placebo. All lost at least 5% of baseline body weight.

- 10% weight loss was achieved by 22.6% and 17.4% of patients receiving lorcaserin 10 mg BID and QD respectively, 9.7% of patients in the placebo group.

- Headache, nausea, and dizziness were the most common lorcaserin-related adverse events.

- U.S. Food and Drug Administration-defined echocardiographic valvulopathy occurred in 2.0% of patients on placebo and 2.0% on lorcaserin 10 mg BID.

- Conclusion: **Lorcaserin (Belviq) administered in conjunction with a lifestyle modification program was associated with dose-dependent weight loss that was significantly greater than with placebo** (Fidler, et al., 2011).

Lorcaserin treatment decreases body weight and reduces cardiometabolic risk factors in obese adults: A six-month, randomized, placebo-controlled, double-blind clinical trial.

- Lorcaserin is a serotonin 2c receptor agonist that promotes weight loss while contributing to the prevention and improvement of type 2 diabetes and improvement of atherogenic lipid profiles, without higher rates of major cardiovascular events.

- We measured, for the first time, lipid particle quantification, lipid peroxidation, appetite-regulating hormones.

- A total of 48 obese participants were enrolled in this six-month, randomized (1:1), placebo-controlled, double-blinded clinical trial.

- Lorcaserin treatment reduced fat mass (P < 0.001), the fatty liver index (P < 0.0001) and energy intake (P < 0.03) without affecting energy expenditure or lean mass.
- Total low-density lipoprotein (LDL) (P < 0.04) and small LDL particles (P < 0.03) decreased, while total high-density lipoprotein (HDL) P < 0.02) increased and heart rate significantly decreased with lorcaserin treatment.
- These data suggest that lorcaserin treatment for six months improves cardiometabolic health in obese individuals, acting mainly through the brain (Tuccinardi, et al.,2019).

Lorcaserin and metabolic disease: weight-loss dependent and independent effects

Weight management pharmacotherapies can improve metabolic diseases through weight-dependent and weight-independent effects. Lorcaserin is a selective 5-hydroxytryptamine (HT) 2C receptor agonist. Serotonin or 5-HT is a neurotransmitter that not only regulates food intake and energy expenditure but also mediates glucose homeostasis. Human data support the hypothesis that lorcaserin-mediated improvement in metabolic parameters may be mediated by both weight loss-dependent and weight loss-independent effects, especially regarding improvements in glycaemic parameters.

Methods:
This retrospective analysis evaluated 6,897 patients with overweight or obesity (with or without diabetes mellitus) across three randomized, placebo-controlled, double-blind, 52-week clinical trials that evaluated lorcaserin 10 mg twice daily. 509 patients from only one of the studies had type 2 diabetes mellitus.

Conclusions:
Across Phase III clinical trials, lorcaserin 10 mg BID improved multiple cardiometabolic parameters through both weight-loss dependent and independent mechanisms.

Discussion
No therapeutic agent that specifically targets serotonergic pathways is yet approved for treatment of DM.
So how might serotonergic agents affect glucose parameters?
Lorcaserin is thought to act upon the arcuate nucleus area of

the hypothalamus via neural areas having energy balance functions (e.g. pro-opiomelanocortin [POMC], agouti-related peptide and cocaine-regulated and amphetamine-regulated transcript). Specifically, lorcaserin is believed to activate POMC neurons, resulting in second-order signaling via melanocortin 4 (MC4) receptors. Central activation of MC4 receptors may reduce appetite and thus contribute to weight loss. Increased MC4-receptor activation may also increase sympathetic nerve activity, which may promote adipose tissue lipolysis. Reductions in adipocyte size and adipose tissue expansion with MC4 activation potentially improves hyperglycaemia. These mechanisms may help explain why weight loss via MC4 activation (as occurs with lorcaserin) may improve glucose homeostasis (Bays, Perdomo, Nikonova, Knoth, & Malhotra, 2018).

5. Contrave

- (bupropion-antidepressant/naltrexone-opioid receptor antagonist) rejected by FDA in 2011 due to increased heart rate and blood pressure in some trials and one death due to myocardial infarction.
- Because it increases catecholamines (dopamine, noradrenaline) bupropion-induced hypertension can occur and was one of the reasons for its rejection in 2011.
- A further safety study allowed approval in **2014**. Not a controlled substance. Decreases appetite and food craving by activating POMC neurons (pro-opiomelanocortin) in the hypothalamus.
- Nausea is the most common side-effect.
- The combination results in a median weight loss of 5.4% (Greenway, et al., 2010) (Halpern, Faria, & Halpern, 2011) (Anderson, et al., 2002).
- **To understand the combination, we focus on the mechanism of action of bupropion.**
- It is a norepinephrine and dopamine reuptake inhibitor used mainly to treat depression and smoking cessation.
- The usual dose for depression and smoking cessation is 300 mg per day.

- The most common side effects of bupropion are insomnia and headache. Seizures are the most serious adverse effect (0.4%).
- In the arcuate nucleus of the hypothalamus, increased levels of both dopamine and norepinephrine fire anorexigenic (decrease appetite) proopiomelanocortin (POMC) neurons leading to appetite suppression (Greenway, et al., 2009). POMC activation leads to a negative autologous feedback of beta-endorphin production, (which triggers pleasure response to food), explaining the early weight loss plateau (Greenway, et al., 2009).
- Bupropion alone leads to a mean weight loss of nearly 3 kg and patients achieve an early plateau of weight stabilization (Anderson, et al., 2002).
- The half-life of bupropion is 21 hours.
- Bupropion does decrease the seizure threshold in people susceptible to seizures but the paper was done in 1989 and one review calculated an absolute risk after two years of exposure of only 0.48% (Davidson, 1989).
- The FDA advises to ask about any seizure history and also warns about use in patients with anorexia or bulimia nervosa, since purging symptoms can reduce seizure threshold and a substantial number of individuals with eating disorders engage in weight loss programs (Horne, et al., 1988).
- The anti-platelet drugs ticlopidine (Ticlid) and Clopidrogel (Plavix) can increase bupropion levels.
- Bupropion is metabolized by the liver and the kidneys. Caution should be exercised in patients with liver damage, severe kidney disease and severe hypertension.

Review of Mechanism of bupropion (from left to right)
Bupropion - arcuate nucleus hypothalamus - increase dopamine/noradrenalin - POMC neuron - alpha-melanocyte stimulating hormone (a-MSH)/beta-endorphin - melanocortin-4-receptors (MC4R) - DECREASE FOOD INTAKE.
Naltrexone is the other component in Contrave.

- It is an opioid antagonist approved for alcohol and opioid dependence with a high affinity for the mu-receptor (key receptor for opioids).
- The dose used for opioid addiction and alcoholism is 50 mg daily. Because naltrexone is a competitive antagonist of 2 opioid receptors, it blocks beta-endorphin signaling, permitting a more pronounced effect of bupropion on anorexigenic neurons (Greenway, et al., 2009).
- Naltrexone is not approved for weight loss as a monotherapy since it induces less than a 5% weight loss long-term. The most common side effect is nausea. Naltrexone should not be used in patients with liver failure or recent opioid use. The European Medicines Agency (EMA) approved naltrexone/bupropion marketed under the name Mysiba in March 2015.
- The dose is 8 mg/90 mg tablet everyday with increasing the dose every week or as tolerated up to 2 tabs BID. **Slow titration is the key since nausea is the overriding side-effect.**
- Personally, I tell patients to increase it slowly as tolerated and I would rather have them be on only two tabs after 6 weeks rather than have them discontinue it when they could not tolerate 3 or 4 tabs per day.
- The full titration dose of naltrexone is only 32 mg compared to the usual 50 mg used for alcoholism and opioid addiction.
- The "12-week rule" still applies but I wait until they have titrated themselves to the best tolerated dose for the individual, and then the 12-week cut-off starts.
- Contrave was studied in about 4,500 obese and overweight patients in total. Two trials showed twice as many patients lost at least 5% with Contrave compared to placebo at one year.

An excellent review of Contrave was done by Georgios A. Christou, and Dimitrios N. Kiortsis in the journal Hormones in 2015 entitled, **The efficacy and safety of the naltrexone/bupropion combination for the treatment of obesity: an update**. Many of the explanations in the last few paragraphs can be attributed to their review article.

Objective: The combination of 32 mg naltrexone and 360 mg bupropion prolonged release (NB32) was recently approved by both the food and drug administration (FDA) and the European medicines agency (EMA) as an adjunct to a comprehensive lifestyle intervention to achieve weight loss.
Design: Randomized controlled trials with naltrexone/bupropion prolonged release were selected through a search based on PubMed.
Results:

- NB32 treatment resulted in 5.0-9.3% weight loss, while the placebo-subtracted weight loss was 3.2-5.2% during 56 weeks of treatment.
- The proportion of treated patients with $\geq 5\%$ weight loss was 45-66%.
- NB32 was associated with a decrease in waist circumference, serum triglycerides and insulin resistance and an increase in high-density lipoprotein-cholesterol (HDL-C).
- The most common side effects were nausea, constipation, headache and vomiting.
- Serious adverse effects, which were very rare, included suicidal thoughts and seizures. In the majority of patients NB32 treatment was well tolerated.

Conclusion:
- Naltrexone/bupropion combination appears to be an effective adjunct to a comprehensive lifestyle intervention in order to achieve weight loss and treat obesity-related comorbidities (Christou & Kiortsis, 2015).

Naltrexone/Bupropion ER (Contrave); Newly Approved Treatment Option for Chronic Weight Management in Obese Adults

- Health care costs for obese patients were on average $1,429 higher than for patients of normal weight.
- Contrave - two active components, naltrexone and bupropion, are both approved by the FDA.

MECHANISM OF ACTION

- the combination is theorized to work synergistically in the hypothalamus and the mesolimbic dopamine circuit to promote satiety, reduce food intake, and enhance energy expenditure.
- Pro-opiomelanocortin (POMC) cells found in the arcuate nucleus of the hypothalamus produce melanocyte-stimulating hormone (alpha-MSH) and beta-endorphin, an endogenous opioid. The alpha-MSH activates the melanocortin-4 receptor (MC4R), leading to decreased food intake, increased energy expenditure, and weight loss.
- Naltrexone, an opioid antagonist, disrupts beta-endorphin inhibitory feedback on POMC cells.

The naltrexone/bupropion combination enhances the effect of POMC signaling more than either drug alone.

- After 12 weeks of treatment with naltrexone/bupropion, a patient should have achieved at least a 5% weight loss since initiation of therapy. If this result is not attained within 12 weeks, then naltrexone/bupropion should be discontinued because it is unlikely that the patient will derive benefit from it.

Renal Impairment Dosing Recommendations

- Mild: No dosage adjustment recommended
- Moderate to severe: One tablet in the morning and evening
- End stage renal disease: Use is not recommended

Hepatic Impairment Dosing Recommendations

Mild to severe: One tablet in the morning

- Patients older than 65 years of age may be more sensitive to naltrexone/bupropion's central nervous system adverse effects. No specific dose adjustments are recommended based solely on age, but using caution is advised.
- Safety and efficacy studies for patients younger than 18 years of age have not been performed, and the drug is not recommended for this age group.
- Naltrexone/bupropion administration is not recommended following a high-fat meal due to a significant increase in systemic exposure.

EFFICACY IN CLINICAL TRIALS

Contrave Obesity Research-I (COR-I) study

1. Contrave Obesity Research-II (COR-II) study

2. Contrave Obesity Research-Intensive Behavior Modification study (COR-BMOD)
3. Contrave Obesity Research-Diabetes study (COR-Diabetes)

These were four 56-week, multicenter, randomized, double-blind, placebo-controlled, phase 3 trials enrolling 4,536 patients to evaluate the efficacy and safety of naltrexone/bupropion.

- In three of the four studies, the patient populations' mean age was 44 to 46 years, the BMI was 36 kg/m^2, more than 85% were women, and more than 68% were Caucasian. The COR-Diabetes trial, however, had a mean age of 54 years and 54% of the participants were female.

- **Patients treated with naltrexone/bupropion 32 mg/360 mg achieved statistically and clinically significant weight reduction when compared with placebo in all four phase 3 studies**.

- Naltrexone/bupropion has been administered to 3,475 patients with more than 2,300 patient-years of exposure.

- Common Adverse Reactions were nausea 32.5% vs 6.7%, constipation 19.2% vs 7.2%, headache 17.6% vs 10.4% compared to placebo.

- Naltrexone/bupropion has been associated with increases in resting heart rate and average blood pressure. In clinical trials, naltrexone/bupropion was not associated with a clinically significant change in blood pressure or electrocardiogram parameters. The number of cardiovascular events reported in clinical trials was considered to be too low to exclude a potential risk (Sherman, Ungureanu, & Rey, 2016).

<u>**Qysmia/Contrave combination-**</u> the FDA has recently approved using the two medicines together to provide more choices and hopefully better results to people that suffer from obesity. This approach using different pharmacological pathways to counteract the complex redundant, adaptive pathways that interact with weight regulation is used all the time regarding diabetes and hypertension. By potentially using lower doses of medicines, less side effects and improved tolerability may happen.

"Combination therapies are a promising new area in obesity treatment, similar to what occurs with diabetes and hypertension. Safety assessment is highly important due to the high number of potential users on a chronic basis" (Halpern & Mancini, 2017).

Is pharmacotherapy enough for urgent weight loss in severely obese patients?

Multiple medications are available presently to help patients with severe obesity. The present diagram summarizes the agents.

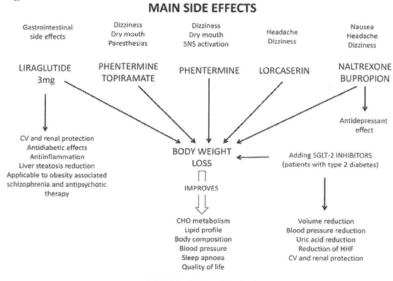

(Gargallo-Vaamonde, Perdomo, de la Higuera, & Frubeck, 2019)

Chapter 26: Case Studies of weight loss patients:

I have followed the patient's below for several years. I initially chose them because of success at early weight loss. I did not remove any patients to show real world issues. Some patients have died.

1. L.H. 58-year-old WM started weight loss program 9/2/14. Medical problems were morbid obesity, OSA, 24 hr. Oxygen use, DM, HTN, anemia, DJD, hypogonadism, and hyperlipidemia. He was on eight medications and required 160 units of insulin per day with a HgbA1c level of 10.3 (257 average glucose). He weighed 430 lbs. (BMI 67.41). Approximately 2 ½ years later he had lost 99 lbs., has a HGBA1c level 7.1 (150), takes a baby aspirin, Invokana, Lipitor, metformin, phentermine, terazosin, Trulicity, Neurontin and wears 2 liters of oxygen 24 hrs. per day along with CPAP at night. He was off insulin. He was as low as 302 lbs. on 7/2016. Despite losing over 100 lbs he slowly regained most of his weight over the next year. He developed anasarca and was noted to have a cardiac ejection fraction of 20%. He continued to struggle with worsening obstructive sleep apnea and finally died from obesity complications October 2018. He was able to keep 50 lbs off for over 4 years. At one time he was self-motivated and working on his house.

2. N.N. 56-year-old WM with DM, HTN, OSA, knee DJD, hypogonadism, smoker. He was on six meds and weighed

344 lbs. (BMI 48) on 12/2013. He has lost 107 lbs. and weighs 237 lbs. as of 2/17/17 with BMI 0f 33.05. He takes a baby aspirin, diclofenac, Flomax, Glucophage, Invokana, Levitra, lisinopril, phentermine, and testosterone. He does not take a statin due to myalgias. His bp is controlled, but his HgbA1c is 8.2 (187) on 12/23/16. His use of testosterone and weight loss has probably delayed knee replacements for several years and has greatly improved his quality of life. His weight 9/2018 was 257.4 lbs. with a HgbA1C 7.9 (177). He has kept off 86 lbs (25% body weight) over 5 years. His situation exemplifies the benefits of weight loss. Without changing his lifestyle, he would be on large doses of insulin and probably weigh 400 lbs.

3. L.P. 72-year-old WM with morbid obesity, DM, HTN, lipids, and DJD. He was on eight meds and injected 92 units of insulin per day with HgbA1c level 6.6 (134). He weighed 284 lbs. (BMI 42.3). About 100 days into phentermine he developed atrial fibrillation/flutter at a rate of 113 beats/minute. Phentermine was stopped, Eliquis started long-term, Coreg increased and he converted to normal sinus rhythm. He restarted phentermine three months later and has continued to lose weight without any cardiac or other issues. As of 2/16/17 he had lost 68 lbs. and weighed 216 lbs., (BMI 30.99). He has had no further issues with rapid a-fib. He takes allopurinol, Coreg, Eliquis, Flomax, gemfibrozil, Lipitor, Maxzide, metformin, phentermine, and vitamin D. Unfortunately, his wife passed away and he regained some of his weight and his HbgA1c climbed to 9.5 (230). He has developed worsening renal function, decreased systolic cardiac function and restarted insulin twice per day. He has been able to keep off over 45 lbs since 2014.

4. B.M. 63-year-old BF on nine meds weighing 403 lbs. (BMI 69) on 9/2012. She has OSA, Anemia, HTN, reflux, asthma and needs both knees replaced. She does not have diabetes. As of 4/17/17 she has lost 120 lbs. and takes 14 medicines including 90 tablets of Narco 10/325 mg every month for severe knee pain. She cannot exercise. Her HgbA1c is 5.4.

She had   surgery remove a hard nodule of adipose tissue behind her right knee and has developed an abscess twice in that area. She struggles with weight and bilateral knee pain. Her most recent weight is 315. She takes 9 prescription medicines.

5.   C.N. 50-year-old WF with DM, sciatica, lipids on no meds and weighs 221 lbs. (BMI 36.3) with HgbA1c 6.9 (143) on 11/2014. Eleven months later she is on 2 meds and has lost 53.5 lbs. with HGBA1C level 5.4 and weighs 167.5 lbs. (BMI 27.5). Lost to follow-up.

6.   B. P. 32-year-old WF with bipolar disorder, HTN, chronic hypoxia, alcoholism, GED graduate with disability for last 5 years living with an alcoholic boyfriend. She weighed 420 lbs. 1/2015 with a BMI 72.5. She did not have diabetes and took Xanax 0.5 mg q12 hrs. prn anxiety, Buspar 10 mg bid, clonidine 0.1 mg tid, Prozac 40 mg qd, and Lopressor 25 mg bid. Took phentermine for less than 3 months (took 84 capsules 30 mg) and stopped due to aggravating anxiety. Her Xanax dose was increased and Xanax extended release 3 mg along with Topamax 50 mg bid were added. After 26 months (3/9/17), she lost 234 lbs. and weighed 187 lbs. with BMI 32. She had been successful at getting out of a bad relationship, stopped binge drinking and was taking extended release Xanax to help with anxiety. Despite all the success she apparently had, she went back to a bad relationship and committed suicide a month after her last visit with my office.

7.   J.W. 35-year-old WM who has been obese his entire life. He has OSA, hgbA1c 6.5 (130), married with two kids. Cannot tolerate CPAP mask. Works fulltime. I also see his parents for weight loss. Takes only oxcarbazepine for trigeminal neuralgia. His weight was 527 lbs. on 12/15/15. He has a very large pannus that hangs down to his knees and he avoids walking in public due to his large pannus. I started him on phentermine 30 mg daily and increased it to 37.5 mg daily 7/22/16. I added Contrave 8/90 mg 3/15/17 to help him lose more weight. As of 5/9/2017 he weighed 400

lbs. and had lost 127 lbs. He had successful panniculectomy that weighed 55 lbs. On 7/2017 his weight was 345 lbs. making his weight loss at 182 lbs. He did not return to my office for continued weight loss.

Obesity and the co-morbidities associated with them can be devastating to the person and family. Both the physical and mental components of obesity need to be addressed. As you can tell from these examples, many patients are chronically-ill with multiple co-morbidities. I also have dozens of healthy patients essentially with only extra weight that did not have any end-organ damage to begin with.

I have had 2 patients on phentermine develop atrial fibrillation. My impression is that this is probably the typical background rate you would find in an older Medicare internal medicine practice. I think phentermine helped promote atrial fibrillation just as a B-blocker decreases the occurrence. Both patients had OSA which promotes arrhythmias due to hypoxia and adrenergic stimulation.

One overlooked group of patients that have potential are obese patients with chronic respiratory failure on oxygen. By decreasing their weight, the work of breathing decreases and their quality of life improves.

Chapter 27: Chocolate Milk

"It used to be that I'd eat to run; the more I ran, the more I needed to eat. But now, I run to eat." Tom Fleming (elite marathon runner)

Chocolate milk and white milk maybe the perfect drinks next to water.

Chocolate milk for recovery from exercise: a systematic review and meta-analysis of controlled clinical trials.

Chocolate milk (CM) contains carbohydrates, proteins, and fat, as well as water and electrolytes, which may be ideal for post-exercise recovery. We systematically reviewed the evidence regarding the efficacy of CM compared to either water or other "sport drinks" on post-exercise recovery markers.

Twelve studies were included in the systematic review.

CM provides either similar or superior results when compared to placebo or other recovery drinks. Overall, the evidence is limited and high-quality clinical trials with more well-controlled methodology and larger sample sizes are warranted (Amiri, Ghiasvand, Kaviani, Forbes, & Salehi-Abargouei, 2018).

The effectiveness of chocolate milk as a post-climbing recovery aid.

Cross-over design to compare water with chocolate milk as recovery aids following high intensity endurance climbing.

Ten male climbers (age: 22±1 years-old, climbed a Tredwall (Brewer Ledge M6) until exhaustion (Tredwall is rotating rock-climbing wall).

The participants consumed either water or chocolate milk 20 minutes after the climb and then again with their evening meal. The exercise protocol was repeated 24 hours after the original climb. The second condition was completed 7 days later. An improved performance was found after the consumption of chocolate milk, with both a greater distance climbed and duration.

Results:

Muscle soreness scores were lower three days after exercise following chocolate milk. Chocolate milk resulted in further sustained climbing, a decrease in muscle soreness, compared to water. A criticism of the study was that water and chocolate milk are not isocaloric so it seems obvious to me that a caloric drink would do better (Potter & Fuller, 2015).

Consumption of dark chocolate attenuates subsequent food intake compared with milk and white chocolate in postmenopausal women.

Chocolate has a reputation for contributing to weight gain. However, the effect of varying concentrations of cocoa in chocolate on energy intake and appetite is not clear.

Objective:

To compare the acute effect of consuming an **isocaloric** dose of dark, milk and white chocolate on subsequent energy intake, appetite and mood in postmenopausal women.

Methods:

Fourteen healthy postmenopausal women (57.6 ± 4.8yr) attended three experimental trials comparing consumption of 80% cocoa [dark chocolate], 35% cocoa [milk chocolate] and cocoa butter [white chocolate] (2099 kJ).

Results:

- Ad libitum energy intake following dark chocolate (1355 ± 750 kJ)

- milk chocolate (1693 ± 969 kJ; P = 0.008)

- white chocolate (1842 ± 756 kJ; P = 0.001)

- Blood glucose and insulin concentrations were transiently elevated in response to white and milk chocolate consumption compared with the dark chocolate (P < 0.05).

Conclusion:

Dark chocolate attenuates subsequent food intake in postmenopausal women, compared to the impact of milk and white chocolate consumption (Marsh, Green, Naylor, & Guelfi, 2017).

International Society of Sports Nutrition Position Stand: protein and exercise (2017)

Key points

- When adequate carbohydrate is delivered, adding protein to carbohydrate does not appear to improve endurance performance over the course of a few days or weeks.

- Adding protein during or after an intensive bout of endurance exercise may reduce feelings of muscle soreness.

- Protein supplementation exerts a small to modest impact on strength development.

- Pooled results of multiple studies using meta-analytic and other systematic approaches consistently indicate that protein supplementation (15 to 25 g over 4 to 21 weeks) exerts a positive impact on performance.

- When combined with a hyperenergetic diet and a heavy resistance-training program, protein supplementation may promote increases in skeletal muscle cross-sectional area and lean body mass.

- When combined with a resistance-training program and a hypo-energetic diet, an elevated daily intake of protein (2 – 3× the RDA) can promote greater losses of fat mass and greater overall improvements in body composition.

- Protein consumption directly after resistance exercise is an effective way to acutely promote a positive muscle protein balance, which if repeated over time should translate into a net gain or hypertrophy of muscle.

- A pre-exercise meal will provide amino acids during and after exercise and therefore it stands to reason there is less need for immediate post-exercise protein ingestion.

- Athletes should consume a meal during the post-workout (or pre-workout) time period since it may either help or have a neutral effect.

- Whey protein provides a distinct advantage over other protein sources including soy (considered another fast absorbing protein) and casein (a slower acting protein source) on acute stimulation of MPS (muscle protein synthesis). Whey proteins appear to be the most extensively researched for pre/post resistance exercise supplementation, possibly because of their higher EAA (essential amino acid) and leucine content, solubility, and optimal digestion kinetics. These characteristics yield a high concentration of amino acids in the blood (aminoacidemia) that facilitates greater activation of MPS and net muscle protein increase, in direct comparison to other protein choices. The addition of creatine to whey protein supplementation appears to further augment these adaptations.

- Muscle protein synthesis increases approximately 30–100% in response to a protein-containing meal to promote a positive net protein balance, and the major contributing factor to this response is the EAA content.

- The anabolic response to feeding is pronounced but transient. During the post-prandial phase (1–4 h after a meal) MPS is elevated, resulting in a positive muscle protein balance. In contrast, MPS rates are lower in a fasted state and muscle protein balance is negative. Protein buildup only occurs in the fed state. The concentration of EAA in the blood regulates protein synthesis rates.

- 30 g of whey protein, 30 g of casein protein, and 33 g of carbohydrate consumed 30-min prior to sleep resulted in an elevated morning resting metabolic rate in young fit men compared to a non-caloric placebo.

- Protein consumption in the evening before sleep might be an underutilized time to take advantage of a protein feeding opportunity that can potentially improve body composition and performance.

- It seems pragmatic to recommend the consumption of at least 20-25 g of protein (~0.25 g/kg/meal) with each main meal with no more than 3–4 h between meals.

- A protein dose of 20–40 g of protein (10–12 g of EAAs, 1–3 g of leucine) stimulates MPS, which can help to promote a positive nitrogen balance.

- The EAAs are critically needed for achieving maximal rates of MPS making high-quality, protein sources that are rich in EAAs and leucine the preferred sources of protein.

- Studies have suggested that pre-exercise feedings of amino acids in combination with carbohydrate can achieve maximal rates of MPS, but protein and amino acid feedings during this time are not clearly documented to increase exercise performance.

- Ingestion of carbohydrate + protein or EAAs during endurance and resistance exercise can help to maintain a favorable anabolic hormone profile, minimize increases in muscle damage, promote increases in muscle cross-sectional area, and increase time to exhaustion during prolonged running and cycling.

- Total protein and calorie intake appear to be the most important consideration while the impact of timing strategies (immediately before or immediately after a workout) appears to be minimal.

- A relative dose of 0.25 g of protein per kg of body weight per dose might operate as an optimal supply of high-quality protein.

- Research indicates that rates of MPS rapidly rise to peak levels within 30 min of protein ingestion and are maintained for up to three hours before rapidly beginning to lower to basal rates.

- The current RDA for protein is 0.8 g/kg/day with multiple lines of evidence indicating this value is not an appropriate amount for a training athlete to meet their daily needs.

- Daily intakes of 1.4 to 2.0 g/kg/day operate as a minimum recommended amount while greater amounts may be needed for people attempting to restrict energy intake while maintaining fat-free mass.

- 40 gms protein per meal are likely needed to maximize MPS responses in elderly individuals.

- Even higher amounts (~70 g) appear to be necessary to promote attenuation of muscle protein breakdown.

- Research has shown that products containing animal and dairy-based proteins contain the highest percentage of EAAs and result in greater hypertrophy and protein synthesis following resistance training when compared to a vegetarian protein-matched control, which typically lacks one or more EAAs.

- The three branched-chain amino acids (BCAAs), leucine, isoleucine, and valine are unique among the EAAs for their roles in protein metabolism, neural function, and blood glucose and insulin regulation. A balanced consumption of the EAAs promotes the greatest increases.

- Multiple human studies have supported the contention that leucine drives protein synthesis.

- The body uses 20 amino acids to make proteins, seven of which are essential.

- EAAs appear to be uniquely responsible for increasing MPS with doses ranging from 6 to 15 g all exerting stimulatory effects. One to three g of leucine per meal appear to be needed to stimulate protein translation machinery.

- Milk protein contains the highest score on the PDCAAS rating system, and in general contains the greatest density of leucine. Milk can be fractionated into two protein classes, casein and whey. (PDCAAS-protein digestibility corrected amino acid scale. Measure of amino acid quality and ease of digestion).

- The faster-digesting whey protein may be more beneficial for skeletal muscle adaptations than the slower digesting casein.

- The addition of milk protein to a post-workout meal may augment recovery, improve protein balance, and speed glycogen replenishment.

- One large egg has 75 kcal and 6 g of protein, but only 1.5 g of saturated fat while one large egg white has 16 kcal with 3.5 g of protein and is fat-free.

- Meat-based diets increase fat-free mass, but they may specifically increase muscle mass. A diet high in meat protein in older adults may provide an important resource in reducing the risk of sarcopenia.

- Two critical variables exist that determine a protein's impact on overall protein production and protein turnover: a) the protein's leucine content and b) the rate at which the protein is digested. In general, the proteins with the greatest leucine content include dairy (9–11%), egg (8.6%), and meat (8%), while sources low in leucine include plant-based proteins. Faster digesting sources of protein include whey and egg whites, soy, and very lean cuts of meat (>95% lean).

- MPS after consumption of whey was approximately 93% and 18% greater than casein and soy, respectively.

- Athletes should seek protein sources that are both fast-digesting and high in leucine content to maximally stimulate rates of MPS at rest and following training.

- Skim milk contains approximately 9 g of protein in a 90-cal eight-ounce serving, making it approximately 40% protein. Full-fat milk is approximately 150 kcal a serving, with 8 g of protein (21%).

(Jäger, et al., 2017)

In summary, increasing protein intake using whole foods as well as high-quality supplemental protein sources can improve the adaptive response to training.

Chapter 28: Testosterone

Many adverse consequences develop with extra weight. One adverse consequence is testosterone deficiency. Until recently, it was thought that testosterone deficiency in middle-aged men and older men mainly affected the quality of life, and it was unlikely to affect morbidity or mortality. Population-based studies indicate that testosterone deficiency predicts future development of type 2 diabetes, metabolic syndrome, cardiovascular events, mobility limitations, frailty, and mortality (Cunningham & Toma, 2011) (Ding, Song, Malik, & Liu, 2006) (Laaksonen, et al., 2004) (Krasnoff, et al., 2010) (Hyde, et al., 2010) (Laughlin, Barrett-Connor, & Bergstrom, Low serum testosterone and mortality in older men, 2008) (Khaw, et al., 2007) (Menke, et al., 2010) (Maggio, et al., 2007). By treating hypogonadism, many metabolic and orthopedic issues can be improved. Because testosterone is key to muscle mass and muscle mass controls a person's basal metabolic rate, one of the best ways to prevent weight gain is maintaining a normal testosterone level. The higher the muscle mass, the higher the metabolic rate, and the lower the tendency to gain weight.

- Unfortunately, decreases in muscle mass is a normal part of the aging process. There is no other tissue that declines more dramatically with aging than skeletal muscle. When muscle mass decreases 30% below the mean of young adults there is an increased risk of functional impairment and disability. Treating a person that has a low testosterone level along with having symptoms of hypogonadism can help prevent and treat obesity. Here are some thoughts about how testosterone effects obesity, weight, cardiovascular risk and other clinical issues.

- Data suggest that T levels in the mid-normal range relate to an optimal CV risk profile at any age, and that T levels either above or below the physiological normal range may increase the risk of atherosclerotic heart disease (Goodman, et al., 2015).
- The average decline in T levels with aging is 1-2% per year.
- Six pounds of muscle are lost per decade, metabolic rate decreases 3% per decade, and 16 pounds of fat are gained per decade starting somewhere between the third and fourth decade.
- If one eats the same amount every year and does not increase energy expenditure either through work or exercise, they will gain weight each year typically starting at 35 years-old.
- A wealth of evidence accumulated over several decades suggests that low T levels increase risk and normal to higher normal levels appear to be beneficial for CV mortality and risk (Morganteler, 2015).
- In men with hypogonadism, long-term testosterone therapy appears to be effective in achieving sustained improvements in all cardiometabolic risk factors and may be effective as an add-on measure in the secondary prevention of cardiovascular events in hypogonadal men with a history of CVD (Haider, et al., 2016).
- In the presence of significant insulin resistance, testosterone replacement therapy increases insulin sensitivity. This effect is evident after 3 months' treatment and maintained for at least up to 12 months. A 12-month study showed that testosterone improved insulin sensitivity by 15%, an effect that is equivalent to that observed by metformin usage, a mainstay of management in type 2 diabetes.
- The three major tissues that account for whole-body insulin resistance are muscle, liver, and fat. Seventy percent of reduced insulin sensitivity is accounted for by striated muscle. It should be no surprise that testosterone improves insulin resistance since 70% is accounted for by muscle.

Chapter 28: Testosterone

- Because of irrational safety concerns about testosterone replacement therapy, only 5% of hypogonadal men receive appropriate treatment in the US.
- If adequate T levels are obtained and the person does not have resolution or improvement in hypogonadal symptoms after 6 months of treatment, then treatment should be discontinued. Monitoring of several parameters are important. A baseline low T level should be obtained along with PSA, DRE (digital rectal exam), HGB or HCT before starting T therapy. Many insurance companies require a second low testosterone level before insurance will pay for treatment. A simple very conservative approach is to check PSA, HGB/HCT, and T level at 3 months, 6 months, 12 months and then annually along with DRE at 6 months, 12 months and annually. PSA recommendations are mainly for men over 40 (Buvat, Maggi, Guay, & Torres, 2013).
- Muscle decay is advocated as a true biomarker of aging.
- After the age of 35 years, a physiological decline of muscle mass occurs at an annual rate of 1-2% with a 1.5% per year reduction in strength, which accelerates around 3% after the age of 60 years.
- As we age chemical reactions become less efficient, more mistakes occur, repair abilities worsen and more energy and effort are needed to maintain the status quo. Anti-inflammation systems decrease and inflammatory mediators increase. Eventually the scales change from an anabolic product to a more progressively catabolic system till the system fails. We can slow down this process by exercise, and calorie restriction superimposed hopefully by favorable genetics.
- The idea that testosterone causes prostate cancer has been conclusively shown to be not true. A 15-yr retrospective study of 150,000 men by Kaplan and Hu found that testosterone replacement therapy was not associated with prostate cancer. Meta-analysis reported no evidence that T administration increases prostate cancer. Case closed.

- In light of increased life expectancy, we find no justification to recommend restricting T therapy based on age.

- With data over the last 13 years, we can comfortably say that low testosterone has negative consequences on many systems of the body and is a biomarker of illness. This was written in 2004.

- Hemoglobin levels in prepubertal boys and girls are similar but increase in boys after age 13 years mirroring changes in T levels. These data suggest that T contributes to the 1-2 g/dl difference between adult men and women.

- Non-prescription Over-the-counter testosterone boosters and products may carry hidden dangers. There's not a lot of scientific evidence for any supplement that claims to boost or promote testosterone. These products have been around since stagecoaches and quackery tonics. A man who thinks he's short on testosterone shouldn't be looking in a health food store for answers, he should go to a doctor's office. (Woolston, 2011)

- Heavy resistance exercise has not shown to elicit the same magnitude of hormonal responses (i.e. muscle mass, protein synthesis) in younger men (30 years old) versus older men (62 years old). The hypertrophic response of muscle to training in older men is blunted when compared with younger counterparts, and this has been attributed to the deficient anabolic hormone profile (Giannoulis, Martin, Nair, Umpleby, & Sonken, 2012).

- Elderly men over 65 years of age with late-onset hypogonadism benefit as much from testosterone treatment as do younger men and that benefit is lost when treatment is discontinued.

- Many people are treated with testosterone without measuring a level. That would be like treating women for "presumed hypothyroidism" without adequate bloodwork, commencing with maximal dose thyroxine and then concluding that thyroid replacement was highly dangerous (Hackett G., 2016).

- Modest reductions in skeletal muscle mass with aging do not cause functional impairment and disability: however, when skeletal muscle mass relative to body weight is 30% below the mean of young adults, an increase risk of functional impairment and disability is found. The development of sarcopenia in the elderly is not the result of one single change occurring during aging but is a consequence of multisystem changes.

- Falls are the leading cause of fatal and non-fatal injuries for older Americans. One-fourth of Americans aged 65+ fall each year. One out of five falls cause a serious injury such as broken bones or a head injury. One-fourth of seniors who fracture a hip from a fall will die within six months of the injury. The most profound effect of falling is the loss of independent living.

- I am thinking of opening up the first organic anti-aging clinic for both men and women with a complete guarantee associated with every prescription. Patients can line up outside my office and I promise each and every office visit will only last 5 minutes and cost only $25. I will have a clinic on more corners then Starbucks and after 2 years offer a public offering on the stock market and sell for a billion dollars. I will guarantee elevated Growth Hormone levels and also guarantee feeling happier. My secret will be mass produced scripts prescribing more sleep and more regular exercise since that is a great way that has been well-documented and supported in peer-reviewed medical journals to increase Growth Hormone levels. It will also decrease catabolic hormones and promote more anabolic hormones.

- About two thirds of male patients with advanced cancer and more than 70% with cancer cachexia have low testosterone levels compared to 6% of males in the general population. By improving performance scores with testosterone, a person may improve his survival chances since many chemotherapies will be adjusted based on low performance scores. The potential benefit seems to far exceed the minimal risk.

- The Endocrine Society guidelines recommend measuring testosterone levels in patients requiring long-term opioid therapy.

- The Endocrine Society has concluded "Evidence supports the short-term efficacy and safety of high physiological doses of testosterone treatment of postmenopausal women with sexual dysfunction due to hypoactive sexual desire disorder (HSDD) (2015).

Chapter 29: 10,000 steps

It's a little like wrestling a gorilla. You don't quit when you're tired, you quit when the gorilla is tired. Robert Strauss (author)

"Happy feet": evaluating the benefits of a 100-day 10,000 step challenge on mental health and wellbeing.

Evidence is beginning to highlight the value of walking, particularly focusing on the Japanese mark of obtaining 10,000 steps per day. Workplace based step challenges have become popular.
This study investigated the impact of a 100-day, 10,000 steps program on signs of depression, anxiety and stress as well as general well-being using standardized psychological scales.
Discussion
This study demonstrated that engaging in a workplace step program improved stress levels by 8.9%, signs of depression by 7.6%, anxiety by 5.0% and well-being by 2.1% from baseline. This reinforces the benefits of this type of exercise regimen as playing a small yet significant role in improving mental as well as physical health.

With most adults spending at least half of their life working, the workplace is an important setting for promoting mental health and well-being change. 10,000 step challenges may significantly and meaningfully improve mental health and well-being through simple and inexpensive work-based interventions (Hallam, Bilsborough, & de Courten, 2018).

The effect of two different health messages on physical activity levels and health in sedentary overweight, middle-aged women.

12-week study evaluated whether a 10,000 steps per day message was more effective than a 30 minute a day message in increasing physical activity in low active, overweight women.
Methods:
Thirty participants were randomized into 2 groups: Group 1 was asked to undertake 30 minutes of walking/day, whereas Group 2 was asked to accumulate 10,000 steps/day.
Results:
The 10,000 steps and the 30 minutes groups' daily average number of steps per day were significantly higher than baseline at week 6 and at week 12.
At week 12, the 10,000 steps group were taking an average of 4616 steps per day more (43% increase) than at baseline and the 30 minutes group were taking an average of 2761 steps per day more (35% increase) than at baseline.
There was a significant difference in the number of steps with the 10,000 steps group versus 30 minutes group at 12 weeks (p = 0.045).
Conclusions:
This study found that low active, overweight women undertook significantly more physical activity when they had a daily 10,000 step goal using a pedometer, than when they were asked to achieve 30 minutes of walking/day. Therefore, we suggest that **a public health recommendation of "10,000 steps/day", rather than the "30 min/day" could be applied to promote increased physical activity in sedentary middle-aged women** (Pal, Cheng, & Ho, 2011).

Steps, moderate-to-vigorous physical activity, and cardiometabolic profiles.

6000 Canadian adults (41.5 years, SD 14.9) were evaluated by multiple parameters and different levels of activity. The relative benefits of meeting the current moderate-to-vigorous intensity physical activity (MVPA) consisting of 150 min/wk or 10,000 steps/day. The cardiometabolic markers were blood pressure, lipid levels, Homeostatic Model Assessment of Insulin Resistance (HOMA-IR), hemoglobin A1c, C-reactive protein (CRP), and body mass index (BMI). Activity were divided above and below 150 min/wk and steps were separated into 5000-7499 (low active), 7500-9999 (somewhat active), greater than/equal 10,000 (active), and less than 5000 (inactive).

- BMI and A1c are more favorable across a 150 min/week MVPA threshold than across a 10,000 steps/day threshold.

- Important cardiometabolic improvements emerge at $\geq$ 7500 step/day.

Given that most benefits to markers of health were at the $\geq$7500 step/day threshold and that there was some additional benefit across the 150min/week MVPA threshold compared to a 10,000 steps/day threshold, we suggest aiming for $\geq$7500 steps/day and then advancing to a 150min/MVPA goal (Hajna, Ross, & Dasgupta, 2018).

Objectively Measured Daily Steps and Subsequent Long-Term All-Cause Mortality: The Tasped Prospective Cohort Study.

- Self-reported physical activity has been inversely associated with mortality. The objective is to determine the prospective association of daily step activity on mortality among adults

- Cohort study of adults residing in Tasmania, Australia between 2000 and 2005 who participated in one of three cohort studies (n = 2,576 total participants).

- Daily step activity by pedometer at baseline at a mean of 58.8 years of age, and for a subset, repeated monitoring was available 3.7 (SD 1.3) years later (n = 1 679). All-cause mortality (n = 219 deaths) was ascertained. 90% of participants were followed-up over ten years.

- Higher daily step count at baseline was linearly associated with lower all-cause mortality. Risk was altered little by removing deaths occurring in the first two years.

- Increasing baseline daily steps from sedentary to 10 000 steps a day was associated with a 46% lower risk of mortality in the decade of follow-up. In addition, those who increased their daily steps over the monitoring period had a substantial reduction in mortality risk, after adjusting for baseline daily step count or other factors (Dwyer, et al., 2015).

Daily step count and all-cause mortality in a sample of Japanese elderly people: a cohort study.
This study examined the relationship between pedometer-assessed daily step count and all-cause mortality in a sample of elderly Japanese people.

Methods
Participants included 419 (228 males and 191 females) physically independent, community-dwelling 71-year-old Japanese people. The number of steps per day was measured by a waist-mounted pedometer for seven consecutive days at baseline. Participants were divided into quartiles based on their average number of steps per day followed over a mean period of 9.8 years (1999-2010) for mortality.

1. first quartile, < 4503 steps/day   hazard ratio 1.0
2. second quartile, 4503-6110 steps/day   hazard ratio 0.81
3. third quartile, 6111-7971 steps/day   hazard ratio 1.26
4. fourth quartile, > 7972 steps/day   hazard ratio 0.46

Results
Seventy-six participants (18.1%) died during the follow-up period. Participants in the highest quartile had a significantly lower risk of death compared with participants in the lowest quartile (Yamamoto, et al., 2018).

How many steps/day are enough? Preliminary pedometer indices for public health.
A value of 10000 steps/day is gaining popularity with the media and in practice and can be traced to Japanese walking clubs and

a business slogan 30+ years ago. 10000 steps/day appears to be a reasonable estimate of daily activity for apparently healthy adults and studies are emerging documenting the health benefits of attaining similar levels. **Preliminary evidence suggests that a goal of 10000 steps/day may not be sustainable for some groups, including older adults and those living with chronic diseases. Another concern about using 10000 steps/day as a universal step goal is that it is probably too low for children, an important target population in the war against obesity.** Based on currently available evidence, we propose the following preliminary indices be used to classify pedometer-determined physical activity in healthy adults:

- <5000 steps/day may be used as a 'sedentary lifestyle index'
- 5000-7499 steps/day is typical of daily activity excluding sports/exercise and might be considered 'low active'
- 7500-9999 likely includes some volitional activities (and/or elevated occupational activity demands) and might be considered 'somewhat active'
- >or=10000 steps/day indicates the point that should be used to classify individuals as 'active'
- Individuals who take >12500 steps/day are likely to be classified as 'highly active' (Tudor-Lock & Bassett, 2004)

Walking cadence and mortality among community-dwelling older adults.

- Older adults are encouraged to walk ≥100 steps/minute for moderate-intensity physical activity (i.e., brisk walking).
- It is unknown if the ability to walk ≥100 steps/minute predicts mortality.
- 100 steps/minute is equivalent to 3 miles per hour which is normal speed for walking.
- A population-based cohort study among 5,000 older adults from the Third National Health and Nutrition Survey (NHANES III; 1988-1994). Median follow-up was 13.4 years. Average participant age was 70.6 years old.

Measurements:
- Walking cadence (steps/minute) was calculated using a timed 2.4-mile walk.

- Walking cadence was divided at ≥100 steps/minute versus <100 steps/minute.

Results:

- Among 5,000 participants, 3,039 (61 %) walked ≥100 steps/minute During follow-up, 3,171 subjects died.
- Ability to walk ≥100 steps/minute predicted a 21 % reduction in all-cause mortality.
- Each ten-step increase in walking cadence predicted a 4 % reduction in all-cause mortality.
- In secondary analyses, ability to walk ≥100 steps/minute predicted reductions in cardiovascular-specific mortality, cancer-specific mortality, and mortality from other causes.

Conclusion:

The ability to walk ≥100 steps/minute predicts a reduction in mortality among a sample of community-dwelling older adults (Brown, Harhay, & Harhay, 2014).

Walking four times weekly for at least 15 min is associated with longevity in a cohort of very elderly people.

A 10-year cohort study was conducted with 152 self-caring and mobile people, mean age 80 years.

Results:

- During the 10-years of follow-up, 96 (63%) died. Old age, chronic diseases, smoking, depression, CD4/CD8 ratio and coffee consumption were significantly predictors of mortality.

- Over-all survival was highest for subjects walking at open air for 4 times weekly for at least 15 min in comparison to subjects walking less than 4 times weekly (40% versus 22%).

Elderly people walking at open air for four times weekly had 40% decreased risk of mortality that individuals who walked less than four times weekly [relative risk (RR)=0.53; p=0.01] (Fortes, et al., 2013)

Chapter 29: 10,000 steps

.

Chapter 30: Exercise

"The good ones pretend they don't train hard; the bad ones say they train like Olympic champions. They're never completely fit and never completely well. If an athlete ever admits to being ready for competition, without the slightest injury, raring to go and sure to win, you know it's time to send for the jacket with the laces up the back" Pat Butcher – British running journalist.

"PattiSue" Plumer, is an American former middle-distance and long-distance runner who ran in the 1988 Seoul and 1992 Barcelona Olympics. She wrote "Workouts are like brushing my teeth; I don't think about them. I just do them. The decision has already been made."

What can I say about exercise? The benefits of exercise are profound and everyone agrees. Exercise is a key component of general health, weight loss and maintenance of weight. People who succeed at maintaining a healthy weight make exercise a large part of their life. Unfortunately, many people do not l exercise. Exercise is usually defined as planned or structured physical activity and involves repetitive bodily movements. It has a start and a finish. People do not have to formally exercise but need to increase their

Obesity: A Clinical Review

physical activity. Physical activity simply means any movement which burns calories. One does not need to exercise 40 minutes continuously, but many can do physical activity 10 minutes at a time, 4 times per day. Developing lifelong positive behaviors promotes success. Physical activity and exercise may generate a net effect on energy balance much greater than the direct energy cost of the activity alone. Many studies of human subjects indicate beneficial effects lasting up to 48 hours.

If exercise is so great, then why do so few people partake? The answer is easy- it is hard. When was the last time you say a runner on the street smiling? What is more fun having a bowl of ice cream or breathing hard and sweating? I have some patients tell me that they do not mind exercising as long as they don't have to sweat. If someone is not brought up exercising, then exercising is like learning a foreign language.

I exercise for many reasons. One reason is to prepare myself to handle an illness both physically and mentally when it happens. One day I will be weak and frail. How a person responds to an illness or surgery speaks volumes about their health. For instance, one person is released from the hospital in 2 days from a knee replacement while another person, the same age, may go to a skilled nursing facility for 2 weeks. Many patients do not have insight about how difficult major or minor surgery can be. Sometimes, I wish I could say that surgery is like a man or woman coming at you with a very sharp knife while you are asleep and the person is very good with the knife too. Of course, this is just a silly analogy but it still amazes me how unrealistic some people are. I also exercise to maintain muscle mass. Exercise releases endogenous endorphins that make people feel good and is a very strong stimulus for growth hormone which gives me the irrational idea that I will live forever. One of the problems with getting older is the idea of feeling invincible goes away. As you get older you lose that feeling. It sometimes returns after a good workout but becomes less and less often. When I exercise,
I see an old man that no longer flows like liquid but looks and feels like a stick figure. Instead of being smooth and flowing like a ballet dancer, I am more like a stiff-legged person. I don't float like a butterfly or sting like a bee, I putter like a turtle and sweat like a pig. I'm just buying time till my next nuisance injury that makes me

slower than I already feel. The idea that I am in better shape than 98% of people my age provides no comfort at all. I get discouraged at times but always remember to never quit. It is like the old Woody Allen phrase "I feel life is divided into the horrible and the miserable. That's the two categories. The horrible are like, terminal cases, you know, blind people, crippled. I don't know how they get through life. It's amazing to me. And the miserable is everyone else. So, you should be thankful that you're miserable, because that's very lucky, to be miserable."

Dr. James Gibney wrote an article how fuel works in our bodies. It is beautifully written and flows very well. That is not a description of my body anymore. Embrace the paragraph.

The ability to perform exercise requires combustion of metabolic fuels, transforming chemical into kinetic and thermal energy. Glucose is the preferred fuel source for short-term high-intensity activity, whereas FFAs (free fatty acids) become increasingly important during more prolonged activity. O2 delivery to muscles depends upon adequate ventilation and 02 transport to hemoglobin, circulatory distribution by an adequate cardiac output and peripheral circulation, dilatation of the muscle capillary network, and extraction of 02 by the muscle fibers with either storage in myoglobin or immediate combustion. Growth Hormone (GH) could improve exercise performance through increased delivery of substrate and oxygen to exercising muscle, increased muscle strength, or a combination of these variables. GH could also improve exercise performance through indirect mechanisms, including changes in body composition or more efficient thermoregulation. (Gibney, Healy, & Sönksen, 2007)

Resistance training with weights will not promote clinically significant weight loss but is very helpful for ADLs (activities of daily living) and helps maintain muscle mass. Resistance training has been shown to increase HDL by 8-21%, decrease LDL by 13-23% and reduce TG by 11-18%. Statistics show 25% of individuals do no physical activity and 50% do insufficient physical activity. A simple test to assess the intensity of exercise is the "talk test." Low intensity allows one to talk comfortably or sing. Moderate intensity allows fragmented talk and high intensity exercise the person is not able to speak. People that exercise want to procrastinate or make excuses like everyone else but they still exercise because they deeply believe the benefits outweigh the hassle.

A 2012 article entitled **Exercise acts as a drug; the pharmacological benefits of exercise** by J Vina in the British Journal of Pharmacology expresses some insights.

- The beneficial effects of regular exercise for the promotion of health and cure of diseases have been clearly shown. Exercise is so effective that it should be considered as a drug. As with any drug, dosing is very important. More attention needs be paid to the dosing and to individual variations between patients. **The philosopher Plato (427-347 BC) said "Lack of activity destroys the good condition of every human being while movement and methodical physical exercise saves and preserves it."** (Myers, et al., 2004; Vina, Sanchis-Gomar, Martinez-Bello, & Gomez-Cabrera, 2012)

- Modest increments in energy expenditure due to physical activity (about 1000 kcal per week) or an increase in physical fitness of 1 MET (metabolic equivalent) is associated with lowering mortality by about 20% (Myers, et al., 2004).

- Both resistance and aerobic training have been shown to be of benefit for the control of diabetes; however, resistance training may have greater benefits for glycemic control than aerobic training (Dunstan, et al., 2005).

- Wen, et al., (2011) noted that 15 minutes a day or 90 minutes a week of moderate-intensity exercise is of benefit in terms of life expectancy, even for subjects with cardiovascular risks. Moderate-intensity activities are those in which heart rate and breathing are raised; but, still, it is possible to speak comfortably. This occurs around 4-6 METS and brisk walking at 3 mph is one such activity.

- A dose-response relation appears to exist, such that people who have the highest levels of physical activity and fitness are at lowest risk of premature death (Warburton, Nicol, & Bredin, 2006). Having said that, less active men who participate in vigorous activity were more likely to have a myocardial infarction during exercise than the most active men (Thompson, et al., 2007). "You don't run before you walk."

- In the pharmacological treatment of many conditions, physicians typically start with a dose of a drug believed to be the minimum effective dose. The intensity of aerobic training should also be titrated in healthy people. As with medicines, special considerations should be taken when prescribing exercise for people with special needs such as elderly, children, pregnant women, overweight or obese patients and patients with chronic diseases.

- Exercise causes a significant reduction in cancer rates, specifically colon and breast cancer (Shephard & Futcher, 1997) (Pederson, 2006).

- Exercise acts as an antioxidant, because training increases the expression of antioxidant enzymes (Gomez-Cabrera, Domenech, & Viña, 2008).

- An interesting study in the International Journal of Sports Medicine looked at high intensity exercise in 2011. It is widely held among the general population and even among medical professionals that moderate exercise is a healthy practice but long-term high intensity exercise is not. The specific amount of physical activity necessary for good health remains unclear.

- F. Sanchis-Gomar and others studied the longevity of 834 Tour de France cyclists from France (465), Belgium (173), and Italy (196), between 1930 and 1964 with death rates up till December 31, 2007 compared with the pooled general population of France, Belgium, and Italy for comparative ages. A very significant increase in average longevity (17%) of the cyclists were noted compared to the general population. The age at which 50% of the general population died was 73.5 years compared to 81.5 years in Tour de France participants. (Sanchis-Gomar, Olaso-Gonzalez, Corella, Gomez-Cabrera, & Vina, 2011)

Consecutive days of exercise decrease insulin response more than a single exercise session in healthy, inactive men.

- It is reported that a single bout of exercise can lower insulin responses 12-24 h post-exercise; however, the insulin responses to alternate or consecutive bouts of exercise is unknown.

- the purpose of this study was to examine the effect of exercise pattern on post-exercise insulin and glucose responses following a glucose challenge.

- Ten male participants (n = 10, mean ± SD, Age 29.5 ± 7.7 years; BMI 25.7 ± 3.0 kg/m^2) completed three exercise trials of walking for 60 min at ~ 70% of VO$_{2max}$.

- The trials consisted of: three consecutive exercise days (3CON), three alternate exercise days (3ALT), a single bout of exercise (SB), and a no exercise control (R).

- Twelve to fourteen hours after the last bout of exercise or R, participants completed a 75 g oral glucose tolerance test (OGTT) and blood was collected at 30 min intervals for the measurement of glucose, insulin, and C-peptide.

- Calculated incremental area under the curve (iAUC) for glucose and C-peptide was not different between the four trials. Insulin iAUC decreased 34.9% for 3CON compared to R (p < 0.01).

- **Three consecutive days of walking at ~ 70% VO$_{2max}$ improved insulin response following an OGTT compared to no exercise. It is possible, that for healthy males, the effect of a single bout of exercise or exercise bouts separated by more than 24 h may not be enough stimulus to lower insulin responses to a glucose challenge** (Castleberry, et al., 2019).

A randomized controlled trial on the effectiveness of 8-week high-intensity interval exercise on intrahepatic triglycerides, visceral lipids, and health-related quality of

life in diabetic obese patients with nonalcoholic fatty liver disease.

- It has been reported that aerobic exercise is effective in reducing the characteristics of NAFLD (nonalcoholic fatty liver disease).

- This a randomized controlled trial to ascertain the effectiveness of 8-week high-intensity interval exercise (45-55% VO_{2peak}, 30-60 min × 5 days/week; n = 12) on intrahepatic triglycerides (IHTG), visceral lipids and HRQoL in diabetic obese patients with NAFLD. 32 diabetic obese patients with NAFLD aged 45 to 60 years (21 men and 11 women) were enrolled. They were randomly assigned to 2 groups, 16 patients in each group, high-intensity interval (HII) exercise and control groups.

- There were significant differences between the 2 groups at the end of the study. These study findings exhibited significant improvements in IHTG, VO2peak, visceral lipids, glycohemoglobin, plasma glucose, and all dimensions of HRQoL in the HII group (P <.05),

- Eight-week high-intensity interval aerobic exercise has a beneficial effect on IHTG, visceral lipids, and HRQoL in diabetic obese patients with NAFLD (Abdelbasset, Tantawy, Kamel, Alqahtani, & Soliman, 2019).

Low skeletal muscle mass is associated with the risk of all-cause mortality in patients with type 2 diabetes mellitus.

- Patients with type 2 diabetes mellitus (T2DM) have an increased risk of muscle mass reduction. However, the association between muscle mass and mortality in T2DM remains unknown.

- This was a historical cohort study with the endpoint of all-cause mortality. This study included 163 elderly Japanese men and 141 postmenopausal women with T2DM whose body compositions were evaluated using dual-energy X-ray absorptiometry. Low muscle mass was defined as a skeletal muscle mass index (SMI) of $<7.0 \, \text{kg/m}^2$ for men and $<5.4 \, \text{kg/m}^2$ for women.

- During the 6-year follow-up period, 32 men and 14 women died.

- T2DM duration, glycated hemoglobin, serum creatinine, fasting C-peptide, body mass index, and lean body mass were associated with the risk of mortality in men [hazard ratio (HR)] = 1.81and women = 4.53.

- Neither fat mass nor bone mineral content was associated with mortality.

- Low SMI was associated with increased mortality in women (HR = 5.97), and men (HR = 2.38).

- Low muscle mass was independently associated with all-cause mortality in patients with T2DM. The preservation of skeletal muscle mass is important to protect patients with T2DM from increased mortality risk (Miyake, Kanazawa, Tanaka, & Sugimoto, 2019).

Cross-sectional relationships of exercise and age to adiposity in 60,617 male runners.

- Cross-sectional analyses of 64,911 male runners between 18 and 55 years old who provided data on their body mass index (97.6%) and waist circumference (91.1%).

- Increases in BMI with age were greater for men who ran under 16 km/wk (7.27 miles/wk) than for relatively longer distance runners.

- These data suggest that age and vigorous exercise interact with each other in affecting men's adiposity and are consistent with the proposition that vigorous physical activity must increase with age to prevent middle-age weight gait (Williams & Pate, 2005).

Relationships of age and weekly running distance to BMI and circumferences in 41,582 physically active women.

Cross-sectional analyses were conducted of 41,582 female runners.

Results:

- Vigorous exercise diminished the apparent increase in adiposity with age.

- The increase in average BMI with age was greatest in women who ran less than 3.6 miles/wk.

- Intermediate in women who ran 3.6 to 14.0 miles/wk.

- Least in those who averaged over 14.5 miles/wk.

- Before age 45, waist circumference rose for those who ran 0 to 3.2 miles/wk.

- Waist circumference showed no significant relationship to age for those who ran 3.6 to 17.7 miles/wk.

- Declined in those who ran 18 miles/wk or more.

- Age related-increases in hip and chest circumferences before 45 years old were significantly less in women who ran longer weekly distances.

Discussion:

Exercise may mitigate age-related increases in adiposity and that age affects exercise-induced reductions in adiposity. This study emphasizes the degree of activity required to maintain healthy adipose levels. Walking 3 times per week is just not enough (Williams & Satariano, 2005).

Effect of Moderate to Vigorous Physical Activity on All-Cause Mortality in Middle-aged and Older Australians.

A prospective cohort study looking at all-cause mortality in 204,542 Australian adults aged 45 through 75 years old over an 8-year period looking at death rate and amount of moderate to vigorous exercise activity.

1. Low time 10-149 minutes/week. Death rate 4.81%
2. Moderate time 150-299 minutes/week. Death rate 3.17%
3. Large time 300 minutes/week or more. Death rate 2.64%

There was an inverse dose-response relationship between proportion of vigorous activity and mortality. (Gebel, et al., 2015)

Locomotive Syndrome: Definition and Management.

Locomotive syndrome is a condition of reduced mobility due to impairment of locomotive organs. The Japanese Orthopedic Association proposed the term in 2007. The average Japanese life expectancy in the year 2014 was 80.5 years for men and 86.8 years for women. Common issues among people aged 70-74 years old include fear of falling (81.7%), not being able to stand without arm support (81.1%), not being able to ascend stairs without using rail or wall for support (81.3%), slow gait speed (71.7%), and refraining from going out (50%). The three main components of the locomotive syndrome are:

1. Bones, joints, intervertebral disks
2. Muscular system
3. Nervous system.

The orthopedic conditions contributing to the locomotive syndrome have high prevalence rates in patients above 40 years:

1. Lumbar spondylosis 81.5% males, 65.6% females
2. Knee osteoarthritis 42.6% males, 62.4% females
3. Osteoporosis 12.4% males, 26.5% females.
4. Sarcopenia 13.8% males, 12.4% females.

The number of orthopedic surgical treatments requiring hospitalization dramatically increases after the age of 50 years. While physical interventions are effective in people with mild to moderate disability, their utility is limited in people with severe disability, emphasizing the importance of early detection of the locomotive syndrome and early intervention. (Nakamura & Ogata, 2016).

Exercise can be very helpful in this situation by promoting supportive muscle mass and increasing the number of years that we have a healthy orthopedic reserve.

Antioxidants for preventing and reducing muscle soreness after exercise: a Cochrane systematic review.

Determine whether antioxidant supplements and antioxidant-enriched foods can prevent or reduce delayed-onset muscle soreness after exercise.

- 50 studies with a total of 1089 participants (961 were male and 128 were female) with an age range of 16-55 years.

- The antioxidant dosage was higher than the recommended daily amount.

- The majority of trials (47) had design features that carried a high risk of bias.

Conclusions
- There is moderate to low-quality evidence that high-dose antioxidant supplementation does not result in a clinically relevant reduction of muscle soreness after exercise of up to 6 hours or at 24, 48, 72 and 96 hours after exercise.

- There is no evidence available on subjective recovery and only limited evidence on the adverse effects of taking antioxidant supplements (Ranchordas, Rogerson, Soltani, & Costello, 2018).

Physical exercise as a preventive or disease-modifying treatment of dementia and brain aging.
A rapidly growing literature strongly suggests that exercise, specifically aerobic exercise, may attenuate cognitive impairment and reduce dementia risk. The idea of neuroplasticity is an evolving concept that has important implications in disease prevention and treatment. Meta-analysis and randomized controlled trials have shown the following:

1. Midlife exercise significantly reduced later risks of mild cognitive impairment and dementia.
2. Among patients with dementia or mild cognitive impairment, 6-12 months of exercise documented better cognitive scores compared with sedentary controls.
3. Aerobic exercise in healthy adults were associated with significantly improved cognitive scores.
4. One year of aerobic exercise in seniors was associated with significantly larger hippocampal volumes and better spatial memory.
(hippocampus-center of emotion, memory, autonomic nervous system).

5. Physically fit seniors had significantly larger hippocampal or gray matter volumes compared with unfit seniors.

6. Brain cognitive networks studied using functional magnetic resonance imaging display improved connectivity after 6 to 12 months of exercise.

Besides a brain neuroprotective effect, physical exercise may also attenuate cognitive decline via mitigation of cerebrovascular risk, including the contribution of small vessel disease to dementia. Exercise should not be overlooked as an important therapeutic strategy. (Ahlskog, Geda, Graff-Radford, & Petersen, 2011)

Health risk behaviors among high school and university adolescent students.

Investigate health risk behaviors of a large adolescent sample (730 adolescents, 294 males and 436 females), residing in different areas of Greece. High school students and University newcomers, aged 14-21 years (17.8±4.5 years), self-reported health risk behaviors via an anonymous, closed-type, validated questionnaire.

The lower the frequency of exercise, the higher the consumption of psychoactive substances (P=0.022). This article speaks for itself (Tsitsimpikou, et al., 2018).

Exercise attenuates the association of body weight with diet in 106,737 runners

The high prevalence of obesity in Western societies has been attributed in part to high-fat low-CHO (carbohydrate) food consumption. However, people have also become less active, and inactivity may have increased the risk for weight gain from poor dietary choices. Analyses were performed to test whether diet-weight relationships were attenuated by vigorous exercise.

Methods

Age- and education-adjusted cross-sectional regression analyses of 62,042 men and 44,695 women recruited for the National Runners' Health Study were conducted.

Conclusions

Vigorous exercise may mitigate diet-induced weight gain, albeit not guaranteeing protection from poor dietary choices. As one gets older exercising is no guarantee that weight gain will not occur (Williams, Exercise attenuates the association of body weight with diet in 106,737 runners, 2011).

Does physical activity attenuate, or even eliminate, the detrimental association of sitting time with mortality? A harmonized meta-analysis of data from more than 1 million men and women.

It is unclear whether physical activity attenuates or even eliminates the detrimental effects of prolonged sitting. We examined the associations of sedentary behavior and physical activity with all-cause mortality.

Methods:

Systematic review, searching six databases. All study data reported daily sitting time and TV-viewing time into four standardized groups each, and physical activity into quartiles (in metabolic equivalent of task [MET]-hours per week).

Findings:

Of the 16 studies included in the meta-analysis, 13 studies provided data on sitting time and all-cause mortality. These studies included 1,005,791 individuals. Daily sitting time was not associated with increased all-cause mortality in those in the most active quartile of physical activity. Watching TV for 3 hours or more per day was associated with increased mortality regardless of physical activity, except in the most active quartile, where mortality was significantly increased only in people who watched TV for 5 hours/day or more

Interpretation:

High levels of moderate intensity physical activity (i.e. about 60-75 min per day) seem to eliminate the increased risk of death associated with high sitting time. However, this high activity level attenuates, but does not eliminate the increased risk associated with high TV-viewing time (Ekelund, et al., 2016).

Exercise patterns, ingestive behaviors, and energy balance.

Aerobic training is superior to resistance training for weight loss, although resistance training helps preserve lean body mass better. Weight loss does not differ among different intensities when energy expenditure is matched by adjusting duration.

Differing patterns of physical activity exhibited by normal weight, overweight, and obese people during weekdays and weekend days are consistent with their weight status; leaner people are more physically active (Li, O'Connor, Zhou, & Campbell, 2014). Essentially the energy you exert and the calories you eat are key.

Cardiorespiratory, enzymatic and hormonal responses during and after walking while fasting

In terms of fat breakdown, we conclude that performing a low intensity aerobic exercise in a fasting condition does not seem to offer an advantage, as compared with performing the same exercise under a feeding condition. Moreover, based on Cortisol (C) levels, we also concluded that if a primary goal is to burn fat while, simultaneously, maintaining muscle mass, performing a low intensity aerobic exercise under a fasting condition might not be the best choice (Vilaca-Alves, et al., 2018).

Is There Evidence that Runners can Benefit from Wearing Compression Clothing?

A computerized research of several electronic databases. RESULTS: Compression garments exerted no statistically significant mean effects but did show small positive benefits. Multiple variables were looked at as noted below.

- Running performance, time to exhaustion, running economy, perceived exertion, markers of muscle damage and inflammation, post-exercise leg soreness and the delay in onset of muscle fatigue, any other variables (Engel, Holmberg, & Sperlich, 2016).

I look at this study with the conclusion that compression clothing is a positive beneficial maneuver. Something does not have to be statistically significant to be beneficial. If I can improve my marathon time by 3 minutes, that is not statistically significant but may be the difference between qualifying for the Boston Marathon or not.

Does Muscle Mass Affect Running Times in Male Long-distance Master Runners?

Master athletes are defined as athletes of 35 years of age and older. A gradual loss of muscle fibers begins at the age of about 50 years and continues to the age of about 80 years where about 50% of the fibers are lost from the limb muscles. It has also been shown that body fat is a strong predictor variable for endurance performances such as cycling, triathlon, and running. The percentage of body fat and training characteristics, not skeletal muscle mass, were related to running times for master runners of all distances. Body fat seems to be the most important anthropometric variable in endurance athletes as has already been shown for half-marathoners, marathoners, and triathletes (Knechtle, Rust, Knechtle, & Rosemann, 2012).

Another study, entitled **Lifelong Physical Activity Regardless of Dose Is Not Associated with Myocardial Fibrosis**, refuted the suggestion that long-term intensive physical training may be associated with adverse cardiovascular effects, including the development of myocardial fibrosis. 92 seniors (mean age 69 years, 27% women) free of major chronic illnesses who engaged in stable physical activity over 25 years were classified into 4 groups by the number of sessions per week of aerobic activity.

Group 1   less than two 30 minutes sessions per week.
Group 2   2-3 sessions/week.
Group 3   4-5 sessions/week.
Group 4   6-7 sessions/week.

All subjects underwent cardiopulmonary exercise testing and cardiac magnetic resonance imaging, including late gadolinium enhancement assessment of fibrosis. Cardiac imaging demonstrated increasing left ventricular end-diastolic volumes, end systolic volumes, stroke volumes, with increasing doses of lifelong physical activity.
A lifelong history of consistent physical activity, regardless of dose ranging from sedentary to competitive marathon running, was not associated with the development of focal myocardial fibrosis (Abdullah, et al., 2016).

A prospective cohort study looking at all-cause mortality in 204,542 Australian adults aged 45 through 75 years old over an

8-year period looking at death rate and amount of moderate to vigorous exercise activity was published in JAMA 2015.

    1. Low time 10-149 minutes/week. Death rate 4.81%

    2. Moderate time 150-299 minutes/week. Death rate 3.17%

    3.Large time 300 minutes/week or more. Death rate 2.64%

There was an inverse dose-response relationship between proportion of vigorous activity and mortality (Gebel, et al., 2015).

Few strategies have been effective in treating the rapid rise in obesity worldwide. A study presently being conducted by will focus on preventing excessive weight gain rather than weight reduction:

Evaluating a small change approach to preventing long term weight gain in overweight and obese adults.

Individuals will reduce overall energy balance by 100-200 kcal per day by reducing calorie intake and/or increase daily step count by 2000 per day (2000 steps are about 100 kcals). The primary outcome is change in body weight and body composition. 320 primarily white (305) overweight and obese men and women are randomized to Usual care or Small change approach. The intervention is two years with a one-year follow-up (Ross, Hill, Latimer, & Day, 2016).

In some people, the reality may be to prevent more weight gain rather than weight loss. Although not as glamorous as weight loss, this could be very helpful for millions.

Antioxidants for preventing and reducing muscle soreness after exercise: a Cochrane systematic review.

To determine whether antioxidant supplements and antioxidant-enriched foods can prevent or reduce delayed-onset muscle soreness after exercise.

Results

In total, 50 studies were included in this review which included a total of 1089 participants (961 were male and 128 were female) with an age range of 16-55 years. All studies used an antioxidant dosage higher than the recommended daily amount. The majority of trials (47) had design features that carried a high risk of bias due to selective reporting and poorly described allocation concealment, potentially limiting the reliability of their findings.

Conclusions

There is moderate to low-quality evidence that high-dose antioxidant supplementation does not result in a clinically relevant reduction of muscle soreness after exercise of up to 6 hours or at 24, 48, 72 and 96 hours after exercise. There is no evidence available on subjective recovery and only limited evidence on the adverse effects of taking antioxidant supplements (Ranchordas, Rogerson, Soltani, & Costello, 2018).

Cross-sectional relationships of exercise and age to adiposity in 60,617 male runners.

To assess in men whether exercise affects the estimated age-related increase in adiposity, and whether age affects the estimated exercise-related decrease in adiposity.

Methods:

Cross-sectional analyses of 64,911 male runners who provided data on their body mass index (97.6%) and waist circumference (91.1%).

Results:

Between 18 and 55 yr old, the decline in BMI with weekly distance run was significantly greater in men 25-55 yr old than in younger men. Declines in waist circumference with distance were also significantly greater in older than younger men. Increases in BMI with age were greater for men who ran under 16 km/wk than for relatively longer distance runners. Waist circumference increased with age at all running distances, but the increase diminished by running further.

Conclusion:

These data suggest that age and vigorous exercise interact with each other in affecting men's adiposity and are consistent with the proposition that vigorous physical activity must increase with age to prevent middle-age weight gain (Williams & Pate, Cross-sectional relationships of exercise and age to adiposity in 60,617 male runners., 2005).

Discrepancy between self-reported and actual caloric intake and exercise in obese subjects.

Some obese subjects repeatedly fail to lose weight even though they report restricting their caloric intake to less than 1200 kcal per day. We studied two explanations for this apparent resistance to diet—low calorie burning (physical activity) and underreporting of caloric intake--in 224 consecutive obese subjects. Group 1 consisted of nine women and one man in whom we measured indirect calorimetry and analysis of body composition for 14 days. Group 2, subgroups served as controls consisted of 67 women and 13 men with no history of diet resistance.

Results:

Total energy expenditure and resting metabolic rate with diet resistance (group 1) were within 5 percent of the predicted values for body composition, and there was no significant difference between groups 1 and 2 in the ability to burn calories and exercise. In contrast, **the subjects in group 1 underreported their actual food intake by an average (+/-SD) of 47 +/- 16 percent and overreported their physical activity by 51 +/- 75 percent.** Although the subjects in group 1 had no distinct psychopathologic characteristics, they perceived a genetic cause for their obesity, used thyroid medication at a high frequency, and described their eating behavior as relatively normal (Lichtman, et al, 1992)

Over the last three years I have noticed how patients absolutely abhor physical activity and exercise. Many people do not grow up with exercise playing a part of their lives and now it's like learning a foreign language. Age does not matter either, I could be talking to a first-year college student or a 45-year-old bank executive. I tell people that walking is the best physical activity and is essential for any quality of life. When people stop walking, they turn to rust and become sarcopenic. Sarcopenia is probably the biggest reason for falls as we age. It is a synonym for frailty or adult failure to thrive. It is defined as having decreased upper extremity muscle mass that is two or more standard deviations below a healthy adult 18-40-year-old along a low walking speed below 1.8 mph in a 4-minute walking test. Normal walking speed is 3.1 mph. A tortoise does not beat the rabbit if he falls all the time. Many people will self-motivate themselves when they start seeing weight loss and that is the best part of my day.

Chapter 31: I'm too weak or old to exercise

"I usually take a two-hour nap from one to four"
Yogi Berra

Exercise is a challenge for everyone but especially for older people with sarcopenia or people with chronic illnesses like obesity and severe arthritis.

Whole-body vibration training in obese subjects: A systematic review

- Lifestyle modifications consisting of diet and exercise has mostly been an unsuccessful strategy for treating obesity and sarcopenic obesity.
- In the last two decades, whole-body vibration training (WBVT) has emerged as an alternative exercise modality for strength training.
- WBVT improved body composition, muscle strength and cardiovascular function in various populations, including obese individuals. Sinusoidal vibrations stimulate the primary endings of the muscle spindles, which in turn activate α-motor neurons and induce rapid eccentric-concentric involuntary contractions; this mechanism is known as tonic vibration reflex.
- This systematic review aimed at defining the outcomes of WBVT on obese individuals.
- The sample size of obese participants ranged from n = 7 to n = 40 (mean age range: 20 to 59 years). A total of 321 subjects were involved. We included 18 papers published

2010–2017 from Medline, Scopus, Web of Science, PEDro and Scielo until July 2018. Sixteen out of 18 papers focused on obese women.

- WBVT mainly consisted in a series of exercises performed on the platform, namely squats (at different degrees of knee flexion) and calf-raises. Interventions consisted of three sessions/week lasting 6 to 12 weeks in 13/18 studies. Vibration frequency was mostly between 25 and 40 Hz, with a peak-to-peak displacement (amplitude) of 1–2 mm. Exercises bouts lasted 30 to 60 seconds, with a work/rest ratio from 1:1 to 1:2.

- Vibration therapy is standardized for prolonged occupational exposure but not for physical therapy. Daily exposure was "unsafe" in 7/18 studies according to American National Standards Institute (looks at industrial vibration safety issues).

- 10 weeks of WBVT produced significant weight/fat mass reduction, leg strength improvements, and enhanced glucose regulation when added to hypocaloric diet.

Summary of evidence

- Participants' body weight, BMI, fat mass, arterial stiffness decreased in the majority of studies with an increase in hip/lumbar spine bone mineral density. Fluid movement produced by vibration is anabolic to bone.

- Exercise helps decrease blood pressure. Remember decreasing systolic and diastolic BP by 5–10 mmHg corresponds to 30–40% reduction in the risk of death due to stroke and other cardiovascular complications.

- Leg muscle strength improved following 6 to 12 weeks of WBVT in untrained pre- and post- menopausal obese women by 8% to 18% and even up to 40%.

- No study revealed muscle mass loss. Conversely, an increase of lean mass and reduction in LDL and triglycerides was observed by Miyaki et al.

- Yang et al. found an enhanced dynamic stability in terms of a larger decline in fall rate in WBVT (-45%) than in the placebo group (-25%).

- Six to twelve weeks of WBVT in obese individuals generally led to a reduction in fat mass and cardiovascular improvements.
- Clearly, the reaction to vibration is not only biomechanical as WBVT elicits the combined response of the musculoskeletal, cardiovascular, endocrine and nervous systems.
- Three factors may contribute to fat mass reduction: (i) the acute exposure to vibration activates the central sympathetic nervous system, whose innervation of white adipose tissue triggers lipolysis;(ii) WBVT enhances glycemic control by improving insulin action and glucose regulation; (iii) WBVT promotes GH release, which stimulates metabolism and is usually reduced in obese subjects.
- Bellia et al. found a 35% increase of insulin sensitivity following 8 weeks of WBVT with static squats; additional effects on metabolic regulation were an increase of adiponectin and a decrease of leptin levels.
- In patients with type-2 Diabetes Mellitus, insulin-mediated glucose uptake in the skeletal muscle improved, probably due to increase in femoral artery blood flow.
- The mechanical oscillatory contractions during vibration serve as an active muscle pump and increase stroke volume, probably enhancing venous return and preload.
- Total peripheral resistance to blood flow increases during body vibration. As a compensation, more capillaries are opened to keep a necessary level of cardiac output.
- Improved leg muscle blood flow can contribute to muscle mass increase in older adults. This positively affects balance control.
- Results by Vissers et al., showed that patients treated with WBVT succeeded in maintaining a weight loss of 10% at 12 months
- WBVT stimulates reflexive muscle contractions "in a safe and gentle manner.
- Six papers explicitly reported no unfavourable symptoms or adverse effects resulting from the vibration stimulus

Isolated cases of lower leg phlebitis, mild knee pain and back pain after two weeks of training were reported.

- Muir et al. proposed that vibrations can be considered reasonably safe on a basis of 15 minutes of exposure/day if enclosed within the boundaries of 30–50 Hz and 2.25–7.98 g (intensity of vibration).

Conclusion

- Whole-body vibration training is a promising adjuvant intervention therapy for obese women.
- WBVT could be a useful mode of exercise for deconditioned obese people with poor motivation: when combined with dietary intervention or prescribed as alternative to traditional exercise training, WBVT is as effective as aerobic and resistance exercise in reducing fat mass and moderating the deficit of the relative muscle strength. Lastly, WBVT may be effective in vascular health promotion and prevention in young obese women (Zago, Capodaglio, Ferrario, Tarabini, & Galli, 2018).

Light Intensity Physical Activity and Sedentary Behavior in Relation to Body Mass Index and Grip Strength in Older Adults: Cross-Sectional Findings from the Lifestyle Interventions and Independence for Elders (Life) Study.

- Light intensity activities, such as walking or light housework, contribute to energy expenditure and may therefore contribute to lowering fat mass levels by improving energy balance to energy expenditure.
- 1,635 participants with 67% women aged 70-89 years old with heightened risk of mobility/disability yet able to walk 400 meters in 15 minutes without sitting, leaning or assistance from a walker or another person wore an accelerometer for seven consecutive days to assess energy expenditure.

The study showed that greater time spent in light intensity activity and lower sedentary times (for example watching TV) were associated with lower BMI (Bann, et al., 2013).

Chapter 31: I'm too weak or old to exercise

Short-term water-based aerobic training promotes improvements in aerobic conditioning parameters of mature women.

- Aging is accompanied by a decrease in aerobic capacity. Therefore, physical training has been recommended to soften the effects of advancement age.
- The aim of this study was to assess the effects of a short-term water-based aerobic training of mature women. Twenty-two women (65.91) were submitted to a five-week water-based interval aerobic training.
- It is concluded that a water-based aerobic interval training only five weeks is able to promote improvements in aerobic capacity of mature women (Costa, et al., 2017).

Physical exercise as a preventive or disease-modifying treatment of dementia and brain aging

A rapidly growing literature strongly suggests that exercise, specifically aerobic exercise, may attenuate cognitive impairment and reduce dementia risk. The idea of neuroplasticity is an evolving concept that has important implications in disease prevention and treatment. Meta-analysis and randomized controlled trials have shown the following:
1. Significantly reduced risk of dementia associated with midlife exercise.
2. Midlife exercise significantly reduced later risks of mild cognitive impairment.
3. Among patients with dementia or mild cognitive impairment 6-12 months of exercise documented better cognitive scores compared with sedentary controls.
4. Aerobic exercise in healthy adults were associated with significantly improved cognitive scores.
5. One year of aerobic exercise in seniors was associated with significantly larger hippocampal volumes and better spatial memory.

6. Physically fit seniors had significantly larger hippocampal or gray matter volumes compared with unfit seniors.

7. Brain cognitive networks studied using functional magnetic resonance imaging display improved connectivity after 6 to 12 months of exercise.

Besides a brain neuroprotective effect, physical exercise may also attenuate cognitive decline via mitigation of cerebrovascular risk, including the contribution of small vessel disease to dementia. Exercise should not be overlooked as an important therapeutic strategy (Ahlskog, Geda, Graff-Radford, & Petersen, 2011).

Exercise Training and Nutritional Supplementation for Physical Frailty in Very Elderly People.

Randomized, placebo-controlled trial comparing progressive resistance exercise training, multi-nutrient supplementation, both interventions and neither interventions in 100 frail nursing home residents with an average age of 87 years old (range72 to 98) over a 10-week period.

Muscle strength increased 113%, gait velocity increased by 11.8%, stair-climbing power by 28.4% compared to less than 5% increase or decline in non-exercisers.

In contrast, multi-nutrient supplementation alone without exercise was not helpful. Several studies have shown acquisition of maximal strength, even in patients of advanced age and those with chronic disease the superiority of high-intensity, dynamic resistance training for them. The aging musculoskeletal system retains its responsiveness to progressive resistance training, and most important, the correction of disuse is accompanied by significant improvement in the levels of functional mobility and overall activity (Fiatarone, et al., 1994).

The acute effect of maximal exercise on plasma beta-endorphin levels in fibromyalgia patients.

Chapter 31: I'm too weak or old to exercise

This study aimed to investigate the effect of strenuous exercise on β-endorphin (β-END) level in fibromyalgia (FM) patients compared to healthy subjects.
 30 FM patients and 15 healthy individuals. All study participants underwent a treadmill exercise test using modified Bruce protocol (M. Bruce). The goal of the test was achieving at least 70% of the predicted maximal heart rate (HR Max). The serum levels of β-END were measured before and after the exercise program. Measurements were done while heart rate was at least 70% of its predicted maximum.

Results:

The mean of exercise duration in the FM and control groups were 24.26 and 29.06 minutes, respectively, indicating a shorter time to achieve the goal heart rate in FM patients ($P < 0.003$). Compared to healthy subjects, FM patients had lower serum β-END levels both in baseline and post-exercise status (Mean 122.07 μg/ml and 246.55 μg/ml in the control group versus 90.12 μg/ml and 179.80 μg/ml in FM patients, respectively; $P < 0.001$).

Conclusions:

We found that fibromyalgia patients had lower levels of β-END in both basal and post-exercise status. Exercise increased serum β-END levels in both groups but the average increase in β-END in fibromyalgia patients was significantly lower than in the control group. Fibromyalgia patients have a blunted surge response of beta-endorphins to exercise. This lower opioid tone (beta-endorphins are naturally-occurring opioids) may be a key factor in the development of chronic allodynia (triggering of a pain response from stimuli which does not normally provoke pain) and the increased sensitization to peripheral stimuli seen in fibromyalgia patients (Bidari, Ghavidel-Parsa, Rajabi, Sanaei, & Toutounchi, 2016).

Chapter 32: Obesity Paradox

"No one goes there nowadays, it's too crowded"
Yogi Berra

The obesity paradox is the concept that obesity may be protective and associated with greater survival in certain groups of people.

Accuracy of Body Mass Index to Diagnose Obesity in the US Adult Population.

Body mass index (BMI) is the most widely used measure to diagnose obesity. However, the accuracy of BMI in detecting excess body adiposity in the adult general population is largely unknown.

Methods:

A cross-sectional design of 13,601 subjects (age 20-79.9 years; 49% men) from the Third National Health and Nutrition Examination Survey. Bioelectrical impedance analysis was used to estimate body fat percent (BF%). We assessed the diagnostic performance of BMI using the World Health Organization reference standard for obesity of BF%>25% in men and>35% in women. We tested the correlation between BMI and both BF% and lean mass by sex and age groups adjusted for race.

Results:

- BMI-defined obesity (> or =30) was present in 19.1% of men and 24.7% of women

- BF%-defined obesity was present in 43.9% of men and 52.3% of women.

- The diagnostic performance of BMI diminished as age increased.

- In men, BMI had a better correlation with lean mass than with BF%
- In women, BMI correlated better with BF% than with lean mass.
- In the intermediate range of BMI (25-29.9), BMI failed to discriminate between BF% and lean mass in both sexes.

Conclusions:

- The accuracy of BMI in diagnosing obesity is limited, particularly for individuals in the intermediate BMI ranges, in men and in the elderly.
- A BMI cutoff of> or =30 has good specificity but misses more than half of people with excess fat.
- These results may help to explain the unexpected better survival in overweight/mild obese patients (obesity paradox) (Romero-Corral, et al., 2008).

The Obesity Paradox and Heart Failure: A Systematic Review of a Decade of Evidence.

There is scientific consensus that obesity increases the risk of cardiovascular diseases, including heart failure. **However, among persons who already have heart failure, outcomes seem to be better in obese persons as compared with lean persons: this has been termed the obesity paradox, the mechanisms of which remain unclear.**

This study systematically reviewed the evidence of the relationship between heart failure mortality (and survival) and weight status. Search of the PubMed/MEDLINE and EMBASE databases was done. The initial search identified 9879 potentially relevant papers, out of which ten longitudinal studies met the inclusion criteria.

All ten studies reported improved outcomes for obese heart failure patients as compared with their normal weight counterparts; worse prognosis was demonstrated for extreme obesity (B M I > 40 kg/m2). The findings of this review will be of significance in informing the practice of asking obese persons with heart failure to lose weight. (Oga & Eseyin, 2016).

Prognostic value of body mass index and body surface area on clinical outcomes after transcatheter aortic valve implantation.

- Inverse associations between Body Mass Index (BMI) and Body Surface Area (BSA) with mortality in patients after Transcatheter Aortic Valve Implantation (TAVI) have been reported.
- This "obesity paradox" is controversial, and it remains unclear which parameter, BMI or BSA, is of greater prognostic value.
- The aim of this study was to investigate the association of BMI and BSA on 30 day and 1-year mortality using Society of Thoracic Surgeons (STS) risk factors after TAVI.

Methods

- This prospective, observational study consisted of 917 consecutive patients undergoing TAVI at our center from 2011 to 2014.
- The median age of the patients was 82.6 years, with a mean STS Predicted Risk of Mortality (STS-PROM) of 6.6% ± 4.3.
- Throughout the study period (mean follow-up time was 297 days), 150 (16.4 %) patients died; 72 (7.9 %) patients died within 30 days of TAVI.
- After risk adjustment, the association between body constitution and 30-day mortality was not significant for either measure.
- BMI but not BSA, was significantly associated with 1-year survival.
- There was no association between stroke, vascular complications, or length of stay with BMI or BSA.

Conclusion

BMI was associated with survival at 1-year after TAVI. Despite the trend towards implementing BSA in risk score calculation, BMI may be more suitable for the assessment of TAVI patients (Arsalan, et al., 2016).

Prognostic value of body mass index in transcatheter aortic valve implantation: A "J"-shaped curve

- Obesity in patients with established cardiovascular disease has previously been identified as an indicator of good prognosis, a phenomenon known as the "obesity paradox." The prognostic significance of BMI in patients with severe aortic stenosis (AoS) undergoing TAVI is a matter of current debate, as published studies are scarce and their results conflicting.

- This is an observational, retrospective study involving 770 patients who underwent TAVI for AoS. The cohort was divided into three groups based on their BMI: normal weight ($\geq$18.5 to <25kg/m^2), overweight ($\geq$25 to <30kg/m^2) and obese ($\geq$30kg/m^2).
- The predictive effect of BMI on all-cause mortality 3 years following TAVI intervention was analyzed using a Cox regression.

Results:
155 patients died during follow-up.
The overweight group (n=302, 38.97%), experienced a lower mortality rate compared to the normal weight and obese groups (15.9% vs 25.7% and 21.0%, respectively).
Conclusion:
BMI is a predictive factor of all-cause mortality in AoS patients undergoing TAVI. This relationship takes the form of a "J-shaped" curve in which overweight patients are associated with the lowest mortality rate at follow-up (González-Ferreiro, et al., 2016).

The obesity paradox in patients undergoing transcatheter aortic valve implantation: is there any effect of body mass index on survival?
- A total of 148 consecutive patients undergoing TAVI were compared in regard to all-cause mortality at 30-day and 12 months.
Results:
- Obesity was diagnosed in 37 (25.2%) patients, 73 (49.7%) patients were overweight, and 37 (25.2%) had normal weight. Prevalence of lower frailty as assessed by five-metre

walk test was confirmed in obese patients as compared to other groups.

- There was no difference between the groups in terms of 30-day all-cause mortality (p = 0.15).
- 12-month all-cause mortality was lowest in obese patients.
- Increase in BMI was independently associated with lower all-cause mortality after TAVI (Tokarek, et al., 2019)

"Obesity paradox" in transcatheter aortic valve implantation

- To determine whether body mass index (BMI) is associated with mortality in transcatheter aortic valve implantation (TAVI).
- MEDLINE and EMBASE were searched through September 2015 using PubMed and OVID.
- Our search identified 11 eligible studies including 10,196 patients undergoing TAVI.
  Conclusion:
  Overweight or obesity may be associated with better 30-day survival but this "obesity paradox" may not extend that survival benefit past 6 months., (Takagi & Umemoto, 2017).

One explanation for the better statistics for overweight patients compared to others is the idea that being overweight in the elderly population is usually considered a sign of relatively good health and losing weight in this group is usually not recommended unless many comorbidities exist. Any person with a very shortened lifespan should not lose weight. Due to the higher metabolic demands and comorbidities usually noted in patients with severe aortic stenosis, a person that can maintain excess weight under this stressed environment may have a survival advantage. The survival advantage is more short-term then long-term. Essentially the person is running a race all the time and passing a stress test daily.

Chapter 33: Liposuction

Invasive and non-invasive surgical procedures to remove unwanted fat are becoming more common. Does liposuction help with metabolic disorders such as diabetes, insulin resistance, hypertension and hyperlipidemia? Here are a few articles.

Absence of an effect of liposuction on insulin action and risk factors for coronary heart disease.

Liposuction has been proposed as a potential treatment for the metabolic complications of obesity.

Methods:

We evaluated the insulin sensitivity of liver, skeletal muscle, and adipose tissue as well as levels of inflammatory mediators and other risk factors for coronary heart disease in 15 obese women before and 10 to 12 weeks after abdominal liposuction.

Results:

- Those with normal oral glucose tolerance lost 9.1 kg of fat
- Those with type 2 diabetes lost 10.5+ kg of fat

Liposuction

- Did not significantly alter the insulin sensitivity of muscle, liver, or adipose tissue
- Did not significantly alter plasma concentrations of C-reactive protein, interleukin-6, tumor necrosis factor alpha, and adiponectin.
- Did not significantly affect other risk factors for coronary heart disease (blood pressure and plasma glucose, insulin, and lipid concentrations) in either group.

Conclusions:

Abdominal liposuction does not significantly improve obesity-associated metabolic abnormalities.

Decreasing adipose tissue mass alone will not achieve the metabolic benefits of weight loss (Klein, et al., 2004).

Large-volume liposuction and prevention of type 2 diabetes: a preliminary report.

- The study enrolled 31 patients with a body mass index (BMI) exceeding 30 over a 1-year period. 16 of the 30 patients returned for a follow-up visit 3 to 12 months postoperatively.
- The average aspirate was 8,455 ml without dermolipectomy (tummy tuck) and 5,795 ml with dermolipectomy.
- The average blood sugar level dropped 18% and the average weight loss was 9.2%. The average drop in BMI was 6.2%, and HbA1C showed a decrease of 2.3%.
- The patients with the best weight loss had the best reduction in blood sugar level and blood pressure. One dehiscence, two wound infections, and three seromas were reported.
- Liposuction alone did not improve obesity but helped to motivate some of the patients to lose weight. These patients had the best results.
- **Liposuction may provide the stimulus to improve overall health** (Nareste, Nareste, Buckspan, & Ersek, 2012).

Cryolipolysis for Fat Reduction and Body Contouring: Safety and Efficacy of Current Treatment Paradigms

- Data from the American Society for Aesthetic Plastic Surgery indicate that liposuction replaced breast augmentation as the most popular surgical procedure in 2013.
- Clinical studies have reported a 21.7 percent incidence of minor complications as well as a 0.38 percent incidence of major complications.
- Liposuction remains an invasive procedure and carries the inherent risks associated with surgery.
- Cryolipolysis is one of the most recent forms of noninvasive fat reduction to emerge. **The concept that**

lipid-rich tissues are more susceptible to cold injury than the surrounding water-rich tissue. **Cryolipolysis, introduced in 2007, is performed by applying an applicator to the targeted area set at a specific cooling temperature for a preset period of time.** This targets adipocytes while sparing the skin, nerves, vessels, and muscles.

- Initial preclinical and clinical studies have demonstrated the efficacy of cryolipolysis for subcutaneous fat layer reduction.

- **Studies have suggested that the addition of posttreatment manual massage may enhance the effectiveness of a single cryolipolysis treatment, and that multiple treatments may lead to further improvement.**

- A systematic review of the MEDLINE and Cochrane databases yielded a final number of 19 articles.

- Common treatment areas included the abdomen, brassiere rolls, lumbar rolls, hip rolls/flanks, inner thighs, medial knee, peritrochanteric areas, arms, and ankles.

- Common complications noted after cryolipolysis included erythema, bruising, swelling, sensitivity, and pain. These side effects are generally resolved within a few weeks after treatment. No persistent ulcerations, scarring, paresthesias, hematomas, blistering, bleeding, hyperpigmentation or hypopigmentation, or infections have been described.

- With more than 450,000 procedures performed thus far, cryolipolysis is becoming one of the most popular alternatives to liposuction for spot reduction of adipose tissue.

- It is believed that vacuum suction with regulated heat extraction impedes blood flow and induces crystallization of the targeted adipose tissue when cryolipolysis is performed. The temperatures induced in cryolipolysis have no permanent effect on the overlying dermis and epidermis.

- **Ultimately, crystallization and cold ischemic injury of the targeted adipocytes induce apoptosis of these cells and a pronounced inflammatory response, resulting in their eventual removal from the treatment site within** the following several weeks. Histological studies show that within 3 months, macrophages are mostly responsible for clearing the damaged cells and debris.

- Multiple studies have demonstrated that cholesterol, triglycerides, low-density lipoprotein, high-density lipoprotein, aspartate transaminase/alanine transaminase, total bilirubin, albumin, and glucose remained within normal limits during and after cryolipolysis.

- **Contraindications to cryolipolysis include cold-induced conditions such as cryoglobulinemia, cold urticaria, and paroxysmal cold hemoglobinuria. Cryolipolysis should not be performed in treatment areas with severe varicose veins, dermatitis, or other cutaneous lesions.**

- A second successive course of cryolipolysis treatment can lead to further fat reduction, although the extent of improvement was not as dramatic as the first treatment. **The optimal temperature is 4°C.**

- **One hypothesis for potentially improved efficacy with manual massage is that manual massage caused an additional mechanism of damage to the targeted adipose tissue immediately after treatment, perhaps from tissue-reperfusion injury.**

- **A nerve biopsy taken at 3 months after treatment showed no long-term changes to nerve fibers, concluding that temperature and duration of cryolipolysis have no permanent effect on nervous tissue.**

- Rare side effects include vasovagal reaction and paradoxical adipose hyperplasia. Jalian et al. estimated an incidence of 0.0051 percent, or approximately one in 20,000, for paradoxical adipose hyperplasia (Ingargiola, Motakef, Chung, Vasconez, & Sasaki, 2015).

Chapter 34: Inflammation, Inflammaging and Microbiome Dysbiosis

Chronic, low-grade inflammation is recognized as a major characteristic of aging. This phenomenon is so pervasive that the term inflammaging has been coined to emphasize that many major age-related disabilities, including cancers, susceptibility to infections, and dementia have immunopathogenic components. Inflammaging appears to be much more complex than previously thought, and a variety of tissues and organs participate in producing inflammatory stimuli. The list is extensive and includes the immune system, but also adipose tissue, skeletal muscle, liver, and the gut. The gut is of unique importance, because it is the body's largest immune organ and contains trillions of bacteria that can release inflammatory stimuli into the portal and systemic circulation. Two reviews provide excellent summaries:

Gut microbiome and metabolic syndrome

The human intestine contains approximately 100 trillion microorganisms comprising up to 1,000 different species of bacteria, yeasts, and parasites, weighting approximately 2 kg and carrying at least 100 times as many genes as the whole human genome. This microbiological population renews itself every 3 days and has an active biomass similar to that of a major human organ. It is estimated that around 20-25% of the world's population has metabolic syndrome, and people with the condition are twice as likely to die from and three times as likely to have a heart attack or stroke compared with people without the syndrome. It has been proposed that the gut microbiota is an important environmental factor involved in the regulation of body weight and energy homeostasis. **One hypothesis is obese and lean individuals have distinct different microbiota with measurable differences in their ability to extract energy from their diet and to store it in fat tissue. Microbiota alteration by using pro- and prebiotic dietary supplements is a potential nutritional target in the management of obesity and obesity-related disorders**. A probiotic is described typically as a bacterial supplement consisting of Lactobacillus acidophilus, Lactobacillus casei, and bifidobacteria. Prebiotics are non-digestible fiber compounds that pass undigested through the upper part of the gastrointestinal tract and stimulate the growth and/or activity of gut microbiota that colonizes the large intestine by feeding them. **There is increasing evidence that the gut microbiota plays a significant role in glucose homeostasis, the development of impaired fasting glucose, type 2 diabetes, and insulin resistance.** According to the International Diabetes Federation's estimates, about 382 million people around the world had diabetes in 2013, and this figure was expected to increase by 55% to 592 million by 2035. It is recognized that the anti-inflammatory function of probiotics assists in treating low grade inflammation. It has been shown that modification of intestinal microbiota by probiotics may have a role in the maintenance of a healthier gut microbiota and could be a potential adjuvant in the treatment of insulin resistance and type 2 diabetes. Because of the positive findings in animal trials of probiotics for controlling fasting glucose and insulin resistance, there has been increasing interest in human studies. Several studies suggest that oral probiotics have useful effects on total cholesterol and LDL cholesterol for subjects with high, borderline, and normal cholesterol levels. Roux-en-Y gastric bypass has been shown to significantly change the gut microbiota and Lactobacilli given to morbidly obese patients having Roux-en-Y gastric bypass had significantly greater weight loss and increased B12 levels. Many vitamins are created by colonic bacteria (Mazidi, Rezaie, Kengne, Mobarhan, & Ferns, 2016).

Chapter 34: Inflammation, Inflammaging and Microbiome Dysbiosis

Gut Dysbiosis and Muscle Aging: Searching for Novel Targets against Sarcopenia

- A growing body of evidence suggests that the innumerable microorganisms that populate the mammalian gastrointestinal tract (gut microbiota) are tightly linked to the aging process of their host.

- The human gut microbiota exists in a symbiotic and commensal relationship with 10–100 trillion microbial cells, mostly bacteria but also yeast, virus/phages, fungi, archaea (single-celled microorganisms different from bacteria) microeukaryotes, protozoa, helminths (worms), and parasites.

- The gut represents the largest contributor to the human microbiota. **The human gastrointestinal tract harbors about 10^{14} bacterial cells, which is ten times the number of human cells in the body. Despite a high degree of interindividual variability in gut microbiota composition, there is a remarkable similarity in the basal gene metabolic activities across individuals.**

- Gut microbiota is involved in the production of micronutrients, such as essential vitamins and cofactors; regulation of the immune system; transformation of xenobiotics; breakdown of complex lipids, proteins, and polysaccharides into metabolite intermediates [e.g., short-chain fatty acids (SCFA)]; and waste product detoxification and finally represents a barrier against the spread of pathogens.

- Contributing to bile acid metabolism and recirculation; absorption of calcium, magnesium, and iron; regulation of fat storage; and activation of bioactive compounds.

- As the largest endocrine organ, the gut releases hormones by means of enteroendocrine cells. Besides its barrier-like role that protects the host from pathogen colonization, the intestinal microbiota also participates in the development and homeostasis of the host immune system.

- **70% of the body immune cells reside in the gut-associated lymphoid tissue.** The interaction between gastrointestinal cells and commensal bacteria fosters

309

immunological tolerance or inflammatory responses to pathogens by regulating immune homeostasis in the gut. This crosstalk between microbiota and gut mucosal cells modulates the production of various cytokines and chemokines. These can be proinflammatory or anti-inflammatory.

- Most gut microbial changes observed during aging are attributable to diet composition. Furthermore, reduced intestinal motility unfavorably affect gut fermentative processes in advanced age.
- Dysbiosis has also been related to obesity, inflammatory bowel disease, type 1 and type 2 diabetes, and nonalcoholic steatohepatitis.
- Diet is indicated as the main culprit responsible for metabolic diseases linked to gut dysbiosis.
- The administration of pre- and probiotics has been recommended to mitigate some of the age-related alterations in the intestinal microbiota associated with several gastrointestinal and respiratory diseases.
- Probiotics defined as "live microorganisms" confer a health benefit on the host" exert their beneficial effects on the host by improving gut barrier function, immunomodulation, and production of neurotransmitters.
- The downside of probiotic usage includes the potential risk of inducing gastrointestinal side effects, an unfavorable metabolic profile, excessive immune stimulation, and systemic infections in susceptible individuals.
- Fermented nondigestible compounds, referred to as prebiotics, favor the proliferation of health-promoting bacteria that may positively affect muscle health. These findings suggest that *Lactobacillus* and *Bifidobacterium* may influence gut-muscle communication and regulate muscle size.
- The administration of symbiotic, comprising the probiotic *Bifidobacterium longum* and an inulin-based prebiotic component, has also been demonstrated to have an effect on the age-related changes in the intestinal microbiota.

- Pre- and/or probiotic supplementation may prevent age-related muscle loss by increasing the abundance of *Bifidobacterium* and butyrate producers in old individuals.

- Gut microbiota plays a crucial role in maintaining the balance of pro- and anti-inflammatory responses. Aged gut microbiota may elicit an inflammatory response and display lower capability of counteracting adverse microbes or removing their metabolites.

- Age-related differences in the gut microbiota composition have been suggested to relate to the progression of diseases and frailty in old age.

- *Faecalibacterium prausnitzii, represents more than 5% of bacteria in intestine,* exhibits a positive role in muscle function.

- Prebiotic supplementation (inulin plus fructooligosaccharides) has been shown to increase muscle strength and endurance in frail older adults, thereby highlighting the potential of prebiotic supplementation as a treatment for age-associated deficits in muscle function (Picca, et al., 2018).

The contributory role of gut microbiota in cardiovascular disease.

The human gut harbors more than 100 trillion microbial cells, far outnumbering the human host cells of the body. We are the minority shareholders in our body. Homo sapiens DNA is estimated to represent less than 10% of the total DNA within our bodies, due to the staggeringly large numbers of microbes that reside in and on us, primarily within our gut. The major taxa present in gut microbiota consist primarily of 2 major bacterial phyla, Firmicutes and Bacteroidetes, whose proportions appear to remain remarkably stable over time within individuals and their family members. However, the composition of the remaining gut microbiota is remarkably diverse and dynamic, with both acute and chronic dietary exposures significantly affecting the overall microbial community. **There has been a long-standing understanding of the contribution of dysbiosis (abnormal changes in**

intestinal microbiota composition) to the pathogenesis of some diseases of altered intestinal health. Gut microbial communities differ in vegetarians and vegans compared with omnivores. Gut microbiota act as a filter for our largest environmental exposure-what we eat. Technically speaking, food is a foreign object that we take into our bodies in kilogram quantities every day. The microbial community within each of us significantly influences how we experience a meal. Differences in gut microbiota composition are associated with the development of complex metabolic disorders such as obesity and insulin resistance. Several studies have shown that 3 metabolites of dietary phosphatidylcholine that gut microbiota interact with may be linked to cardiovascular disease in humans. The three are choline, betaine, and TMAO (trimethylamine-N-oxide) with TMAO being the main culprit. In a study of over 4,000 subjects undergoing elective cardiac angiography, elevated TMAO levels predicted major adverse cardiac events such as death, myocardial infarction, and stroke over a 3-year period. Patients in the upper quartile for TMAO levels (compared with the lowest quartile) had a significant 2.5-fold increased risk of experiencing a major adverse cardiac event (MI, stroke, or death), independent of traditional cardiovascular risk factors, renal function, and medication use, as well as overall poorer event-free survival (Tang & Hazen, 2014).

The Effects of Vegetarian and Vegan Diets on Gut Microbiota.

- The difference in gut microbiota composition between individuals following vegan or vegetarian diets and those following omnivorous diets is well documented. A plant-based diet appears to be beneficial for human health by promoting the development of more diverse and stable microbial systems (Tomova, et al., 2019).

Chapter 35: Vagus Nerve & VBloc

"Pacemakers for everyone. I want to invent one to prevent procrastination".

Mechanistic relationship between the vagal afferent pathway, central nervous system and peripheral organs in appetite regulation.

The hypothalamus is the center of food intake and energy metabolism regulation. Information signals from peripheral organs are mediated through the circulation or the vagal afferent pathway and input into the hypothalamus, where signals are integrated to determine various behaviors, such as eating. Numerous appetite-regulating peptides are expressed in the central nervous system and the peripheral organs, and interact in a complex manner. Of such peptides, gut peptides are known to bind to receptors at the vagal afferent pathway that extend into the mucosal layer of the digestive tract, modulate the electrical activity of the vagus nerve, and subsequently send signals to the solitary nucleus and furthermore to the hypothalamus.

All peripheral peptides other than ghrelin suppress appetite, and they synergistically suppress appetite through the vagus nerve. In contrast, the appetite-enhancing peptide, ghrelin, antagonizes the actions of appetite-suppressing peptides through the vagus nerve, and appetite-suppressing peptides have attenuated effects in obesity as a result of inflammation in the vagus nerve. Implantable devices that electrically stimulate the vagus nerve are being investigated as novel treatments for obesity in basic and clinical studies (Ueno & Nakazato, 2016).

Effect of Vagal Nerve Blockade on Moderate Obesity with an Obesity-Related Comorbid Condition: The ReCharge Study.

Vagal nerve blockade (vBloc) therapy was shown to be a safe and effective treatment for moderate to severe obesity. This report summarizes the safety and efficacy of vBloc therapy in the prespecified subgroup of patients with moderate obesity.
Methods:
The ReCharge Trial is a double-blind, randomized controlled clinical trial of participants with body mass index (BMI) of 40–45 or 35–40 kg/m2 with at least one obesity-related comorbid condition. Participants were randomized 2:1 to implantation with either a vBloc or sham device with weight management counseling. Eighty-four subjects had moderate obesity (BMI 35–40 kg/m2) at randomization.
Results:
- Fifty-three participants were randomized to vBloc and 31 to sham. Qualifying obesity-related comorbidities included dyslipidemia (73 %), hypertension (58 %), sleep apnea (33 %), and type 2 diabetes (8 %).
- The vBloc group achieved a significant percentage excess weight loss of 33 % compared to 19 % with sham at 12 months.
- Common adverse events of vBloc through 12 months were heartburn/dyspepsia and implant site pain; the majority of events were reported as mild or moderate.
Conclusions:
vBloc therapy resulted in significantly greater weight loss than the sham control among participants with moderate obesity and comorbidities with a well-tolerated safety profile (Morton, et al., 2016).

Two-Year Outcomes of Vagal Nerve Blocking (vBloc) for the Treatment of Obesity in the ReCharge Trial.

The ReCharge Trial demonstrated that a vagal blocking device (vBloc) is a safe and effective treatment for moderate to severe obesity. This report summarizes 24-month outcomes (n = 103).

Methods:

After 12 months, participants randomized to vBloc continued open-label vBloc therapy. Weight loss, adverse events, comorbid risk factors, and quality of life (QOL) will be assessed for 5 years.

Results:

- At 24 months, 123 (76 %) vBloc participants remained in the trial. Participants who presented at 24 months (n = 103) had a mean excess weight loss (EWL) of 21 %
- 58 % of participants had ≥5 % total weight loss and 34 % had ≥10 % total weight loss.
- Significant improvements were observed in mean LDL (-16 mg/dL) and HDL cholesterol (+4 mg/dL), triglycerides (-46 mg/dL), HbA1c (-0.3 %), and systolic (-11 mmHg) and diastolic blood pressures (-10 mmHg).
- QOL measures were significantly improved.
- Heartburn/dyspepsia and implant site pain were the most frequently reported adverse events.
- Serious adverse event rate was 4.3 %.

Conclusions:

vBloc therapy continues to result in medically meaningful weight loss with a favorable safety profile through 2 years (Apovian, et al., 2017).

Chapter 36: Bariatric Surgery Descriptions

Bariatric surgery resulted from many surgical insights over time but notably from the observation that patients lost weight after undergoing partial stomach removal for ulcers. The medical profession also realized that obesity, especially morbid obesity played a devastating role on the people afflicted with it and something needed to be done. The term Bariatric comes from the Greek word "bari or baros" meaning heavy weight, burden or load. It also appeared in ancient Hebrew text indicating "fat "or fleshy". The term Roux-en-Y was named after the pioneering Swiss surgeon, Dr. César Roux who lived from 1857 to 1934. The "Y" is a description of the upper two arm segments that come together to form the fork in the "Y" of gastric bypass surgery. In 1926, Dr Roux performed the first case of a successful removal of a pheochromocytoma in Europe. The same operation was first done about seven months later in the US by Dr. Charles Mayo (member of Mayo Clinic family).

This term "bariatric" dates back to the writings of Drs. Mason and Ito, who initially developed this procedure in the 1960s.

Gastric Plication.
- Gastric plication techniques include endoscopic sleeve gastroplasty, primary obesity surgery endolumenal, transoral gastroplasty, and plication with the Articulating Endoscopic Circular (ACE) stapler.
- Currently, primary obesity surgery endolumenal is under review by the US Food and Drug Administration, and

endoscopic sleeve gastroplasty is gaining acceptance.

Gastric Sleeve Plication

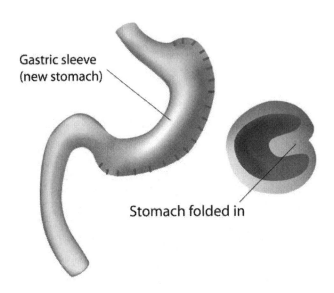

Gastric sleeve (new stomach)

Stomach folded in

(Kumar, 2017)

Laparoscopic gastric plication for the treatment of morbid obesity by using real-time imaging of the stomach pouch.

- Bariatric surgery is a continuously evolving field. Laparoscopic greater curvature plication is a new investigational procedure. The problem is that during gastric plication the exact dimensions and volume of the pouch are not known so frequently it is too large or too tight thus compromising the results. The aim of the study was to identify the parameters that can improve the procedure.

Methods:

- We performed laparoscopic greater curvature plication in 75 obese patients during 2013-2015. The last 25 patients underwent surgery using real-time imaging of the stomach pouch and gastric geometry. With this new

318

approach we obtained the desired volume of
the gastric remnant and we avoided strictures, obstruction
or irregular shape of the pouch, problems that otherwise
could have compromised the outcomes.

Results:

- We found an increased excess weight loss of 55% at six
  month and 65% over a 12-month follow-up period. There
  were no major complications (gastric outlet obstructions or
  leaks) and less minor complications (nausea and vomiting)
  than in the patients operated with
  classic gastric plication procedure.

Conclusion:

- The target population is represented by the obese patients
  who want to obtain similar results to those
  after gastric bypass and sleeve gastrectomy but are
  concerned about removing a part of their stomach.
  Laparoscopic gastric **plication** is a newer minimally
  invasive weight-loss **surgery** technique that reduces the size
  of the stomach capacity to approximately three ounces
  (Borz, et al., 2017).

Bariatric Surgery Procedures

Bariatric surgical procedures cause weight loss by restricting the
amount of food the stomach can hold, causing malabsorption of
nutrients, or by a combination of both gastric restriction and
malabsorption. Bariatric procedures also cause hormonal changes.
Most weight loss surgeries today are laparoscopic
The most common bariatric surgery procedures are gastric bypass,
sleeve gastrectomy, adjustable gastric band, and biliopancreatic
diversion with duodenal switch. Each surgery has its own
advantages and disadvantages.

Roux-en-Y Gastric Bypass – often called gastric bypass – is
considered the 'gold standard' of weight loss surgery. There are 2
components to the procedure. First, a small stomach pouch
approximately one ounce or 30 cc. is created by dividing the top of
the stomach from the rest of the stomach. Next, the first portion
of the small intestine (duodenum) is divided, and the bottom end
of the divided small intestine is brought up and connected to the
newly created small stomach pouch. The procedure is completed

by connecting the top portion of the divided small intestine to the small intestine further down so that the stomach acids and digestive enzymes from the bypassed stomach and first portion of small intestine mix with food.

Roux-en-Y Gastric Bypass

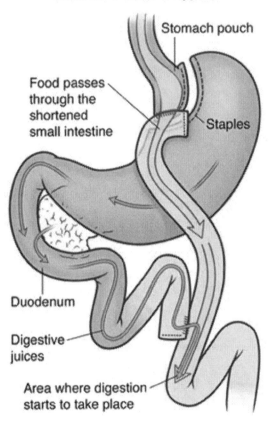

Advantages
- Produces significant long-term weight loss (60 to 80 percent excess weight loss)
- Restricts the amount of food that can be consumed
- Produces favorable changes in gut hormones (esp. ghrelin) that reduce appetite and enhance satiety

Disadvantages
- Is technically a more complex operation than gastric banding or sleeve gastrectomy.
- Can lead to deficits in vitamin B12, iron, calcium, and folate

Sleeve Gastrectomy

The Laparoscopic Sleeve Gastrectomy – often called the sleeve – is performed by removing approximately 80 percent of the stomach. The remaining stomach is a tubular pouch that resembles a banana.

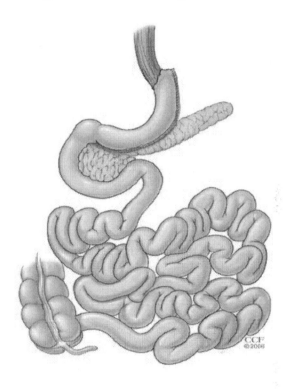

Advantages
- Restricts the amount of food the stomach can hold
- Induces rapid and significant weight loss Weight loss of >50% for 3-5+ year data.
- Requires no foreign objects (i.e. gastric band), and no bypass or re-routing of the food stream (RYGB)
- Causes favorable changes in gut hormones that suppress hunger, reduce appetite and improve satiety

Disadvantages
- Is a non-reversible procedure
- Has the potential for long-term vitamin deficiencies

Adjustable Gastric Band

- The Adjustable Gastric Band – often called *the band* – involves an inflatable band that is placed around the upper portion of the stomach, creating a small stomach pouch above the band, and the rest of the stomach below the band.

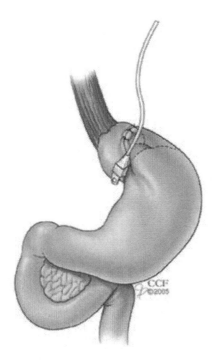

- Reducing the size of the opening is done gradually over time with repeated adjustments or "fills."

Advantages

- Reduces the amount of food the stomach can hold
- Involves no cutting of the stomach or rerouting of the intestines
- Is reversible and adjustable
- Has the lowest rate of early postoperative complications and mortality among the approved bariatric procedures
- Has the lowest risk for vitamin/mineral deficiencies

Disadvantages

- Slower and less early weight loss than other surgical procedures

- Greater percentage of patients failing to lose at least 50 percent of excess body weight compared to the other surgeries
- Requires a foreign device to remain in the body
- Can result in possible band slippage or band erosion into the stomach.
- Can have mechanical problems with the band, tube or port.
- Can result in dilation of the esophagus if the patient overeats
- Highest rate of re-operation

Biliopancreatic Diversion with Duodenal Switch (BPD/DS) Gastric Bypass

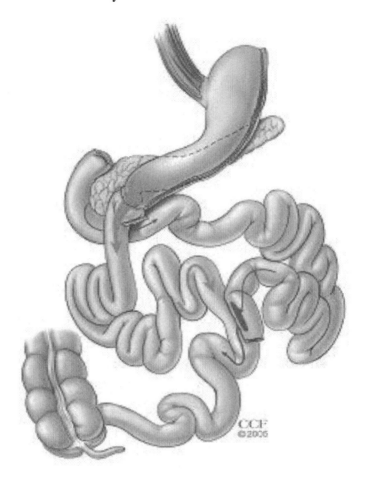

- The is a procedure with two components. First, a smaller tubular stomach pouch is created, very similar to the sleeve gastrectomy. Next, a large portion of the small intestine is bypassed.

The Procedure

- The duodenum, or the first portion of the small intestine, is divided just past the outlet of the stomach. A segment of the distal (last portion) small intestine is then brought up and connected to the outlet of the newly created stomach, so that when the patient eats, the food goes through a newly created tubular stomach pouch and empties directly into the last segment of the small intestine. Roughly three-fourths of the small intestine is bypassed by the food stream.

- The bypassed small intestine, which carries the bile and pancreatic enzymes is reconnected to the last portion of the small intestine so that they can eventually mix with the food stream. There is a significant amount of small bowel that is bypassed by the food stream.
- Additionally, the food does not mix with the bile and pancreatic enzymes until very far down the small intestine. This results in a significant decrease in the absorption of calories and nutrients (particularly protein and fat).

Advantages
- Results in greater weight loss than RYGB, LSG, or AGB.
- Allows patients to eventually eat near "normal" meals
- Reduces the absorption of fat by 70 percent or more
- Causes favorable changes in gut hormones to reduce appetite and improve satiety

Disadvantages
- Has higher complication rates and risk for mortality than the AGB, LSG, and RYGB.
- Has a greater potential to cause protein deficiencies and long-term deficiencies in a number of vitamin and minerals.

Held from 1977-1982, the Bariatric Surgery Colloquium Meetings were some of the first gatherings of bariatric surgeons. The first one was on April 28-29, 1977 and was entitled Gastric Bypass Workshop. Dr. Edward E. Mason, the inventor of the gastric bypass surgery opened up the conference. Some of his comments are;

- "You will notice that we had some rain this morning and this is welcome in Iowa because it makes the corn grow. We feed the corn to the pigs and pigs to people and then we get more gastric bypass candidates."
- "The risk of sudden death begins to show up in people who weigh over 120% of this average population weight. As weight increases the difference in the incidence of sudden death is striking. There is a fourfold increase in risk."
- "When we started doing gastric bypasses in 1966 we were afraid to operate on people that weighed 400 to 500 lbs."
- "They operate by the time-honored principle that God only gave you so many heart beats and if you waste them

doing silly things like exercise you haven't got enough left when it really counts, such as at meal times."

Obesity is a disease that can be fatal. Why the insurance companies will charge extra or not even give insurance to people that are grossly obese and then turn around and refuse to pay for an operation that treats that condition is beyond me. This is not cosmetic surgery. This is a disease. It is potentially lethal.

Chapter 37: Bariatric Surgery

"The Cadillac of weight loss" (baby boomer joke)

Bariatric surgery is the most successful tool for obesity treatment but is reserved for patients that are moderately or severely impacted by obesity and meet selection criteria. Most programs require failure from a medically supervised weight loss program for 6 months first. Bariatric programs have dieticians, behavior therapists, physical therapists, psychological assessments, and very frequent follow-ups to increase the chances of success. **Indications for surgery are a BMI of 40 or greater or a BMI of 35 with co-morbidities.** The FDA has approved gastric banding for a BMI of 30 with co-morbidities. The three most common procedures are gastric banding, Roux-en-Y gastric bypass and Sleeve gastrectomy. All are done laparoscopically and take usually less than 2 hours to complete. Gastric-banding is outpatient surgery and the other two require 1-3 days hospitalization. Gastric-banding was very popular at one time but presently it is done less than 3% of the time. Some programs are starting outpatient sleeve gastrectomy. It is important that bariatric surgeons and obesity specialist physicians work together since bariatric surgery is not 100% successful at weight loss and weight regain is an important issue. Bariatric surgery has a 10-20% primary failure rate (no successful initial weight loss).

Routine bariatric labs are usually B12, calcium, vitamin D, iron studies and are drawn at 3 months, 6 months, 12 months and then annually. Vitamins C, A, K, E are usually not deficient. Routine medicines are 2 multivitamins, calcium citrate 1200-2000 mg, (better absorption with citrate compared with carbonate), vitamin D 3,000 mg, iron sulfate 325 mg, and B12 0.5 mg daily. The approximate costs of various bariatric surgical procedures in Indiana in 2019 were Roux-en-Y gastric bypass $ 24,000, Laparoscopic Banding $15,000, Sleeve gastrectomy $ 19,000, and Duodenal switch $ 27,000. Out-of-pocket expense if insurance covers it is about $3500.

Treatment of Adult Obesity with Bariatric Surgery.

In 2013, approximately 179,000 bariatric surgery procedures were performed in the United States, including the laparoscopic sleeve gastrectomy (42.1%), Roux-en-Y gastric bypass (34.2%), and laparoscopic adjustable gastric banding (14.0%). On average, weight loss of 60% to 70% of excess body weight is achieved in the short term, and up to 50% at 10 years. Remission of type 2 diabetes mellitus occurs in 60% to 80% of patients two years after surgery and persists in about 30% of patients 15 years after Roux-en-Y gastric bypass. Other obesity-related comorbidities are greatly reduced, and health-related quality of life improves. The Roux-en-Y procedure carries an increased risk of malabsorption sequelae, which can be minimized with nutritional supplementation and surveillance. **Overall, these procedures have a mortality risk of less than 0.5%. Cohort studies show that bariatric surgery reduces all-cause mortality by 30% to 50% at seven to 15 years post-surgery compared with patients with obesity who did not have surgery. Dietary changes, such as consuming protein first at every meal, and regular physical activity are critical for patient success after bariatric surgery** (Schroeder, Harrison, & McGraw, 2016).

American Society for Metabolic and Bariatric Surgery estimation of metabolic and bariatric procedures performed in the United States in 2016

Bariatric surgery, despite being the most successful long-lasting treatment for morbid obesity, remains underused as only approximately 1% of all patients who qualify for surgery actually undergo surgery.

Objective:

The objective of this study was to determine metabolic and bariatric procedure trends since 2011 and to provide the best estimate of the number of procedures performed in the United States in 2016.

Result:

Compared with 2015, the total number of metabolic and bariatric procedures performed in 2016 increased from approximately 196,000 to 216,000. The sleeve gastrectomy trend is increasing, and it continues to be the most common procedure. The Roux-en-Y gastric bypass and gastric banding procedure continue to decrease every year. The percentage of revision procedures and biliopancreatic diversion with duodenal switch procedures increased slightly. Finally, intragastric balloons placement emerged as a significant contributor to the cumulative total number of procedures performed.

Conclusion:

There is increasing use of metabolic and bariatric procedures performed in the United States from 2011 to 2016, with a nearly 10% increase noted from 2015 to 2016 (English, et al., 2018).

Recent estimates by the ASMBS (American Society for Metabolic and Bariatric Surgery) show the following:

Estimate of Bariatric Surgery Numbers, 2011-2017

Published June 2018

	2011	2012	2013	2014	2015	2016	2017
Total	158,000	173,000	179,000	193,000	196,000	216,000	228,000
Sleeve	17.80%	33.00%	42.10%	51.70%	53.61%	58.11%	59.39%
RYGB	36.70%	37.50%	34.20%	26.80%	23.02%	18.69%	17.80%

Band	35.40%	20.20%	14.00%	9.50%	5.68%	3.39%	**2.77%**
BPD-DS	0.90%	1.00%	1.00%	0.40%	0.60%	0.57%	**0.70%**
Revision	6.00%	6.00%	6.00%	11.50%	13.55%	13.95%	**14.14%**
Other	3.20%	2.30%	2.70%	0.10%	3.19%	2.63%	**2.46%**
Balloons	—	—	—	—	0.36%	2.66%	**2.75%**

The ASMBS total bariatric procedure numbers are based on the best estimation from available data (BOLD, ACS/MBSAQIP, National Inpatient Sample Data and outpatient estimations).

A 39-hospital collaborative group looking at 44,000 patients undergoing bariatric surgery from 2008 to 2013 revealed sleeve gastrectomy rose from 6% to 67%, Roux-en-Y dropped from 58% to 27%, adjustable banding fell from 35% to 5% (Reames, Finks, Bacal, Carlin, & Dimick, 2014).

Only one percent of medically eligible patients undergo bariatric surgery. Most pre-bariatric surgery patients go on a very low-calorie diet before surgery to prepare them for calorie reduction and also to reduce the liver volume to make surgery technically easier. A low-calorie diet can decrease the liver by almost 30% within 2 weeks. Sleeve gastrectomy has become the most common procedure and gastric-banding is decreasing dramatically. (Blackburn Course in Obesity Medicine, 2014)

Bariatric surgery risk is divided into peri-operative (first 30 days) and long term. Pulmonary embolism is the most common reason for death. Peri-operative death is 1 in 500, anastomotic leak 1%, wound infection 2%, DVT/PE 2% and nausea/vomiting/dehydration about 20%. Long-term complications are peptic ulcer disease 3-5%, small bowel obstruction 1%, internal hernia 0.8%, surgical stenosis 2% and vitamin/nutrient deficiency 10-25%. Marginal ulcers occur in up to 20% of Roux-en-Y gastric bypass patients. Gallstone formation and kidney stone formation increase with any rapid weight loss. Most programs do not do prophylactic cholecystectomies.

A rare but very hard complication to treat is post bypass hyper-insulinemic hypoglycemia. Increased GLP-1 secretion has been postulated to contribute to the mechanism mediating the refractory hypoglycemia. It is rare before one year postop, and generally has an onset 2-4 years after surgery. Treatment is frequent small meals. Acarbose 25 mg TID (inhibits alpha glucosidase that cleaves glucose from carbohydrates and delays carbohydrate absorption) can be added. Diazoxide (inhibits insulin release) is then added to decrease the overzealous pancreas (diazoxide is usually used to treat rare insulinomas). A pancreatic resection would be the last resort. (Blackburn Course in Obesity Medicine, 2014)

An uncommon statistic expressed is the five-fold increased successful suicide rate following gastric bypass surgery. This seems more realistic after realizing that 20-60% of bariatric surgery patients have psychopathology. **Mood disorders, anxiety disorders, and eating disorders can be aggravated with bariatric surgery.** There still is no procedure for surgically excising the psychosocial influences promoting weight regain after surgery. Depression and shifting calories to more carbohydrate dense foods and drinks are the most common reason for weight regain (sorry Starbucks). **In general, about 60-70% of patients lose at least 50% excess weight at 10 years. Bariatric surgery is not only for adults but has been successful in adolescents. All organizations involved in bariatric surgery agree that 150 minutes per week (30 minutes 5x/week) is insufficient for prevention of weight regain after bariatric surgery. It needs to be 60-90 minutes per day.**

<u>**Bariatric surgery improves the employment rate in people with obesity: 2-year analysis**</u>.
Beyond medical complications, people with obesity experience dramatic impairment of quality of life, including adverse workplace effects. Obesity results in weight-based discrimination and a high rate of unemployment because of work disability, absenteeism, loss of productivity, and cost. <u>Objectives</u>:

Compare the employment rate before and 2 years after obesity surgery and the difference in weight loss between worker and nonworker patients.

Results:

- Preoperatively, 158 of 238 were employed
- Postoperatively 199 of 238 were employed (P < .0001).
- There was no difference in weight loss between the worker and nonworker patients.

Conclusion:

This study supports the finding that bariatric surgery also has a positive impact on the professional sphere, providing the opportunity for unemployed patients to return to work (Mancini, et al., 2018).

Meta-analysis of the effectiveness of laparoscopic adjustable gastric banding versus laparoscopic sleeve gastrectomy for obesity.

- Laparoscopic adjustable gastric banding (LAGB) and laparoscopic sleeve gastrectomy (LSG) are common weight loss procedures.
- We systematically searched the PubMed, Embase, and the Cochrane Library through January 2018.
- Thirty-three studies with 4109 patients were included.
- Greater decreases in excess weight with LSG at 6 months, 12 months, 24 months and 36 months than in patients who received LAGB.
- There were no significant differences in the 3-month outcomes between the 2 groups.
- T2DM patients after LSG experienced more significant improvement or remission of diabetes.
- The 2 groups did not significantly differ regarding improvement or remission of hypertension.

Conclusion:

LSG is a more effective procedure than LAGB for morbidly obese patients, contributing to a higher %EWL and greater improvement in T2DM (Li, et al., 2019).

Five Years, Two Surgeons, and over 500 Bariatric Procedures: What Have We Learned?

Standardization, expediting the postoperative period while maintaining safe outcomes are important goals.

Methods:

All laparoscopic sleeve gastrectomies (LSG) and gastric bypasses (LGB) were performed over a 5-year period.

Results:

A total of 545 LSGs and LGBs were performed between 2012 and 2016. Improvements were noted in nearly every field over time, including faster Foley removal, decreased length of hospital stay, decreased use of patient-controlled analgesics (PCAs), and faster advancement of diet.

 Conclusions:

Nearly every aspect of postoperative care has been deescalated while decreasing length of stay and cost to the hospital. All of these has occurred without any increase in complications, re-operations, or re-admissions (Shea, et al., 2017).

Variation in Clinical Characteristics of Women versus Men Preoperative for Laparoscopic Roux-en-Y Gastric Bypass: Analysis of 83,059 Patients.

- The objective of our study was to identify clinical differences between morbidly obese women and men seeking LRYGB.
- Data from 83,059 patients who were about to undergo LRYGB was analyzed in two groups: women (n = 65,325) and men (n = 17,734).
- Cardiopulmonary comorbidities, older age, diabetes, gout, dyslipidemia, abdominal hernia, liver disease, alcohol/ tobacco use/ substance abuse are higher for men (P < 0.0001).
- Women had asthma, somatic pain, gastroesophageal reflux disease, cholelithiasis, abdominal panniculitis, back pain, musculoskeletal pain, mental health disorders, depression, and impaired psychological status more often (P < 0.0001).
- This advanced knowledge may aid management of LRYGB patients. By raising the index of suspicion for weight-related comorbidities, management of non-bariatric surgical

patients may also be facilitated (Schwartz, Bashian, Kushnir, Nituica, & Slotman, 2017).

Racial Comparisons of Postoperative Weight Loss and Eating-Disorder Psychopathology Among Patients Following Sleeve Gastrectomy Surgery.

- This study aimed to examine racial differences in postoperative eating-disorder psychopathology.
- Participants were 123 patients (n = 74 non-Hispanic White and n = 49 non-Hispanic Black) who underwent sleeve gastrectomy surgery within the previous 4 to 9 months and reported regular LOC eating during the previous month.
- Black and White patients did not differ significantly in LOC eating frequency, onset time of postoperative LOC eating, eating-disorder psychopathology, depressive symptoms, or physical or mental health-related quality of life.
- White patients were significantly more likely to meet criteria for lifetime binge-eating disorder than Black patients.
- Black patients were significantly more likely to skip breakfast and dinner and engage in night eating than White patients (Ivezaj, Fu, Lydecker, Duffy, & Grilo, 2019).

Is bariatric surgery effective for co-morbidity resolution in the super-obese patients?

- The purpose of this study was to compare co-morbidity remission and weight loss of super-obese patients with a body mass index (BMI) ≥50 with bariatric patients who have a BMI of 30 to 49.9.

Methods:
- A retrospective analysis was done on obese patients with a diagnosis of ≥1 co-morbidity (T2D, OSA, HTN, or HLD) who had undergone either a sleeve gastrectomy or a Roux-en-Y gastric bypass.
- The patients were stratified based on their preoperative BMI class, BMI of 30 to 49.9 versus BMI ≥50.

Results:
- Of the 930 patients, 732 underwent sleeve gastrectomy and 198 underwent Roux-en-Y gastric bypass.

- **The 6-month remission rates for patients with a BMI of 30 to 49.9(n = 759) versus super-obese patients (n = 171) were:**
- 46.0% and 36.7% for T2D
- 75.0% and 73.2% for OSA
- 35.0% and 22.0% for HTN
- 37.0% and 21.0% for HLD (lipids)
- **The 1-year remission rates for patients with a BMI of 30 to 49.9 versus super-obese patients were**
- 54.2% and 45.5% for T2D
- 87.0% and 89.7% for OSA
- 37.4% and 23.9% for HTN
- 43.2% and 34.6% for HLD
- There was no difference in the mean percent total weight loss for patients with a preoperative BMI of 30 to 49.9 versus the super-obese at the 6-month (21.4%, 20.9%) and 1-year (28.0%, 30.7%) follow-ups.
- Both procedures were very successful for obese and super-obese patients (Hariri, et al., 2018).

Analysis of Laparoscopic Sleeve Gastrectomy Learning Curve and Its Influence on Procedure Safety and Perioperative Complications.

The learning curve for performing Laparoscopic sleeve gastrectomy (LSG) is reviewed.

Methods:

Retrospective study included patients submitted to LSG at an academic teaching hospital. Five hundred patients were included (330 females, median age of 40).

Patients were divided into groups every 100 consecutive patients. Primary endpoint was determining the LSG learning curve's stabilization point, using operative time, intraoperative difficulties, intraoperative adverse events (IAE), and number of stapler firings.

Results:

Based on perioperative morbidity, the learning curve was stabilized at the 100th procedure.

The morbidity rates in the groups were G1, 13%; G2, 4%; G3, 5%; G4, 5%; and G5, 2%.

The reoperation rate in G1 was 3%; G2, 2%; G3, 2%; G4, 1%; and G5, 0%

Conclusion:

The institutional learning process stabilization point for LSG in a newly established bariatric center is between the 100th and 200th operation. Initially, the morbidity rate is high, which should concern surgeons who are willing to perform bariatric surgery (Major, et al., 2018).

Risk Factors for Prolonged Length of Hospital Stay and Readmissions After Laparoscopic Sleeve Gastrectomy and Laparoscopic Roux-en-Y Gastric Bypass.

Laparoscopic sleeve gastrectomy (LSG) and laparoscopic gastric bypass (LRYGB) are the most commonly performed bariatric procedures. There are patients whom the length of stay (LOS) remains longer than targeted without any obvious complications. This study aimed to assess potential risk factors for prolonged LOS and readmissions.

Methods:

Prospective observation of bariatric patients in a tertiary referral university teaching hospital. Exclusion criteria were occurrence of perioperative complications, prior bariatric procedures, and lack of necessary data.

Results:

- Median LOS was 3 (2-4) days.
- LOS > 3 days occurred in 145 (29.47%) patients
- 79 after LSG (25.82%) and 66 after LRYGB (35.48%).
- Factors significantly prolonging LOS were low oral fluid intake, high intravenous volume of fluids administered on the day of surgery, and every additional 50 km distance from habitual residence to bariatric center.
- These patients were the ones without obvious complications but were not stable enough to leave with 3 days (Major, et al., 2018).

Laparoscopic Sleeve Gastrectomy Outcomes in Patients with Polycystic Ovary Syndrome.

- Polycystic ovary syndrome (PCOS) is a common disease among the bariatric population.

- The purpose of this study was to examine per cent excess body weight loss (%EWL) and diabetes control in patients who have PCOS compared with those without PCOS.
- A total of 550 female patients underwent Sleeve Gastrectomy (SG).
- PCOS patients had similar age (36.3 vs 36.2 years), preoperative BMI (47.2 vs 47.2), preoperative HgbA1c (6% vs 5.8%), conversion rate to gastric bypass, and other associated comorbidities compared with non-PCOS comparisons.
- There was no difference in %EWL at 12-month (49.7% vs 53.1%) or 24-month (43% vs 49.8%) postoperative intervals.
- There was no difference in absolute change of HgbA1c at 12 months (-0.47% vs -0.67%).
- SG has equivalent short-term results in %EWL and reduction in HgbA1c for patients who have PCOS and those who do not (Yheulon, et al., 2019).

Roux-en-Y Gastric Bypass Versus Sleeve Gastrectomy for Super Super Obese and Super Obese: Systematic Review and Meta-analysis of Weight Results, Comorbidity Resolution.

Roux-en-Y gastric bypass (RYGB) and sleeve gastrectomy (SG) used for super obesity (body mass index >50) and super- super obesity (body mass index >60) remain controversial. A meta-analysis summarized the evidence with Medline and PubMed literature search. Twelve studies were identified.

- RYGB achieved higher %EWL (excess wgt loss) at 12 months, but no significant difference at 24 months. Resolution of diabetes mellitus and dyslipidemia reached a statistical significance; however, there was no significant difference in hypertension (Wang, et al., 2019).

Outcomes of Roux-en-Y gastric bypass versus sleeve gastrectomy in super-super-obese patients (BMI ≥60 kg/m2): 6-year follow-up at a single university.

- Compare laparoscopic sleeve gastrectomy (SG) and laparoscopic Roux-en-Y gastric bypass (RYGB). Evaluate

SG for super-super obesity (SSO-body mass index >60) patients.

- We retrospectively reviewed the data outcomes of 210 SSO patients who underwent SG or RYGB between January 2000 and December 2011 at a University hospital in Paris, France. The 6-year follow-up data were analyzed and compared.

Conclusions:

- SG and RYGB can be proposed as primary procedures for SSO patients.
- At 4 years, there was no significant difference between procedures regarding EWL%.
- At 6 years, SG group preserves a satisfactory rate of remissions or alleviated diabetes/hypertension.
- **We propose SG as the primary procedure and reserve RYGB as a revision option for super-super obesity** (Arapis, et al., 2019).

Does the future of laparoscopic sleeve gastrectomy lie in the outpatient surgery center? A retrospective study of the safety of 3162 outpatient sleeve gastrectomies.

Determine whether same-day discharge LSG is safe when performed in an outpatient surgery center.

Methods:

The medical records of 3162 patients who underwent primary LSG procedure by 21 surgeons at 9 outpatient surgery centers from January 2010 through February 2018 were retrospectively reviewed.

Results:

- 3,162 patients were managed with enhanced recovery after surgery protocol.
- Mean age was 43.1 years and BMI 42.1 kg/m2.
- Co-morbidities were sleep apnea (14.4%), type 2 diabetes (13.5%), gastroesophageal reflux disease (24.7), hypertension (30.4%), and hyperlipidemia (17.6%).
- Mean total operative time was 56.4 ± 16.9 minutes (skin to skin).

- One intraoperative complication (.03%) occurred.
- Hospital transfer rate was 0.2%.
- 30-day follow-up rate was 85%.
- 30-day readmission rate 0.6%, reoperation 0.6%, reintervention 0.2% and emergency room visit rate 0.1%.
- 30-day mortality rate was 0%.
- Short-term complication rate was 2.5%.

Conclusion:
Same-day discharge seems to be safe when performed in an outpatient surgery center in selected patients. It would appear that outpatient surgery centers are a viable option for patients with minimal surgical risks (Surve, et al., 2018).

Weight Loss Medications in Young Adults after Bariatric Surgery for Weight Regain or Inadequate Weight Loss: A Multi-Center Study.

- A retrospective cohort study of weight loss medications in young adults aged 21 to 30 after Roux-en-Y gastric bypass (RYGB) and sleeve gastrectomy (SG) between November 2000 and June 2014.
- Data were collected from patients who used topiramate, phentermine, and/or metformin postoperatively.
- Patients taking medications at weight loss plateau lost 41.2% of total body weight from before surgery versus 27.1% after weight regain (p = 0.076).
- Topiramate, phentermine, and metformin are promising weight loss medications for 21 to 30 years-old.
- RYGB patients achieve more weight loss on medications but both RYGB and SG patients benefited using weight loss medications.
- Median total body weight loss from pre-surgical weight may be higher in patients that start medication at postsurgical nadir weight (Toth, et al., 2018).

Endoscopic sleeve gastroplasty versus laparoscopic sleeve gastrectomy: a case-matched study.

Endoscopic sleeve gastroplasty (ESG) reduces the gastric lumen to a size comparable to that of laparoscopic sleeve gastrectomy (LSG). Our retrospective study compared the 6-month weight loss outcomes and adverse events of ESG with LSG in a case-matched cohort.

Results:
- A total of 54 ESG patients were matched to 83 LSG patients by age, sex, and body mass index (BMI). The proportion of patients with GERD at baseline was similar in the 2 groups.
- **6-month follow-up %TBWL (compared with baseline).**
- ESG group TBWL 17.1%.
- LSG group - TBWL 23.6%.
- ESG patients had significantly lower rate of adverse events - 5.2%.
- LSG patient adverse events - 16.9%.
- New-onset GERD was significantly lower in the ESG group - 1.9%, LSG group - 14.5%.

Conclusions:
ESG, a minimally invasive same-day procedure, achieved less weight loss at 6 months than LSG, with the caveat that LSG caused more adverse events and new onset GERD than ESG. Both procedures seem to be very successful (Fayad, et al., 2019).

Pros and cons of gastric bypass surgery in individuals with obesity and type 2 diabetes: nationwide, matched, observational cohort study.
- The most effective method for ensuring long-term weight reduction in individuals with obesity as well as beneficial effects on mortality, cardiovascular disease (CVD) and cardiovascular (CV) risk factors is bariatric surgery, Roux-en-Y gastric bypass (GBP) in particular.

- This is a nationwide observational study based on two quality registers in Sweden (National Diabetes Register, NDR and Scandinavian Obesity Surgery Register, SOReg) and other national databases.
- We matched individuals with T2DM who had undergone GBP with those not surgically treated for obesity.

Participants

- 5321 patients with T2DM in the SOReg and 5321 matched controls in the NDR, aged 18–65 years, with BMI >27.5 and followed for up to 9 years.
- Baseline characteristics GBP- women 60.5%, age 49.0, BMI 42.0, married 47.4%.
- Controls- women 63.8%, age 47.1, BMI 40.9, married 41.9%

Results

- Patients with or without T2DM who underwent GBP had lower risks of all-cause mortality (49%), cardiovascular disease (34%), pulmonary complications, embolism, DVT or liver disease
- Event rates for all-cause mortality were 72.9 and 142.1 per 10 000 person-years in GBP and the control group, respectively.
- Risks for coronary heart disease, acute myocardial infarction and congestive heart failure were also lower after GBP.
- Other benefits were observed after GBP. Hospitalisation for hyperglycaemia was less frequent, and the risks of kidney disease, leg amputation and cancer were lower.
- Long-term the risk of anaemia was 92% higher, malnutrition developed approximately three times as often.
- The risks of hospitalisation due to psychiatric disorders or alcohol abuse increased after GBP (73.1 and 26.5 per 10 000 person-years in GBP and the control group.
- Previous studies have shown that depression, which may improve in the first year following bariatric surgery, tends to progress along with suicide and self-harm, particularly if they are pre-existing conditions.

- In agreement with previous studies, we confirmed a higher event rate of alcohol-related problems that lead to hospitalisation after GBP.
- Additional GI surgery was performed in 17.6% of the GBP group, more than three times as much as in the control group. Additional GI surgery in the GBP group were: abdominal pain, bowel obstruction, gallstones, gallbladder disease, pancreatitis, GI ulcers, reflux, hernia, GI leakage, wound complications and bleeding. Some postoperative complications were common shortly after GBP (leakage, wound complications and ulcer/reflux), while others (hernia, bowel obstruction and gallstone) generally increased after 1–2 years (Liakopoulos, et al., 2019).

Seven-Year Weight Trajectories and Health Outcomes in the Longitudinal Assessment of Bariatric Surgery (LABS) Study. To examine long-term weight change and health status following Roux-en-Y gastric bypass (RYGB) and laparoscopic adjustable gastric banding (LAGB).

Design:
- The Longitudinal Assessment of Bariatric Surgery (LABS) study is a multicenter observational cohort study at 10 US hospitals in 6 geographically diverse clinical centers between 2006 and 2009 and followed up until January 31, 2015.

Results:
- Of 2348 participants, 74% underwent RYGB and 26% underwent LAGB.
- For RYBG, the median age was 45 years, the median BMI was 47, 80% were women, and 15% were nonwhite.
- For LAGB, the median age was 48 years, the BMI was 44, 76% were women, and 10% were nonwhite.
- Follow-up weights were obtained in 1300 of 1569 (83%) eligible for a year-7 visit.
- Seven years following RYGB, LAGB, mean weight loss was 28.4% and 14.9% of baseline respectively with 3.9% and 1.4% regain.

- Dyslipidemia prevalence was lower 7 years following both procedures and diabetes and hypertension prevalence were lower following RYGB only.
- Among those with diabetes at baseline (28% with RYGB; 29% with LAGB), the proportion in remission at 7 years were 60.2% for RYGB and 20.3% for LAGB.
- The incidence of diabetes at all follow-up assessments was less than 1.5% for RYGB.
- Bariatric reoperations occurred in 14 RYGB and 160 LAGB participants.

Conclusion:

RYGB had double the baseline weight loss and triple the diabetes remission weight compared to LAGB (Courcoulas, et al., 2018).

A study by Dr. Thomas H. Inge published 1/14/16 in the NEJM looked at 242 adolescents with a mean age 17 years and a mean BMI 53 who underwent bariatric surgery at 5 centers.

- 161 patients underwent Roux-en-Y and 67 had sleeve gastrectomy. 75% were female and 72% were white.

3 years after surgery:

- Mean weight decreased 27%.
- Remission of diabetes 95%.
- Remission of abnormal kidney function 86%.
- Remission of prediabetes 76%.
- Remission of elevated blood pressure 74%.
- Remission of dyslipidemia 66%.
- 57% developed low ferritin levels and 13% had undergone one or more additional intraabdominal procedures.

In conclusion, clinically meaning weight loss and improvements in key health conditions occurred at the three-year mark for adolescents who underwent gastric bypass surgery or sleeve gastrectomy (Inge, et al., 2016).

Comparison Between Marital Satisfaction and Self-Esteem Before and After Bariatric Surgery in Patients with Obesity

- The current prospective observational study conducted on 69 bariatric surgery patients aimed to compare marital satisfaction and self-confidence before and after bariatric surgery in 2013.

- Despite the improvement of sexual relationship, marital satisfaction scores significantly decreased six months after the surgery. No significant difference was found between self-esteem before and after the surgery.
- Weight loss after bariatric surgery did not improve self-esteem and marital satisfaction six months post operatively. (Ghanbari, et al., 2016).

Sexual functioning and sex hormones in men who underwent bariatric surgery.

Assess changes in sexual functioning, sex hormones, and relevant psychosocial constructs in men who underwent bariatric surgery.

Methods

A prospective cohort study of 32 men from the Longitudinal Assessment of Bariatric Surgery-2 (LABS) investigation who underwent a Roux-en-Y gastric bypass (median body mass index 45.1).

Results:

- Men lost, on average, 33.3% of initial weight at postoperative year 1
- 33.6% at year 2
- 31.0% at year 3
- 29.4% at year 4.

Conclusion:

Men who lost approximately one third of their weight after Roux-en-Y gastric bypass experienced significant increases in total testosterone and SHBG. They did not, however, report significant improvements in sexual functioning, relationship satisfaction, or mental health

344

domains of quality of life. This pattern of results differs from that of women who have undergone bariatric surgery, who reported almost uniform improvements in sexual functioning and psychosocial status (Sarwer, et al., 2015).

A retrospective review by Jennifer Schwartz in Obesity Surgery 2016 entitled "**Pharmacotherapy in Conjunction with a Diet and Exercise Program for the Treatment of Weight Recidivism or Weight Loss Plateau Post Bariatric Surgery**"

An estimated 10-30% of bariatric surgical patients regain their weight postoperatively starting as early as 18 months and as far out as 20 years.

Patients who experienced weight regain or weight plateau after Roux-en-Y gastric bypass (RYGB) or laparoscopic adjustable gastric banding (LAGB) were treated with phentermine or phentermine-topiramate.
Fifty-two patients received phentermine (37.5 mg) while 13 received phentermine/topiramate (3.75 mg/23 mg daily for 2 weeks then 7.5 mg/46 mg daily).
Patients in both groups lost weight. Diet was 1200 kcals/day. Phentermine patients lost 6.35 kg (12.8% excess weight), and those prescribed phentermine/topiramate lost 3.81 kg (12.9% excess weight loss).
Conclusion:
Phentermine and phentermine/topiramate in addition to diet and exercise appear to be viable options for weight loss in post-RYGB and LAGB patients who experience weight regain or weight loss plateau (Schwartz, et al., 2016).

A meta-analysis of observational studies of bariatric surgery in a 2009 study by H. Buchwald in the American Journal of Medicine reported that 78% of 3,188 patients with T2DM had normalization of blood glucose in the absence of diabetic medications (Buchwald, et al., 2005).

A new idea with bariatric surgery is the principle that the metabolic changes that happen with surgery play a more important role than the conventional theory that bariatric surgery works by restricting oral intake (volume of stomach with sleeve is only 60-150 cc). Few patients become underweight after surgery unless a complication ensues. It would be common to expect some overshooting if the mechanism for weight loss were primarily mechanical/restrictive. **The preponderance of evidence indicates that most bariatric procedures alter the physiology of energy balance and metabolic regulation, and that biological mechanisms largely account for the efficacy of these operations.** One example is the dramatic drop in insulin after surgery that cannot be explained simply by the lower caloric usage. Another example involves ghrelin, "the hunger hormone from the stomach." Levels decrease with surgery and increase with routine dieting. Bariatric surgeries involving vertical sleeve gastrectomy reduce plasma ghrelin levels by about 60% in the long term (Bohdjalian, et al., 2010). RYGB decreases GLP-1, PYY, Amylin, and Ghrelin.

A 2013 study by Giovanni Corona in The European Journal of Endocrinology looked at sex hormone levels in patients on a low-calorie diet or bariatric surgery. Twenty-four studies were included, enrolling 479 patients with a mean follow-up of 38 weeks and the mean percent body weight loss was 9.8% in the low-calorie diet and 32.0% with bariatric surgery. Body weight loss was associated with a relevant increase in gonadotropins (LH, FSH), along with bound and unbound testosterone and a decline in estrogen. Androgen rise is greater in those who lost more weight as well as in younger, non-diabetic subjects with a greater degree of obesity. **Male hypogonadism is one of the many adverse consequences of overweight and obesity. Evidence indicates that testosterone deficiency induces increased adiposity while increased adiposity induces hypogonadism** (Corona, et al., 2003).

New research involving left gastric artery embolization (LGAE) to decrease Ghrelin levels was first done in animal trials in 2007 and in humans 2013. In 1973, the first reported instance of left gastric artery embolization was performed not for obesity but to treat a gastrointestinal hemorrhage from a gastric ulcer of the lesser curvature (Prochaska, Flye, Johnsrude, 1973). The blood supply to the stomach has adequate collateral flow to allow left gastric artery embolization. Ghrelin-producing cells in the stomach and proximal duodenum produce more than 90% of ghrelin used by the body. Gastrectomy results in an 80% reduction in plasma levels of ghrelin (Takachi, et al., 2006). It is clear that LGAE decreases Ghrelin by reducing secretory cells in the gastric fundus; however, to our knowledge, no study has yet to evaluate how these alterations in ghrelin affect other gut hormones, including leptin and obestatin. LGAE may play a complementary or adjunctive role, in combination with bariatric surgery.

Early data suggest that targeted embolization of the arterial supply to the gastric fundus may provide a safe effective approach to weight loss in the obese patient (Anton, Rahman, Bhanushali, & Patel, 2016).

To improve quality and patient outcomes, it's important to track surgeries and complications. Readmission statistics are nicely documented in **National prevalence, causes, and risk factors for bariatric surgery readmissions**. A total of 18,296 patients with 10,080 laparoscopic Roux-en-Y gastric bypass, 1,829 laparoscopic adjustable gastric banding, and 6,387 laparoscopic sleeve gastrectomy. 955 (5.22%) were readmitted. Characteristics of readmitted patients compared to patients not needing readmission were:

1. BMI greater than 50 (30.2% vs 24.6%).
2. Longer initial operative time (132 minutes vs 115 minutes).
3. Greater than 4-day initial hospital stay (9.57% vs 3.36%).
4. Higher diabetes rate (31.1% vs 27.7%).
5. COPD (2.63% vs 1.72%).
6. HTN (54.5% vs 50.8%).
7. African-American race

Overall, 40.6% of readmitted patients had a complication. Complications were gastrointestinal-related (45%), dietary (33.5%), and bleeding (6.57%). Resident physician involvement decreased readmission rate (Garg, Rosas, Rivas, Azagury, & Morton, 2016).

Change in Pain and Physical Function Following Bariatric Surgery for Severe Obesity

- Severe obesity is associated with significant joint pain and impaired physical function.. Excess weight bearing can lead to joint damage and pain, resulting in activity restriction and walking limitations.
- This report examines pain and physical function in the first 3 years following bariatric surgery.
- The Longitudinal Assessment of Bariatric Surgery-2 (LABS-2) study is an observational study of 2458 adults who underwent an initial bariatric surgical procedure between March 14, 2006, and April 24, 2009, at 1 of 10 hospitals at 6 US clinical centers.
- Demographics were 78.5 female, median age 47, 86.5% white, median BMI 45.9, and 12.3% smokers. Comorbidities were 33.6 diabetes, obstructive sleep apnea 53.5%, severe knee pain 37.6%, severe hip pain 29.7%, and mobility disability 42.7%
- RYGB was the most common surgical procedure (70.4%); one-fourth (25.0%) of patients underwent LAGB; and less than 5% underwent another procedure (sleeve gastrectomy, banded gastric bypass, or biliopancreatic diversion with duodenal switch).

Measures

Validated health surveys provided objective measures (SF-36, and WOMAC).Results

- Median weight loss of total group at year one-30.5%, year two-30.5%, year three-28.2%.
- For RYGB, weight loss at year one-34.1%, year two-34.1%, and year three-31.5%.
- For LAGB, weight loss at year one-14.0%, year two-16.1% and year three-16.2%.

- Following surgery, survey scores showed improvement in knee pain, hip pain, ability to work at year one compared to baseline but did not improve anymore at year three despite additional weight loss. The prevalence of severe walking limitations at year three was not significantly different from baseline.

Discussion

- Approximately 50% to 70% of adults experienced clinically significant improvements in bodily pain and physical function.

- Approximately three-fourths of participants with severe knee and hip pain or disability experienced clinically significant improvements.

- Bariatric surgery may lead to improvements in work productivity.

- Bariatric surgery patients, as a group, continue to have more pain following surgery than the general US population.

- At year three, approximately 1 in 3 participants took pain medication within the prior week for back pain or leg pain and were dissatisfied with their level of back or leg pain.

- At year three, approximately one-fourth of patients reported limitations with walking several blocks.

- In a cross-sectional analysis, Sanchez-Santos et al reported improved mobility of adults at least 5 years after RYGB compared with controls..

- Raoof et al reported that mean scores for bodily pain and physical function on the SF-36 were better 12 years post-RYGB when compared with those of morbidly obese controls who were awaiting surgery (matched on age and sex).

- Another study, which provided follow-up for 145 LAGB patients for 3 to 8 years, reported that fewer patients had significant knee pain at follow-up vs baseline (38% vs 47%; $P < .01$).

Conclusions

Among a cohort of patients with severe obesity undergoing bariatric surgery, a large percentage experienced improvement compared with baseline in pain, physical function, and walk time over three years. However, the percentage with improvement in pain and physical function decreased between year one and year three following surgery. After reviewing the study, my take-home message is to encourage bariatric surgery earlier to lessen or avoid chronic arthritic disability (King, et al., 2016).

Management of obesity after spinal cord injury: a systematic review.

- Individuals with chronic spinal cord injury (SCI) are susceptible to central and visceral obesity and the metabolic consequences.
- To identify and compare effective means of obesity management among SCI individuals.
- This systematic review prior to April 2017 included PubMed/Medline, Embase, CINAHL Psychinfo and Cochrane databases. From 3,553 retrieved titles and abstracts, 34 articles underwent full text review and 23 articles were selected for data abstraction.

Results:
Bariatric surgery produced the greatest permanent weight reduction and BMI correction followed by combinations of physical exercise and diet therapy (Shojaei, Alavinia, & Craven, 2017).

Chapter 38: Bariatric Surgery in Elderly

In many studies, elderly is defined as 60 years old or greater. I am 59 years old and I do not like that concept. I guess I should follow Yogi Berra's advice and **"Take it with a grin of salt." (should be grain but Yogi is Yogi)**

Midterm outcomes of sleeve gastrectomy in the elderly.

- laparoscopic sleeve gastrectomy (LSG) in patients aged ≥60 years.
- LSG between 2008 and 2014 and achieved ≥24-month follow-up were retrospectively reviewed.

Results:

- 55 patients - mean patient age was 63.9.
- mean preoperative body mass index was 43.
- Perioperative morbidity included 5 cases of hemorrhage necessitating operative exploration.
- 2 cases treated with blood transfusion.
- 1 case of portal vein thrombosis managed with anticoagulation.
- No mortalities.
- Mean follow-up time was 48.6 months.
- Mean percentage of excess weight loss was 66.4 at 12 months, 67.5 at 24 months, 61.4 at 36 months, 66.7 at 37 to 60 months, and 50.7 at 61 to 96 months.
- Statistically significant improvement of type 2 diabetes, hypertension, and dyslipidemia were observed at the latest follow-up ($P < .01$).

Conclusion:
LSG (laparoscopic sleeve gastrectomy) offers an effective treatment of obesity and its co-morbidities in patients aged ≥60 years, albeit with a high perioperative bleeding rate at our center; efficacy is maintained for at least 4.5 years (Froylich, et al., 2018).

Outcomes of Laparoscopic Bariatric Surgery in the Elderly Population.

- There have been limited data on the safety of laparoscopic bariatric surgery in the elderly.
- Data from 2011 to 2015 compared outcomes of laparoscopic Roux-en-Y gastric bypass (LRYGB) and laparoscopic sleeve gastrectomy (LSG) between elderly (≥65 years) and nonelderly (18-64 years) patients.
- There were 41,475 LRYGB cases performed, including 2,010 (4.8%) cases in elderly patients.
- Compared with the nonelderly, elderly patients who underwent LRYGB had higher serious morbidity, but similar 30-day mortality.
- There were 44,550 LSG cases performed, including 2,055 (4.6%) cases in elderly patients.
- Compared with the nonelderly, elderly patients who underwent LSG had significantly higher serious morbidity and higher 30-day mortality.

Laparoscopic bariatric surgery is safe in the elderly population, and is similar between bariatric procedures. However, elderly patients have higher serious morbidity. They should be counseled regarding their higher risk, but should not be denied bariatric surgery based solely on their age (Koh, Inaba, Sujatha-Bhaskar, &Nguyen, 2018).

Outcomes of Laparoscopic Sleeve Gastrectomy and Roux-en-Y Gastric Bypass in Patients Older than 60.

- Evaluate the safety and efficacy of bariatric surgery in patients older than 60 years in a retrospective review at Montefiore Medical Center compared to the younger bariatric population done at the same center.

352

- 30 patients had LSG, and 53 patients had LRYGB. The average age was 63.4 years, average pre-op weight was 122.3 kg (269 lbs.) and the average excess body weight 54.8 kg (120 lbs.).
- Co-morbid conditions were hypertension 90.4%, diabetes 63.9%, hyperlipidemia 50.6%, obstructive sleep apnea 34.9%, and asthma 30.1%.
- The percentage body weight loss at 3 months, 6 months and 12 months were 37%, 51.3 % and 65.2 % respectively.

Conclusion:
Bariatric surgery can be safe and effective for patients older than 60 years of age with a low morbidity and mortality; the weight loss and improvement in comorbidities in older patients were clinically significant. When compared to the younger bariatric population at the same medical center, there was no statistically significant difference in the percent weight loss at 12 months or the number of complications due to surgery (Abbas, et al., 2015).

Bariatric surgery in elderly patients: a systematic review.

- Life expectancy has been steadily increasing regardless of sex and ethnic background in the USA. In Finland, life expectancy of a 60-year-old woman in 2008 was 24.3 years, whereas for a man of the same age, it was 22.8 years.
- In a recent statement, the Italian Society for Bariatric and Metabolic Surgery has extended the indications for bariatric surgery for morbidly obese patients up to 70 years of age.
- Twenty-six articles encompassing 8,149 patients aged 60 years or older were reviewed.
- 14 patients died during 30-day postoperative period (mortality 0.01%).
- At one-year follow-up pooled mean excess weight loss was 53.8%, pooled diabetes resolution was 54.5%, pooled hypertension resolution was 42.5%, pooled lipid disorder resolution 41.2%.

Outcomes and complication rates of bariatric surgery in patients older than 60 years are comparable to those in a younger population, independent of the type of procedure performed (Giordano & M, 2015).

Laparoscopic Weight Loss Surgery in the Elderly: An ACS NSQIP Study on the Effect of Age on Outcomes.

- The aim of this study was to characterize the short-term outcomes of laparoscopic weight loss surgery in the elderly.
- The ACS NSQIP database was queried for obese patients aged ≥40 years undergoing laparoscopic Roux-en-Y gastric bypass or sleeve gastrectomy.
- Patients were subdivided into age groups: 40 to 49, 50 to 59, 60 to 64, 65 to 69, and ≥70 years.
- Fifty-three thousand five hundred thirty-three (53,533) patients were identified. Roux-en-Y gastric bypass was performed in 57.5 per cent of cases and was more common than sleeve gastrectomy in all age groups (P < 0.05).
- Comorbidities increased significantly with increasing age.
- minor complications were 4.6% vs 9.1%; P < 0.0001 between the 40-49 and ≥70 years age groups
- Major complications were 2.2% vs 6.3%; P < 0.0001)
- 30-day mortality (0.1% vs 0.5%; P = 0.0001) between the 40 to 49 and ≥70 years age groups.
- Increased age was independently associated with major complications. Mortality also increased with age. Older patients undergoing laparoscopic weight loss surgery have increased morbidity and mortality (Arnold, et al., 2019).

Morbidity Rates and Weight Loss After Roux-en-Y Gastric Bypass, Sleeve Gastrectomy, and Adjustable Gastric Banding in Patients Older Than 60 Years old: Which Procedure to Choose?

- As life expectancy increases, more elderly patients fit into the criteria for bariatric procedures.
- Evaluate the safety and efficacy of RYGB, LSG, and LAGB, in patients older than 60 years.
- **LAGB (laparoscopic adjustable gastric banding,** 68 patients, mean age 62.7 years old, mean BMI 42.7,

Readmission 7 patients (10.3%), Reoperation rate 10.3%, Procedure mortality 1.4%

- **LSG (laparoscopic sleeve gastrectomy)**, 73 patients, mean age 64.1 years old, mean BMI 44.0, Readmission 3 patients (4.1%), Reoperation rate 1.4%, Procedure mortality 0%.
- **RYGB (Roux-en-Y gastric bypass)**, 212 patients, mean age 62.6 years old, mean BMI 45.2, Readmission 29 patients (13.8%), Reoperation rate 9.5%, Procedure mortality 0%.
- At 6, 12, and 18 months the amount of weight loss was the highest in the RYGB group, followed by LSG and LABG.
- Mean number of comorbidities at the last follow-up significantly decreased in LSG and RYGB patients.

Conclusion:

LSG showed the lowest readmission and reoperation rate, and RYGB had the highest mortality rate. Weight loss and comorbidity resolution were effectively achieved in RYGB and LSG patients (Moon, et al., 2016).

[BARIATRICS IN GERIATRICS - IS AGE AN OBSTACLE FOR BARIATRIC SURGERY?]

- Forty-eight elderly patients (mean age 67.9 years, 60% females) had bariatric surgery between 2009 and 2016. Results:
- Laparoscopic sleeve gastrectomy (LSG, 79%).
- Mini gastric bypass, (MGB, 17%).
- Roux-en-Y gastric bypass (RYGB, 4%).
- Weight decreased significantly (average BMI units lost was 9.4 units, $p<0.001$), and the mean EBWL% was 66.8%.
- Improving co-morbidities: DM-65.2%, HTN-54.3%, hyperlipidemia-40%.
- After a follow-up period longer than 4.2 years the failure rate (EBWL<50%) was 53.3%, however, these patients still presented a lower postoperative weight. All the patients who failed underwent LSG.

<u>Conclusion:</u>
Bariatric surgery is very effective in terms of long-term weight loss in the geriatric patient (Haiat, Leibovitz, & Shimonov, 2018).

Chapter 39: Bariatric Surgery in Adolescents

Should bariatric surgery be performed in adolescents?

Adolescent obesity has markedly increased worldwide and obesity prevention strategies are failing. As a result, effective treatment strategies are urgently needed. As behavioral and pharmacological treatment approaches have only moderate effects in severe obesity, bariatric surgery has begun to emerge as a treatment option. In this debate article, we offer arguments opposing and supporting bariatric surgery in the treatment of severe obesity in adolescents.

Bariatric surgery has superior therapeutic outcomes with respect to weight loss and resolution of comorbid diseases over other existing treatments. However, long-term outcomes after bariatric surgery in adolescents are only just beginning to emerge. Furthermore, the procedures are generally considered irreversible, apart from gastric banding. Most importantly, not all adolescents seem to benefit greatly from bariatric surgery and we are not yet able to reliably identify those who stand to gain the greatest benefit. The authors agree that adolescent bariatric surgery should be offered exclusively within formal adolescent obesity programs, delivered by specialist multidisciplinary child/adolescent obesity teams, and within specialist centers, in order to optimize outcomes and minimize potential detrimental effects. Patients and their family/caregivers must be educated regarding the benefits and risks, potential side effects, expected changes in eating behavior and the lifelong requirement for regular medical follow-up after surgery. Before embarking upon a surgical treatment pathway in adolescents with severe obesity, it may also be beneficial to ensure compliance to treatment is demonstrated, in order to minimize the risk of nutritional deficiencies and associated potential complications (Beamish & Reinehr, 2017).

Energetic Adaptations Persist after Bariatric Surgery in Severely Obese Adolescents

Energetic adaptations induced by bariatric surgery have not been studied in adolescents. Energetic, metabolic and neuroendocrine responses to Roux-en-Y gastric bypass surgery (RYGB) were investigated in extremely obese adolescents.

Design and Methods

At baseline and at 1.5, 6, and 12 months post-baseline, 24-h room calorimetry, body composition and fasting blood biochemistries were measured in eleven obese adolescents relative to five matched controls.

Results

- In RYGB group, mean weight loss was 44 kg at 12 months. Total energy expenditure (TEE), activity EE, basal metabolic rate (BMR), sleep EE and walking EE significantly declined by 1.5 months (p=0.001) and remained suppressed at 6 and 12 months. Decreases in serum insulin, leptin, and T3, gut hormones, and urinary norepinephrine (NE) paralleled the decline in EE. Adjusted changes in TEE, BMR and/or sleep EE were associated with decreases in insulin, HOMA, leptin, TSH, total T3, PYY3–36, GLP2 and urinary NE and epinephrine (p=0.001–0.05).
- Energetic adaptations in response to RYGB-induced weight loss are associated with changes in insulin, adipokines, thyroid hormones, gut hormones and sympathetic nervous system activity, and persist 12 months post-surgery.

The majority of the adaptive thermogenesis occurred by 1.5 months after surgery, along with the decline in FFM (fat free mass) and biochemical change and then remained at the suppressed level at 6 and 12 months after surgery.

- TEE (total energy expenditure) decreased by 24%

- AEE (activity energy expenditure) decreased by 41%
- BMR (basal metabolic rate) decreased by 19%
- Sleep EE (sleep energy expenditure) decreased by 24%
- Walking EE (energy expenditure) decreased by 28%

(Butte, et al., 2015)

What impressed me was how rapid and meaningful changes occurred within the first 45 days. When it comes to weight loss results, studies show that weight loss and health benefits resulting from mini gastric bypass are essentially the same as results seen from the standard Roux-en-Y Gastric Bypass.

The main difference between the standard Roux-en-Y gastric bypass procedure (RYGBP) and the One Anastomosis Gastric Bypass (OAGB) can be seen by comparing the two diagrams opposite. It is clear that in the case of the OAGB there is only one anastomosis, whereas in the RYGBP there are *two* – an upper and a lower.
Because of this the OAGB can be done in less time than the RYGBP and – at least theoretically – with fewer early complications.

A 5-Year Follow-up in Children and Adolescents Undergoing One-Anastomosis Gastric Bypass (OAGB) at a European IFSO Excellence Center (EAC-BS).

- A retrospective review of morbidly obese patients between 13 and 19 years, undergoing a one-anastomosis gastric bypass (OAGB) between 2004 and 2012
  Results:
- A total of 39 patients were included, 8 males (20.5%) and 31 females (79.5%), with a mean age of 17.8. Mean preoperative weight was 114.3 and mean BMI 42.2.
- Preoperative comorbidities include type 2 diabetes mellitus (T2DM) in 7.9% of the patients, hypertension in 10.3%, and dyslipidemia in 23.1%.
- Five years after surgery, mean BMI was 25.9 and total weight loss 32.1.

- Remission rate of T2DM, hypertension and dyslipidemia was 100%.
- All the patients received multivitamin and vitamin D supplementation. Anemia secondary to iron deficiency occurred in one female, requiring intravenous iron supplementation for 1 year and later on oral supplementation (Carbajo, et al., 2019).

Trending Weight Loss Patterns in Obese and Super Obese Adolescents: Does Laparoscopic Sleeve Gastrectomy Provide Equivalent Outcomes in both Groups?

- We evaluated 57 adolescents who underwent laparoscopic sleeve gastrectomy from 2011 to 2017.
- In the morbidly obese (MO) group, 82% were female
- 52% were male in the super obese (SMO)
- 13/34 patients in the obese group achieved > 60% percent excess body weight loss (%EBWL)
- 3/23 super obese patients achieved > 60% EBWL
- The average BMI in the obese group was 29.8 at 1 year and 41.3 in the super obese group.
- There was good comorbidity resolution (about 70%) in both groups after surgery.
  Conclusion:
- **Comorbidity resolution after sleeve gastrectomy is excellent in the adolescent population irrespective of initial BMI.** Consideration should be given to earlier bariatric intervention in SMO adolescents to facilitate return to near normal BMI (Norain, Arafat, & Burjonrappa, 2019).

Bariatric Surgery in Children: Indications, Types, and Outcomes.

- MBS (metabolic and bariatric surgery) is safe in adolescents and has also demonstrated sustainable long-term weight loss and improvement in obesity-associated comorbidities.
- A recent prospective multi-institutional trial demonstrated BMI reductions of 3.8 (8%) to 15.1 (28%) after 3 years

among adolescents undergoing the three most common MBS procedures.

- MBS is associated with remission of type 2 diabetes, prediabetes, hypertension, dyslipidemia, and abnormal kidney function in 65-95% of patients in the study.
- MBS is currently the most successful strategy for significant and sustained weight loss and improvement of associated comorbidities (Thenappan & Nadler, 2019).

Sexual behaviors, risks, and sexual health outcomes for adolescent females following bariatric surgery.

- Adolescents females with severe obesity are less likely to be sexually active, but those who are sexually active engage in risky sexual behaviors.
- Five academic medical centers over 4 years
- Using a prospective observational controlled design, female adolescents undergoing bariatric surgery n (111), mean age 16.95 yrs, mean BMI 50.99; 63.1% white
  - nonsurgical comparators n (68) mean age 16.18 yrs, mean BMI 46.47; 55.9% white.
  - completed the Sexual Activities and Attitudes Questionnaire at pre-surgery/baseline and 24- and 48-month follow-up, with 83 surgical females (mean BMI 39.27) and 49 nonsurgical females (mean BMI 48.56) participating at 48 months.

Results:

- Greater increase in behaviors conferring risk for sexually transmitted infections (STIs) for surgical females (P = .03).
- Half (50% surgical, 44.2% nonsurgical, P = .48) reported partner condom use at last sexual intercourse.
- The proportion of participants who had ever contracted an STI was similar (18.7% surgical, 14.3% nonsurgical).
- Surgical patients were more likely to report a pregnancy (25.3% surgical, 8.2% nonsurgical, P = .02) and live birth (16 births in 15 surgical, 1 nonsurgical), with 50% of offspring in the surgical cohort born to teen mothers (age ≤19 yrs).

Conclusion:

Bariatric care guidelines and practices for adolescent females must emphasize the risks and consequences of teen or unintended pregnancies, sexual decision-making, dual protection, and STI prevention strategies to optimize health and well-being for the long term (Zeller, et al., 2019).

Early weight loss in adolescents following bariatric surgery predicts weight loss at 12 and 24 months.

- Growing evidence supports the efficacy of pediatric bariatric surgery. The aim was to investigate the association between early weight loss at 3 months with longer-term weight loss at 12 and 24 months in adolescent post-surgery.
- A retrospective chart review of bariatric surgery patients (n = 28) was conducted.

Results:
- Percent of excess weight loss (%EWL) at 3, 12, and 24 months were 33.6%, 55.0 %, and 55.1 %, respectively.
- %EWL at 3 months was positively associated with %EWL at 12 and 24 months ($P < 0.05$).

Conclusion:
These findings demonstrate that majority of weight loss among adolescents occurs within the first postoperative year. Greater %EWL by 3 months post-surgery predicts successful and sustained weight loss over time (Chu, et al., 2019).

Weight Loss Surgery Utilization in Patients Aged 14-25 With Severe Obesity Among Several Healthcare Institutions in the United States.

- To show the prevalence of weight loss surgery (WLS) in 14-25 years old between 2000 and 2017 at several prestigious bariatric programs.
- Using the Shared Health Research Information Network (SHRINE) and Research Patient Data Registry (RPDR), 18,000 of 2.5 million patients had severe obesity (0.7%).
- From a total of 1879 patients with obesity, 404 (21.5) underweight WLS.
- 2.5% at Washington University

- 2.3% at Beth Israel Deaconess Medical Center
- 1.5% at Boston Medical Center
- 0.4% at Boston Children's Hospital.
- **Even though WLS has shown to be the most effective treatment, it has been underutilized** (Campoverde Reyes, Misra, Lee, & Stanford, 2019).

A pilot study of laparoscopic gastric plication in adolescent patients with severe obesity.

- Metabolic and bariatric surgery in adolescents is safe with long-term treatment efficacy. However, less than 0.1% of adolescents meeting criteria undergo surgery.
- Four adolescents enrolled and underwent LGP; two withdrew 90 days postoperatively and two were followed through 36 months.
- Pre-procedure body mass index was 41.7-53.7 with decreases in % change of BMI of 17.5% and 39.7% at 36 months after surgery. There were no major complications.
- Minor improvements in psychological comorbidities were also reported.
- LGP can be safely performed in adolescents with severe obesity and achieves modest weight loss (DeAntonio, et al., 2019)

Pre-surgical Weight Loss Predicts Post-Surgical Weight Loss Trajectories in Adolescents Enrolled in a Bariatric Program.

- Forty-eight adolescent bariatric surgery candidates were enrolled in a lifestyle- and behavior-oriented bariatric program consisting of a 3-month pre-surgical outpatient intervention and a 6-month post-surgical follow-up.
- Mean BMI decreased by 1.82 points during the program's pre-surgical intervention phase.
- Optimal post-surgical results were associated with moderate pre-surgical weight loss.

- Inversely associated with maternal history of obesity, early-life weight loss attempts, and comorbid learning disorders.
- It may be possible to identify sub-populations of adolescents undergoing bariatric surgery at risk of achieving sub-optimal long-term results (Fennig, et al., 2019).

Chapter 40: Bariatric Surgery and Suicide/Depression

Bariatric surgery is great for weight loss but does not resolve all issues.

Risk of Suicide After Long Term Follow-up from Bariatric Surgery

- Bariatric surgery has emerged as the treatment of choice for class III obesity and by current criteria is appropriate for over 5% of the obese US population.
- Several prior studies have documented an excess of suicide deaths post bariatric surgery with most events occurring more than one-year post surgery.
- Lifetime history of mood or anxiety disorder has been associated with a significantly smaller decrease in BMI during the first six months following surgery.
- Medical data following bariatric operations performed on Pennsylvania residents between 1/1/1995 and 12/31/2004 were compared with suicides between 9/1/1996 and 12/28/2006 in Pennsylvania.
- 31 suicides for 16,683 operations, mean age 45, 65% female, 94% white, overall rate 6.6/10,000, 13.7/10,000 men, 5.2/10,000 women. The highest age rate for men was 45-54 years old and under 35 years for women.
- 29% suicides within the first two years following surgery.
- 68% within three years.

- Age and sex-matched suicide rates in the US age 35-64 were 2.4/10,000 men and 0.7/10,000 women.
- It is very likely that suicide deaths were also underestimated because some of the deaths were listed as drug overdose, rather than suicide, on the death certificate.
- Estimating conservatively using the 2004 AHRQ (Agency for Healthcare Research and Quality) rates, if the overall suicide rate of the current study(6.6/10,000 person-years) were applicable to the total US bariatric surgery sample, then there would have been approximately 500 suicide deaths between 2004 and 2010 among those who had bariatric surgery in 2004 (Tindle, et al., 2010).

If bariatric surgery were scrutinized like a medication or a medical device, post-marketing studies would be required and the FDA would track this suicide statistic closely.

Risk of completed suicide after bariatric surgery: a systematic review.

28 studies were included with one study (Tindle study-above) chosen as reference figure for comparison.

- 23,885 people were included, 95 suicides occurred for 190,000 person-years of post-bariatric surgery data.
- The suicide rate was 4.1/10,000.
- The suicide rate in the Tindle and colleague study was 6.6/10,000 patient years. (bariatric reference suicide rate)
- The general suicide rate in Pennsylvania for ages 35-64 years old was 2.4/10,000 men and 0.7/10,000 women.

Conclusion- Bariatric surgery patients show higher suicide rates than the general population (Peterhänsel, Petroff, Klinitzke, Kersting, & Wagner, 2013).

Psychological Aspects of Bariatric Surgery as a Treatment for Obesity

- Does bariatric surgery address underlying psychological conditions that can lead to morbid obesity and the effect on eating behaviour postoperatively?

- Despite undisputed significant weight loss and improvements in comorbidities, current literature suggests persistent disorders in psychological outcomes like depression and body image.

- Reframing bariatric approaches to morbid obesity to incorporate psychological experience postoperatively would facilitate understanding of psychological aspects of bariatric surgery. (Jumbe, Hamlet, & Meyrick, 2017).

The long-term effect of bariatric surgery on depression and anxiety.

- This systematic review assessed the effects of bariatric surgery on long-term reductions ($\geq$ 24 months) in anxiety and depressive symptom severity in morbidly obese ($\geq$ 35 BMI) participants.
- Psych INFO, Google Scholar and PubMed databases were systematically searched for prospective cohort studies.
- We reviewed 2058 articles for eligibility; 14 prospective studies were included in the systematic review.
- 13 studies (93%) reported significant reductions in depressive symptom severity 2-3 years after bariatric surgery.
- there were reductions in overall anxiety symptom severity at $\geq$ 24 months follow-up.
- Pre-operative anxiety or depression scores did not predict outcomes of post-operative BMI.
- Post-surgery weight loss did not predict changes in anxiety symptoms.
- Currently available evidence suggests that bariatric surgery is associated with long-term reductions in anxiety and depressive symptoms (Gill, et al., 2019).

Chapter 41: Weight Loss Balloons

"These are not condoms filled with water and dropped from rooftops."

The **2017** Obesity Surgery article by Alan A. Saber and et et al., **Efficacy of First-Time Intragastric Balloon in Weight Loss: A Systematic Review and Meta-analysis of Randomized Controlled Trials,** looked at 20 random-controlled trials involving 1,195 patients.

- Fifteen studies randomized their patients (835) to either IGB or sham procedure
- 4 studies used behavioral modification for non-IGB patients (310)
- 1 study (50) used pharmacotherapy (Sirbutramine - monoamine reuptake inhibitor-approved 1997, removed 2010) in the control group.
- Earlier studies employed air-filled IGBs (7 studies, 266 patients), while more recent studies used IGBs filled with fluid (water or normal saline) (13 studies, 929 patients).
- The studies were published from 1987 to 2015.
- The age ranged from 18-65 years old and the average BMI at IGB insertion range from 27 to 50.4 kg/m2.
- Most studies showed female predominance.
- Duration of IGB were from 12-24 weeks depending on the study.

Fluid-filled IGBs had a significant favorable effect over air-filled IGBs.

Side-effects that were significant compared to non-IGB controls were flatulence, abdominal fullness, abdominal pain, abdominal discomfort, and gastric ulcer.

Conclusion:

Intragastric balloon, in addition to lifestyle modification, is an effective short-term modality for weight loss. However, there is not sufficient evidence confirming its safety or long-term efficacy (Saber, et al., 2017).

Filling the Void: A Review of Intragastric Balloons for Obesity. (2007)

Endoscopic bariatric therapies are predicted to become much more widely used in North America for obese patients who are not candidates for bariatric surgery. Of all the endoscopic bariatric therapies, intragastric balloons (IGBs) have the greatest amount of clinical experience and published data supporting their use. Three IGBs are FDA approved and are now commercially available in the USA (Orbera, ReShape Duo, and Obalon) with others likely soon to follow. They are generally indicated for patients whose BMI ranges from 30 to 40 mg/kg^2 and who have failed to lose weight with diet and exercise. IGBs have been shown to be safe, effective, and relatively straightforward to place and remove. Accommodative symptoms commonly occur within the initial weeks post-placement; however, major complications are rare. Gastric ulceration can occur in up to 10% of patients, while balloon deflation with migration and bowel obstruction occurs in <1% of patients. The effectiveness of the Orbera and ReShape Duo IGBs ranges from 25 to 50% EWL (excess weight loss) after 6 months of therapy. The use of IGBs is likely to grow dramatically in the USA, and gastroenterologists and endoscopists should be familiar with their indications/contraindications, efficacy, placement/removal, and complications (Laing, Pham, Taylor, & Fang, 2007).

Recent Clinical Results of Endoscopic Bariatric Therapies as an Obesity Intervention.

Chapter 41: Weight Loss Balloons

Despite advances in lifestyle interventions, anti-obesity medications, and metabolic surgery, the issue of health burden due to obesity continues to evolve. Interest in endoscopic bariatric techniques has increased over the years, as they have been shown to be efficacious, reversible, relatively safe, and cost effective. Some endoscopic bariatric devices include gastric space-occupying devices, endoscopic suturing or plication devices, endoluminal devices, and aspiration therapy devices. These techniques offer a therapeutic window for some patients who may otherwise be unable to undergo bariatric surgery. (Bazerbachi, Vargas Valls, & Abu Dayyeh, 2017).

Intragastric balloon outcomes in super-obesity: a 16-year city center hospital series.

- Intragastric balloons represent an endoscopic therapy aimed at achieving weight loss by mechanical induction of satiety.
- Our study aimed to evaluate the use of intragastric balloon therapy alone and before definitive bariatric surgery over a 16-year period.
- A large city academic bariatric center for super-obese patients.

Methods:

- Between January 2000 and February 2016, 207 patients underwent ORBERA intragastric balloon placement at esophagogastroduodenoscopy.

Results:

- 129 female and 78 male patients had a mean age of 44.5 years and a mean BMI of 57.3 kg/m^2. Fifty-eight percent of patients suffered from type 2 diabetes.
- Time from initial or first balloon insertion to definitive surgical therapy ranged between 9 and 13 months.
- Seventy-six patients had intragastric balloon alone, and 131 had intragastric balloon followed by definitive procedure.
- At 60 months postoperatively the intragastric balloon alone with lifestyle changes demonstrated an excess weight loss of 9.04% and BMI drop of 3.8.
- intragastric balloon with gastric banding demonstrated an excess weight loss of 32.9% and BMI drop of 8.9.

371

- Intragastric balloon and definitive stapled (sleeve gastrectomy, Roux-en-Y gastric bypass) procedure demonstrated a BMI drop of 17.6 and an excess weight loss of 52.8%.
- Overall, there were 3 deaths (1.4%), 2 within 10 days due to acute gastric perforation secondary to vomiting and 1 cardiac arrest at 4 weeks postoperatively.

Conclusion:
- Intragastric balloons can offer effective weight loss in selected super-obese patients within a dedicated bariatric center offering multidisciplinary support. Balloon insertion alone offers only short-term weight loss; however, when combined with definitive bariatric surgical approaches, durable weight loss outcomes can be achieved. A strategy of early and continual vigilance for side effects and a low threshold for removal should be implemented. Surgeon and unit experience with intragastric balloons can contribute to "kick starting" successful weight loss as a bridge to definitive therapy in an established bariatric surgical pathway (Ashrafian, et al., 2018).

Evaluating the safety of intragastric balloon: An analysis of the Metabolic and Bariatric Surgery Accreditation and Quality Improvement Program.

- Laparoscopic bariatric surgery (LBS) is effective for severe obesity but is invasive and costly. Intragastric balloons (IGBs) are increasingly popular as an alternative to LBS with modest short-term weight loss. However, IGBs are associated with complications and a comparison of the safety of IGB to LBS is warranted.

Objectives:
- Compare the safety profile of IGB with LBS through analysis of the Metabolic and Bariatric Surgery Accreditation and Quality Improvement Program (MBSAQIP) database.
- The MBSAQIP collects data from 791 bariatric surgery centers in the United States and Canada.

Results:
- A total of 145,408 patients were included, of which 144,627 (99.5%) underwent LBS and 781 (0.5%) underwent IGB

therapy. With one-to-one propensity score matching, 684 pairs of IGB and LBS patients were selected.

- IGB (odds ratio 1.97) was independently predictive of 30-day adverse outcomes. This was due to a significantly higher nonoperative reintervention rate in the IGB cohort (4.2% versus 1.0%, P < .001) from early balloon removal (2.8%).

Conclusion:

In this propensity-matched analysis, **IGBs were associated with a higher adverse event rate than LBS, due to a 4-times higher nonoperative reintervention rate. The utility of IGB as a primary weight loss intervention should be reconsidered due to its poor safety profile compared with LBS** (Dang, et al., 2018).

Life-threatening visceral complications after intragastric balloon insertion: Is the device, the patient or the doctor to blame?

- A retrospective literature review of databases to detect the occurrence of serious complications following insertion of a BIB/ORBERA intragastric balloon for weight loss.
- Use of an intragastric balloon (IGB), has a long history of early enthusiasm and late disappointment, successes and failures.
- The most known and most frequently used IGB is the BIB (Bioenterics Intragastric Balloon), which was first made available in Europe in 1991.
- the same balloon under the trade name ORBERA (Apollo Endosurgery Inc, Austin Texas, United States), was FDA approved in the summer of 2015.
- many published results have revealed an average of between 55.6% and 32.1% loss of excess body weight at 6 months after treatment, or around 25% at 1 year.
- 23% of patients maintained the loss for up to 5 years.
- It is also recommended that the balloon be left in place within the stomach for a maximum of 6 months while the

patient is enrolled in a medically supervised weight loss program and receives proton pump inhibitors (PPIs).

- balloon insertion should be carefully considered in cases of a large hiatus hernia, inflammatory bowel disease, increased risk of upper gastrointestinal bleeding, pregnancy, and uncontrolled psychiatric disease or drug/alcohol abuse. Previous bariatric or gastric surgery is also considered a contraindication, although the absolute contraindication is reserved strictly for partial gastrectomy cases.

- **The relatively recent FDA approval for use of the Orbera IGB in the United States has led to increased reports of deaths in obese individuals with a balloon in their stomach.**

- Gastric perforation was the most frequently described complication among the three complications studied: 22 cases.

- Nine of these 22 cases (40.9%) occurred very early after implantation (2 hours up to 3 days) in patients having a relative contraindication for balloon insertion, i.e. previous gastric or bariatric surgery, which obviously modifies stomach compliance. There were seven patients who previously had fundoplication for hernia repair (two of whom finally died), one who had undergone sleeve gastrectomy and one with a history of severe abdominal and thoracic trauma.

- In the present review, the authors note twenty-two cases of gastric perforation, two cases of esophageal perforation and 10 cases of bowel obstruction. For the gastric perforation the endoscopist was responsible in nine cases, the patient in four, and the balloon itself in nine. For the two cases of esophageal perforation, the endoscopists were responsible, while for the 12 cases of bowel obstruction, the patient was responsible for seven and the device for the other five cases.

- **an intact gastric wall is initially considered a crucial prerequisite for balloon placement to avoid tissue ischemia from balloon wall pressure.** Mechanical friction and chemical degradation from gastric acid may break it down, with the PPIs acting prophylactically.

Chapter 41: Weight Loss Balloons

- Individual doctors or even institutions without experience, accreditation or the ability to resolve obesity-related or bariatric surgery-related complications must not undertake such procedures.

- Apollo manufacturers in the United States, since FDA approval, report about 5000 balloons sold between July 2015 and August 2017; the American Society for Metabolic and Bariatric Surgery reports 5744 balloons had been inserted in 2016, while facilities accredited to perform the procedure have placed only 1003 of the devices. Who has placed the other 4741 devices in the United States?

- Patient noncompliance issues include; not taking PPIs, excess consumption of cola and not having balloon removed by 6 months.

- **When a "balloon" patient comes to an emergency department complaining of severe abdominal pain, gastric perforation needs to be ruled out. Should the suspicion arise, the patient should not be allowed to leave without a computed tomography scan, and this makes the difference.**

- It is interesting to refer to a very old study (1998–2001). They reported that 49 of 176 balloons (27.8%) unexpectedly evacuated spontaneously, during vomiting in four patients and in the stools in 45, all cases but two occurring after the theoretical date of the 6-month lifespan of the balloon.

- Nowadays, according to Apollo Endosurgery reports, more than 277,000 balloons have been implanted worldwide, mainly in Brazil, Mexico, and Europe–fewer in Asia. In terms of numbers only, the percentages of serious complications reported are almost nil
The American Society of Gastrointestinal Endoscopy's latest published directives state "...training and skill acquisition with endoscopic bariatric techniques and technologies is mandatory before clinical application is undertaken, and should include didactic as well as hands-on practical education". And, furthermore, "...importantly, any practitioner who is interested in performing an endoscopic bariatric procedure should also be educated in the clinical management of obese patients," that means, have the ability

375

to resolve complications themselves (Stavrou, Tsaousi, & Kotzampassi, 2019).

Emerging Non-Surgical Gastric Devices Gain Approval for Weight Management

- FDA Approves TransPyloric Shuttle Nonsurgical Device for Obesity
- The Food and Drug Administration (FDA) approved the TransPyloric Shuttle (TPS), an intragastric device that when implanted endoscopically was shown to be safe and effective in promoting significant weight reduction in individuals with obesity[1,2].
- Gaining regulatory clearance was supported by results of a nine site, pivotal 2:1 randomized trial.[3] The ENDObesity II study—a double-blind, sham-controlled trial—enrolled 302 obese patients, median age: 43 years who were followed for one year.[3]
- "The patients in the treatment group achieved a 9.5% weight loss as compared with 2.8% in the sham group," said principal investigator, Richard I. Rothstein, MD.
- This pivotal study evolved from the ENDObesity I study that followed 20 patients for six months.4 Many patients were still losing weight when the device was removed, so the trial was designed to look at patients' experience using the device for twice as long.
- "The study cohort was 93% female; 72% Caucasian, 18% African American, 11% other nationalities.
- "The TPS is inserted endoscopically and assembled in the stomach, where it moves into position across the pyloric outlet and intermittently blocks the free flow of food into the intestine.
- There are currently four first-generation intragastric devices approved for use: two water filled balloons (Orbera and Reshape), one gas filled balloon (Obalon) and an aspiration device (Aspire Assist). The TPS differs from inflatable intragastric balloons in that it is made of silicone and is substantially smaller and lighter than the water-filled gastric balloon devices, obviating some of the discomfort experienced in patients who have the bulkier devices.

- More significantly, 39.5% of people treated with TPS lost at least 10% or more weight (compared to 14% with sham; P = .0001).
- Only 2.8% of patients experienced serious adverse events (one patient each with esophageal rupture, upper abdominal pain, gastric ulcer, vomiting, and gastric obstruction), which all resolved without sequelae.
- About 20% of participants exited the study which is in sync with findings from other device studies.
- "We see significant advantages in the use of endoscopic procedures for weight loss, which can mimic the mechanisms and physiologic effects of bariatric surgical procedures but are non-invasive and reversible," Dr. Rothstein told *EndocrineWeb*. "Consider that only ~6% of those who are obese receive treatment of their condition, with only 1% of those eligible for a gastric bypass procedure receiving it, representing a major, as yet, unmet need for ~94% of individuals with obesity. "
- "At present, typically none of the FDA-approved intragastric devices are reimbursed through health insurance; It is mainly a self-pay model much the same as cosmetic surgery procedures," said Dr. Rothstein (Godfrey, Rothstein, & Gonzalez-Campoy, 2019).

Gelesis Granted FDA Clearance to Market PLENITY for Weight Loss

- Gelesis, a biotechnology company developing first-in-class oral, non-systemic, superabsorbent hydrogel device cleared to treat obesity received FDA clearance for PLENITY (Gelesis100).
- PLENITY—taken in capsule form with water before lunch and dinner— is made by cross-linking cellulose and citric acid to form a three-dimensional hydrogel matrix. This new prescription-only option has no limitation on the length of its use for weight management.
- PLENTIY works by releases thousands of non-aggregating particles that when combined with water in the stomach creating small gel particles with firmness similar in consistency to vegetables but with no caloric value.[4] These

particles increase in volume in the stomach and small intestine promoting a feeling of fullness that promises to achieve weight loss.

- In the multicenter, double-blinded, placebo-controlled pivotal trial— Gelesis Loss Of Weight (GLOW)—was initiated to assess for a change in body weight among 436 adults with overweight or obesity (BMI $\geq$ 27 and $\leq$ 40 kg/m2) after six months of treatment with PLENITY.[4]

- The study had two primary endpoints: at least 35% of patients achieving $\geq$ 5% weight loss and placebo-adjusted weight loss with a super-superiority margin of 3%.

- 59% of adults in the treatment group achieving weight loss of at least 5%. The study did not meet the 3% super-superiority endpoint. PLENITY-treated individuals had twice the odds of achieving at least 5% weight loss vs. placebo

- In addition, 26% of the adults who completed the 6-month study achieved an average of about 14% weight loss, which was around 30 pounds.[4]

- The overall incidence of adverse events (AEs) in the treatment group was similar to placebo.

- Overall, this nonstimulant, non-systemic weight management treatment has been shown in clinical studies to be effective, safe and well-tolerated.[4]

- Gelesis plans to initiate a targeted US launch of PLENITY in the second half of 2019 and anticipates PLENITY will be broadly available by prescription in 2020 (Gelesis, 2019).

Chapter 42: Fasting

Fasting has been shown to prolong lifespan and promotes great metabolic benefits. There are many ways to fast. Fasting requires a lot of discipline to deal with the "hunger" complaint intermittently.

Flipping the Metabolic Switch: Understanding and Applying Health Benefits of Fasting

- Calorie restriction (CR), has consistently been found to produce reductions in body weight and extend healthy life span across a variety of species, including non-human primates.
- Studies conducted in overweight humans indicate short-term CR (6-months) can significantly improve several cardiovascular risk factors, insulin-sensitivity, and mitochondrial function.
- The vast majority of humans have significant difficulty sustaining daily CR for long periods of time.
- In recent years, intermittent fasting (IF) has gained popularity as an alternative to continuous CR and has shown promise in delivering similar benefits in terms of weight loss and cardiometabolic health (Anton, et al., 2018).

Definition of terms used to describe different types of eating patterns in this review.

- **Intermittent Fasting (IF)** - fasting for varying periods of time, typically for 12 hours or longer.
- **Calorie Restriction (CR)** - a continuous reduction in caloric intake without malnutrition.

- **Time Restricted Feeding (TRF)** - restricting food intake to specific time periods of the day, typically between an 8 – 12 hours each day.
- **Alternate Day Fasting (ADF)** - consuming no calories on fasting days and alternating fasting days with a day of unrestricted food intake or "feast" day.
- **Alternate Day Modified Fasting (ADMF)** - consuming less than 25% of baseline energy needs on "fasting" days, alternated with a day of unrestricted food intake or "feast" day.
- **Periodic Fasting (PF)** - consists of fasting only 1 or 2 days/week and consuming food ad libitum on 5 to 6 days per week.
- Placing time restrictions on feeding has been shown to have broad systemic effects and trigger similar biological pathways as caloric restriction.
- Intermittent fasting regimens improves cardio-metabolic risk factors (such as insulin resistance, dyslipidemia and inflammation cytokines), decrease visceral fat mass, and produce similar levels of weight loss as CR regimens.
- One key mechanism responsible for many of these beneficial effects appears to be "flipping" of the metabolic switch.
- We define the metabolic switch as the body's preferential shift from utilization of glucose from glycogenolysis to fatty acids and fatty acid-derived ketones. The reason we use the word 'preferential' is because there is now a growing body of research to indicate ketones are the preferred fuel for both the brain and body during periods of fasting and extended exercise.
- This switch represents a shift from lipid synthesis and fat storage to mobilization of fat in the form of free fatty acids (FFAs) and fatty-acid derived ketones.
- For this reason, many experts have suggested IF regimens may have potential in the treatment of obesity and related metabolic conditions, including metabolic syndrome and type 2 diabetes.

- The metabolic switch typically occurs between 12 to 36 hours after cessation of food consumption depending on the liver glycogen content at the beginning of the fast.
- Simultaneously, other cell types may also begin generating ketones, with astrocytes in the brain being one notable example. FFAs are transported into hepatocytes where they are metabolized by β-oxidation to produce the ketones β-OHB and acetoacetate, which may in turn induce mitochondrial biogenesis.
- The ketones are transported in high amounts into cells with high metabolic activity (muscle cells and neurons) to generate ATP. Through these physiological processes, ketones serve as an energy source to sustain the function of muscle and brain cells during fasting and extended periods of physical exertion/exercise.
- When the metabolic switch is flipped, retention of lean mass is increased.
- Profiles of circulating glucose and ketone levels over 48 hours in individuals with a typical American eating pattern or two different IF eating patterns.
- In individuals who consume three meals plus snacks every day the metabolic switch is never 'flipped', and their ketone levels remain very low, and the area under the curve for glucose levels is high compared to individuals on an IF eating pattern.

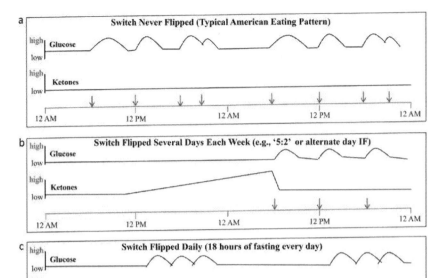

(b) In this example, the person fasted completely on the first day and then at three separate meals on the subsequent day. On the fasting day ketones are progressively elevated and glucose levels remain low, whereas on the eating day ketones remain low and glucose levels are elevated during and for several hours following meal consumption.

(c) In this example the person consumes all of their food within a 6-hour time window every day. Thus, the metabolic switch is flipped on following 12 hours of fasting and remains on for approximately six hours each day, until food is consumed after approximately 18 hours of fasting.

(Modified from Mattson et al 2016).

Fasting in Humans: Historical Perspective

- Historically, fasting has been used as both a religious and a medical practice for thousands of years.
- For example, Benjamin Franklin has been quoted as saying "The best of all medicines is resting and fasting."

Chapter 42: Fasting

- Mark Twain wrote "A little starvation can really do more for the average sick man than can the best medicines and the best doctors. I do not mean a restricted diet; I mean total abstention from food for one or two days."
- These potential benefits, however, must be weighed against potential risks as there have also been numerous adverse effects reported in the medical literature from "therapeutic fasting."
- These include: nausea and vomiting, edema, alopecia and motor neuropathy, hyperuricemia and urate nephropathy, irregular menses, abnormal liver function tests and decreased bone density, thiamine deficiency and Wernicke's encephalopathy, and mild metabolic acidosis. Additionally, several deaths have been reported during or immediately following therapeutic fasting with the etiologies including lactic acidosis, small bowel obstruction, renal failure, and cardiac arrhythmias.
- The adverse events described above have only occurred during or following extended fasts of several weeks or more, and have not been reported in trials of shorter more frequent fasts such as the '5:2' diet, which consists of eating no more than 500 calories on two days per week ADF (alternate day fast) diets, or IF (intermittent fasting) diets.

Fasting Benefits

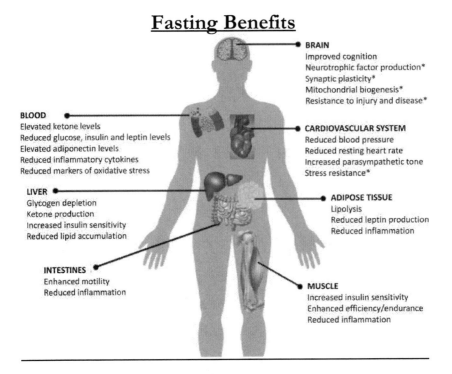

BRAIN
Improved cognition
Neurotrophic factor production*
Synaptic plasticity*
Mitochondrial biogenesis*
Resistance to injury and disease*

BLOOD
Elevated ketone levels
Reduced glucose, insulin and leptin levels
Elevated adiponectin levels
Reduced inflammatory cytokines
Reduced markers of oxidative stress

CARDIOVASCULAR SYSTEM
Reduced blood pressure
Reduced resting heart rate
Increased parasympathetic tone
Stress resistance*

LIVER
Glycogen depletion
Ketone production
Increased insulin sensitivity
Reduced lipid accumulation

ADIPOSE TISSUE
Lipolysis
Reduced leptin production
Reduced inflammation

INTESTINES
Enhanced motility
Reduced inflammation

MUSCLE
Increased insulin sensitivity
Enhanced efficiency/endurance
Reduced inflammation

Avoiding holiday seasonal weight gain with nutrient-supported intermittent energy restriction: a pilot study.

- This pilot randomised controlled study evaluated the effects of a modified 5:2 fast nutrition programme to prevent weight gain in healthy overweight adults during the 6-week winter holiday period between Thanksgiving and New Year.

- For 52 d, twenty-two overweight adults (mean age 41·0 years, BMI 27·3 kg/m²) were assigned to either the nutrition programme (*n* 10; two fasting days of 730 kcal/d of balanced shake and dietary supplements to support weight management efforts, followed by 5 d of habitual diet) or a control group (*n* 12; habitual diet).

- A significant weight loss 1.3 kg (2.2 lbs) from baseline was observed in the nutrition programme. Body weight did not significantly change in the control group. Overall compliance rate was 98 % and no severe adverse events were reported.

- These preliminary findings suggest that this intermittent energy restriction intervention might
support weight management efforts and help promote metabolic health during the winter holiday season (Hirsh, Pons, Joval, & Swick, 2019).

I was surprised that the weight loss was so small. I would have been personally disappointed if I followed this. The control group maintained the same weight despite the holiday season showing us the power of being tracked.

Does eating less make you live longer and better? An update on calorie restriction

According to several authors, a successful approach to healthy aging should be able to counteract the following nine cellular markers of aging:

- telomere erosion
- epigenetic alterations
- stem cells depletion
- cellular senescence
- mitochondrial dysfunction-efficiency decreases and conservation of energy worsens
- genomic instability -mistakes of DNA increase and the ability to repair lessens with age
- proteostasis imbalance – the stability of proteins to degradation lessens with age
- impaired nutrient sensing
- abnormal intercellular communication.

As we age chemical reactions become less efficient, more mistakes occur, repair abilities decline, and more energy and effort are needed to maintain the status quo. Anti-inflammation systems decrease, and inflammatory mediators increase. Eventually the scales change from an anabolic product to a more progressively catabolic system till the system fails. We can slow down this process by exercise, and calorie restriction superimposed hopefully by favorable genetics.

To date, the most robust intervention efficient in warding off the aforementioned cellular markers of aging is calorie restriction (CR) that involves the administration of a well-balanced, nutrient-dense diet that reduces calorie intake by 20%–40%. CR prevents or delays the onset of various age-related diseases such as obesity, type-2 diabetes, neurodegeneration, cardiomyopathy, and cancer.

With aging, the DNA repair capacity decreases causing genome instability. CR has a positive effect on the DNA repair and telomere machinery.

Another mark of cellular aging is related to the crucial functional role performed by proteins inside cells where these molecules integrate all physiological pathways. Therefore, the stability of proteins (proteostasis) indicates the protection of protein structure and function, against environmental and internal stressors, operated by the cell. Vulnerability in proteostasis correlates with age-related changes and longevity rates among species.

Other two hallmarks among CR effects are reduction of oxidative damage and modulation of mitochondrial activity. This means that the diet-reduced calorie intake increases metabolic efficiency and protects against cellular damage and remodeling mechanisms, thereby reducing less efficient metabolism and synthetic pathways. It seems that an evolutionarily conserved response aiming to avoid useless expenditure of energy and to recycle structures for the organisms' survival is activated by CR.

A relevant increase in ROS (reactive oxygen species) level, reduction in antioxidant defenses, and appearance of mitochondrial dysfunction, implying accumulation of oxidative damage to mitochondrial DNA, proteins, and lipids, are usually associated with aging.

The studies about genes influencing lifespan led to the conclusion that human longevity can be influenced by about 25% by genetic factors.

Aging is also characterized by a condition of relevant inflammation, demonstrated by the age-associated rise of several pro-inflammatory factors including TNF-α, interferon-γ, IL-1β, and IL-18. Furthermore, induction of such chronic inflammation during aging can be favored by age-related elevation of oxidative stress that also appears to raise the incidence of age-related diseases. Another feature of aging with pathological consequences is damage accumulated with age leading to chronic inflammation. Such chronic inflammation associated with aging has been identified by the new idea of "inflammaging."

Future applications
Overall, the results from multiple studies show that both reduced calories intake (CR) and the ratio between macronutrients, namely the protein to carbohydrates ratio, positively impact lifespan. A high protein diet in old persons might help people to better cope with a large number of age-related dysfunctions and diseases (Picca, Pesce, & Lezza, 2017).

Chapter 43: "Shut your mouth"

Different ideas and techniques have been tried over time to help people lose weight. The dangers of morbid obesity have been known for hundreds of years. Wiring the jaw has been tried.

Enforced Intermaxillary Fixation (IMF) as a Treatment of Obesity.

Intermaxillary fixation (IMF) using metal cap splints and various linkages was tried in a group of 11 patients as a treatment for obesity. The full cap splints for each dental arch, linked and enforced by special rigid locking devices, proved to be a reliable technique of IMF for periods of up to 3 months. Thereafter, the majority of the patients attempted interference with the IMF linkage or detached the splints.

Eight patients gained weight after removal of the IMF. Two patients were successful in weight stabilization after 2-14 kg weight loss during IMF.

It was concluded that by rigidly enforced IMF for 3 months or longer was an unsuitable treatment mode for the majority of obese patients but could be used as a preparation for other forms of bariatric surgery (Cannel, 1992).

Jaw wiring in the treatment of morbid obesity.

Fourteen patients with intractable morbid obesity had maxillomandibular fixation (MMF) applied in an effort to control their obesity. 10 patients were considered poor risk candidates for bariatric surgery. MMF was applied with the aim of reducing the obesity to a level where a surgical gastric restrictive bariatric procedure could be safely carried out. Eight of the fourteen patients had been rejected for bariatric surgery and two were edentulous. Five had successful weight loss in 16 to 40 weeks (mean percentage overweight lost 84.8, range 39-150) and underwent a gastric restrictive procedure. All five patients have had continuous weight loss after bariatric surgery.

Two patients requested removal of MMF 1 and 2 weeks after application. Three patients, who were candidates for surgery, after successful weight loss over periods from 12 to 28 weeks (mean percentage of overweight lost 45, range 38-50) decided not to proceed with surgical control. All have subsequently regained the lost weight.

Four patients, who had had a previously successful gastric restrictive procedure followed by weight loss, requested MMF in an effort to lose further weight. Over periods from 8 to 16 weeks three of the four had further weight loss (mean percentage of overweight lost 18.3, range 5-30). After removal of MMF all four patients regained some weight. One patient had maintained weight lost with MMF (Ramsey-Stewart & Martin, 1985).

Jaw wiring in treatment of obesity.

17 patients with severe obesity underwent jaw wiring. There were no major complications and patients tolerated the procedure and subsequent minor inconveniences. All patients lost weight at a rate (median 3-25 kg in six months) comparable with that of intestinal bypass surgery and one achieved and maintained her ideal weight. Two-thirds of the patients, however, regained some weight after the wires were removed. Jaw wiring is a simple effective procedure which can be carried out in most hospitals, and has a place in an integrated approach to obesity (Rodgers, et al., 1977).

Chapter 43: "Shut your mouth"

Treatment of massive obesity by prolonged jaw immobilization for edentulous patients.

Twenty massively obese patients who were edentulous in one or both jaws were treated by prolonged jaw immobilization. Dentures were secured under general anaesthesia to the edentulous jaws by various direct wiring methods and the jaws immobilized by interdental wires, where teeth were present, and intermaxillary wires. The wired-in dentures were generally well tolerated with minimal mucosal reaction but with a high incidence of infection around the attachment wires. Patients edentulous in one jaw alone, (11 maxilla, two mandible), managed well and 11 achieved a satisfactory weight loss. The seven patients edentulous in both jaws had considerable difficulty with pain and infection, three having the fixation appliances removed in the immediate post-operative period and only one achieved a satisfactory weight loss.

Thus, prolonged jaw immobilization is an effective means of treating massively obese patients if they are edentulous in one jaw alone but less so if they are completely edentulous (Goss, 1980)

Chapter 44: Eating Disorders

Eating disorders are like Rodney Dangerfield; "they get no respect"

Here are simple descriptions of some eating disorders.

- **Anorexia Nervosa Disorder** - intense fear of gaining weight. BMI underweight, distorted body image. 90% are females age 15-19 years old. Common eating disorder.
- **Binge Eating Disorder (BED)** - eating behavior distresses person, feels shameful, disgusted. Consumes larger amount of food than expected in 2 hours. Frequency is at least 2 days per week for 6 months. Common eating disorder.
- **Bulimia Nervosa Disorder** - binge eating at least once per week for three consecutive months. Purging, vomiting, laxative abuse, diuretic abuse, enemas, obsessive exercise. Shops weight loss clinics. Sexual abuse 25%, females 90%. Majority have normal weight, metabolic alkalosis. Common eating disorder. SSRI's effective.
- **Night Eating Syndrome (NES)** - combination eating disorder, sleep order, mood disorder. Idea that food is needed to sleep. Consumes 25-50% daily calories after evening meal. Up to 40% engage in binge eating. Highly responsive to sertraline (Zoloft).
- **Nocturnal Sleep Eating Disorder** - sleep disorder not eating disorder. Circadian rhythm disorder. Semiconscious state or sleep walking. Involuntary eating while asleep, consumption of peculiar, inedible, sometimes toxic material. May be associated with hypnotics (i.e. Ambien)

Addictive Eating and Its Relation to Physical Activity and Sleep Behavior

- This study aims to investigate the relationship between food addiction with physical activity and sleep behavior.
- Australian adults were invited to complete an online survey.
- The sample comprised 1344 individuals with a mean age of 39.8, of which 75.7% were female.
- Twenty-two percent of the sample met the criteria for a diagnosis of food addiction as per the Yale Food Addiction Scale (YFAS 2.0) criteria, consisting of 0.7% with a "mild" addiction, 2.6% "moderate", and 18.9% classified as having a "severe" food addiction.
- Food-addicted individuals had significantly less physical activity (1.8 less occasions walking/week, 32 min less walking/week, 58 min less moderate to vigorous physical activity /week; $p < 0.05$), sitting for longer on weekends (83 min more on weekends/week; $p < 0.001$), poorer-quality sleep (snore, fall asleep while driving, and more days of daytime falling asleep; $p < 0.05$) compared to non-food-addicted individuals (Li, Pursey, Duncan, & Burrows, 2018).

Food addiction: a valid concept?

Arguments against food addiction (Paul C. Fletcher)
- The application of the term "food addiction" in humans is based on a set of features, held to resemble substance addictions. It carries the claim that this resemblance occurs because certain foods have effects on the brain comparable to those of addictive drugs.
- The central features of substance addiction do not plausibly translate to food and consumption.
- The assertion that foods have pharmacological effects on the brain demands strong and convincing evidence, which has not been found.
- Food addiction, as an explanation for the often-distressing cravings, loss of control, and overconsumption experienced by many, particularly in relation to highly palatable foods, has been with us for many years.

Chapter 44: Eating Disorders

- While one study shows that 88% meeting criteria for food addiction are obese, it is important to note that food addiction is defined by behavioral patterns and experiences relating to eating rather than by weight status.

- The addictive substance remains undiscovered—a problem that cannot be considered trivial. The model rests on a central assertion that either some category of foods, or some specific nutrients, exert a direct effect on the brain, enacting changes that ultimately hijack reward-related behaviors. Some have argued that sugar is the culprit though, as a whole, the evidence for sugar addiction remains deeply unconvincing.

- The current view is that food addiction is distinct even from the eating disorder that perhaps it most resembles: binge-eating disorder.

- The overlap between food addiction and binge-eating disorder is striking. One conclusion from this might be that food addiction is not distinct from the symptom of binge eating. For example, eating increased amounts of food and obtaining less pleasure from eating is taken as evidence of tolerance, while anxiety, dysphoria, and unspecified "physical symptoms" during abstinence from certain foods are viewed as withdrawal symptoms.

- Reviewing the literature from 5 years ago, functional magnetic resonance imaging and positron-emission tomography studies should not be used as a basis for making claims about food addiction. Reviewing the field now, there is no more support for food addiction.

- A person prone to binges or overeating in general feels powerful cravings to consume; they often see little option but to succumb to these cravings, and this capitulation is a matter of shame and guilt. The language of addiction- "this is a biological drive that I alone cannot control"—fits well with this subjective experience, and it brings a means of communicating distress and helplessness. The science narrative that is offered that food, like a drug, has affected a person's brain such that their inhibitory control centers do not work properly, and their reward centers are malfunctioning, is simple and readily accepted.

Arguments in favor of food addiction (Paul J. Kenny)
"My drug of choice is food. I use food for the same reasons an addict uses drugs: to comfort, to soothe, to ease stress."
—Oprah Winfrey

- Some overweight individuals struggle to control their food intake even when their health and well-being depend on it in a manner that is analogous or even homologous to those affected by SUD (substance use disorder) who struggle to control their drug use. Consequently, a history of overconsumption of energy-dense palatable food can remodel brain motivation circuits in a manner that renders some overweight individuals persistently vulnerable to the desirable properties of such food, which negatively impacts their health and well-being.

- Food addiction, as currently diagnosed using the YFAS (Yale Food Addictive Scale- gold standard) and related scales, is considered distinct from obesity.

- Three of the most important clinical features of SUDs are feelings of deprivation when the substance is withheld, a propensity to relapse during periods of abstinence, and consumption that persists despite awareness of negative health, social, financial, or other consequences. Hence, overweight individuals who are unable to exert control over their behavior, despite awareness of the negative consequences, demonstrate the same core failure to control consumption as those suffering from SUDs.

- There is now a preponderance of human functional imaging data showing that energy-dense palatable food can stimulate changes in the activity of many of the same brain structures and circuits known to be impacted by drugs of abuse. For example, palatable food stimulates reward-relevant activity in the striatum. In addition to the striatum, the activity of other brain areas thought to play an important role in drug addiction, such as prefrontal cortical regions and the amygdala, is similarly altered by consumption of palatable food and development of obesity.

- Currently, all that can be concluded from these imaging studies is that palatable food and drugs of abuse can impact the function of similar regions of the brain. These findings suggest that common underlying brain processes are likely involved in overeating and drug use.

- Another argument often used against the notion of a food-directed use disorder is the question of which ingredient in food is the responsible agent. The underlying assumption here is that only those food items that contain this agent will support addiction-relevant behaviors. Recently, arguments have been made for the involvement of refined sugars. My own view is that it is not necessarily a single macronutrient but rather the combinations of macronutrients that when combined alter brain motivation circuits. For example, a recent study in humans found that blended food had a greater impact on the activity on brain areas involved in reward than the single-nutrient food items and may shift dietary preferences toward these highly rewarding, calorie-laden options.

- Addiction should not be viewed as a single unitary disorder, but as a constellation of related syndromes that share similar but not entirely overlapping brain and behavior abnormalities, the most conspicuous of which is a failure to control consumption.

- For example, cocaine use disorder is characterized by cycles of binge consumption interspersed by periods of abstinence. By contrast, tobacco use disorder is characterized by remarkably stable and highly regular patterns of daily use, with no overt signs of intoxication, and binge-like consumption not a general feature of the habit. It is difficult to argue that a tobacco smoker is any less "addicted" than someone who binges on cocaine. Large-scale genome-wide association studies (GWAS) in humans are beginning to identify genetic variants that are robustly associated with complex traits or phenotypes, such as cannabis use, problematic alcohol use, levels of tobacco smoking, and measures of adiposity. Ultimately, drug addiction could provide a useful model for aspects of food overconsumption, just as consumption of foods and other natural rewards serves a useful purpose to better understand drug addiction (Fletcher & Kenny, 2018).

Food Addiction in Sleeve Gastrectomy Patients with Loss-of-Control Eating.

- Food addiction and binge eating share overlapping and non-overlapping features; the presence of both may represent a more severe obesity subgroup.
- Loss-of-control (LOC) eating, a key marker of binge eating, is one of the few consistent predictors of suboptimal weight outcomes post-bariatric surgery.
- This study examined whether co-occurring LOC eating and food addiction represent a more severe variant post-bariatric surgery.
- One hundred thirty-one adults sought treatment for weight/eating concerns approximately 6 months post-sleeve gastrectomy surgery.
Conclusion:
- **17.6% of post-operative patients with LOC eating met food addiction criteria on the YFAS (Yale Food Addiction Scale).**
- Co-occurrence of LOC and food addiction following sleeve gastrectomy signals a more severe subgroup with elevated eating disorder psychopathology, problematic eating behaviors, greater depressive symptoms, and diminished functioning (Ivesaj, Wiedermann, Lawson, & Grilo, 2019).

Food addiction and preoperative weight loss achievement in patients seeking bariatric surgery.

- Evidence suggests that food addiction (FA) is prevalent among individuals with obesity seeking bariatric surgery (BS), but there is no evidence about whether FA is a predictor of weight loss (WL). We aimed to analyze the prevalence of FA in patients with obesity seeking BS and to examine whether FA could predict WL before surgery.
- The study included 110 patients with obesity.
- The prevalence of food addiction was 26.4%. Those who met YFAS 2.0 criteria showed less weight loss after dietary intervention.
- **Food addiction is prevalent with obesity** (Guerrero Pérez, et al., 2018).

Effects of Lisdexamfetamine Dimesylate on Functional Impairment Measured on the Sheehan Disability Scale in Adults with Moderate-to-severe Binge Eating Disorder

- *Diagnostic and Statistical Manual of Mental Disorders, Fifth Edition* (DSM-5) recognizes binge eating disorder (BED) as a distinct eating disorder. **Lisdexamfetamine Dimesylate is Vyvanse.**

- The short-term efficacy, safety, and tolerability of lisdexamfetamine dimesylate (LDX) in adults with moderate-to-severe BED have been examined in two placebo (PBO)-controlled, double-blind, Phase III studies.

- **Participant disposition and demographics.** 383 participants were randomized in Study 1 (PBO, n=191 and LDX, n=192) and 390 participants were randomized in Study 2 (PBO, n=195 and LDX, n=195). Eligible participants were 18 to 55 years of age.

- Dose-optimized LDX (50mg and 70mg) produced statistically greater reductions in binge-eating days per week than did placebo.

- Similarly, LDX (50mg and 70mg) demonstrated efficacy versus placebo in a Phase II, double-blind, fixed-dose study in adults with moderate-to-severe BED, as demonstrated by greater decreases in binge-eating days per week.

- In these short-term studies, the safety and tolerability profile of LDX was similar to its established safety profile for the treatment of attention deficit hyperactivity disorder (ADHD).

- Treatment-emergent adverse events reported by 10 percent or more of participants were dry mouth, decreased appetite, insomnia, and headache.

- Across all three short-term BED studies, observed small increases in blood pressure and heart rate were also consistent with the established safety profile of LDX for ADHD (Sheehan, et al., 2018).

Lisdexamfetamine: chemistry, pharmacodynamics, pharmacokinetics, and clinical efficacy, safety, and tolerability in the treatment of binge eating disorder.

- The indications for lisdexamfetamine (LDX), a central nervous system stimulant, were recently expanded to include treatment of moderate to severe binge eating disorder (BED).

- Expert opinion: LDX is the first medication with United States Food and Drug Administration approval for the treatment of BED. It is an inactive prodrug of d-amphetamine that extends the half-life of d-amphetamine to allow for once daily dosing.

- D-amphetamine acts primarily to increase the concentrations of synaptic dopamine and norepinephrine.

- **In clinical trials, LDX demonstrated statistical and clinical superiority over placebo in reducing binge eating days per week at doses of 50 and 70 mg daily.** Commonly reported side effects of LDX include dry mouth, insomnia, weight loss, and headache, and its use should be avoided in patients with known structural cardiac abnormalities, cardiomyopathy, serious heart arrhythmia or coronary artery disease. As with all CNS stimulants, risk of abuse needs to be assessed prior to prescribing (Ward & Citrome, 2018).

Safety of pharmacotherapy options for bulimia nervosa and binge eating disorder

- Eating disorders, such as binge eating disorder (BED), bulimia nervosa (BN) and anorexia nervosa (AN), are often stigmatized as a lifestyle choice and their pathologies are frequently trivialized.

- However, one large-scale population-based study, which is often cited, estimates the prevalence to be 0.6% for AN, 1.0% for BN, and 2.8% for BED. Women are more at risk and midlife women have an estimated lifetime prevalence of 15.3% for an eating disorder.

- Cognitive behavioral therapy (CBT), as well as intrapersonal therapy (IPT), are considered standard effective therapies for eating disorders.

- For AN, there is strong evidence to suggest that the addition of fluoxetine or other selective serotonin reuptake inhibitor (SSRI) antidepressants to a CBT regimen does not provide an additional therapeutic benefit beyond CBT.
- Currently, there is no FDA-approved medication for the treatment of AN.

This review includes the safety evaluation of the FDA-approved treatments for BN and BED, fluoxetine (Prozac) and lisdexamfetamine (Vyvanse), respectively.

- Fluoxetine (Prozac) was FDA approved for the treatment of major depressive disorder in 1987 and is also approved for obsessive compulsive disorder and acute treatment of panic disorder with or without agoraphobia. Fluoxetine was approved for acute treatment and maintenance of BN in 1994.
- The effectiveness of fluoxetine to treat BN has been determined by several randomized placebo-controlled studies.
- A multi-center study conducted by Fluoxetine Bulimia Nervosa Collaborative Study Group of BN women (n = 387) assessed bingeing and vomiting frequency following an 8-week course of fluoxetine (20 mg/day and 60 mg/day) compared with placebo. Fluoxetine (60 mg/day) effectively reduced binge eating and vomiting episodes per week for the first 7 weeks. From the last observation carried forward analysis, fluoxetine (60 mg/day) reduced binge eating episodes by 67% and vomiting episodes by 56% from pretreatment, whereas placebo resulted in a 33% reduction in binge eating and 5% reduction in vomiting episodes. The lower dose fluoxetine (20 mg/day) only produced a significant reduction in vomiting, which was a 26% reduction from pretreatment.
- Another multi-center study by Goldstein and colleagues evaluated fluoxetine (60 mg/day) compared with placebo over a 16-week time period in BN subjects (n= 398; 96.2% women). The 16-week fluoxetine demonstrated a significant 50% decrease in binge eating and vomiting episodes from pretreatment.
- The long-term maintenance of controlling BN relapse with fluoxetine (60 mg/day) was examined in a 52-week

randomized trial by Romano and colleagues. At 3 months, there was a statistically significant decrease in relapse to bulimic behaviors (or discontinuation rate) between the fluoxetine (19%) and placebo (37%) groups (p< 0.04). Similar rates between treatments were observed at 6 months and 12 months, but they were not statistically different.

- Overall, these studies demonstrate that fluoxetine is effective for treating BN and can improve relapse outcomes in patients.

- In the Fluoxetine Bulimia Nervosa Collaborative Study Group of BN women, the most commonly reported adverse events was insomnia in the 20 mg fluoxetine (17.8%) and 60 mg fluoxetine (23.2%) groups that were significantly different (p < 0.001) from placebo (7.8%). Tremor was also reported in 20 mg fluoxetine (3.1%) and 60 mg fluoxetine (9.03%) that were significantly when compared with placebo (0%).

- In the 16-week multicenter study conducted by Goldstein and colleagues reported adverse events with fluoxetine (60 mg) that were significantly (p < 0.05) different from placebo, included insomnia 34.5% with fluoxetine vs. 18.6% , nausea 30.4% vs. 12.7%) asthenia 21.3% vs. 6.9%) , anxiety 17.6% vs. 8.8%) , tremor 14.2% vs. 2.0%), dizziness 12.5% vs, 3.9%) , yawning 12.2% vs. 0%) , sweating 9.5% vs. 2.0%), and decreased libido 6.4% vs. 1.0%) .

- Decreased libido and anorgasmia are potential side effects associated with fluoxetine.

Lisdexamfetamine dimesylate for the treatment of BED

- The trade name for lisdexamfetamine dimesylate is Vyvanse. In the United States, the FDA approved Vyvanse for the maintenance of attention deficit hyperactive disorder (ADHD) in 2007 for children (6–12 years old) and in adults in 2008.

- In 2015, lisdexamfetamine was approved by the FDA as the only medication available for the maintenance of moderate to severe BED. Efficacy for BED was determined by a phase-II and two phase-III studies.

- The phase II trial consisted of a multicenter randomized, placebo-controlled trial of BED subjects (n = 260; 81.5% female).
- There was a significant (p < 0.005) reduction in binge frequency at study completion (at end of week 11) in BED subject receiving 50 mg/day and 70 mg/day compared with placebo..
- The 30 mg/day (−3.5 mean binge eating/week from baseline) dose of lisdexamfetamine was not different from placebo.
- The phase III trials were randomized placebo-controlled multicenter studies. BED subjects (n =383, for study 1; n = 390 for study 2) received 50 mg/day or 70 mg/day lisdexamfetamine based on their tolerability. At study completion (week 11–12), lisdexamfetamine resulted in a significant mean reduction in binge eating for both studies (p < 0.001).
- A 12-month open label extension study of lisdexamfetamine treatment was conducted in BED subjects (n = 599; 87% female) from Phase II and Phase III trials. The mean duration of lisdexamfetamine exposure was 284.3 days and the optimal dosing was 29.9% for 50 mg/day and 64.9% for 70 mg/day. At week 52, subjects had 1.14 binge eating days for the past 28 days with lisdexamfetamine compared with 16.68 binge eating days at pre-treatment baseline.
- A randomized placebo-controlled 26-week study was conducted in lisdexamfetamine responders in women with BED (n = 275). The primary endpoint was time to binge-eating relapse. The relapse rate was for lisdexamfetamine was 3.7%, whereas the relapse rate was 32.1% in the placebo group.
- Clinical half-life is about 17 hours. A similar pharmacokinetic profile was observed in an older population of subjects.
- A reanalysis of the data from the 12-week phase III trials by McElroy and colleagues determined the time course for the efficacy of lisdexamfetamine for binge eating in BED subjects (n= 724). Beginning on week 1, there was

significant suppression (p < 0.01) of binge eating response in the lisdexamfetamine group.

- The most commonly (> 10% of subjects) reported side effects were dry mouth, decreased appetite, insomnia, and headache. Reduction in baseline body weight and trend for heart rate to increase over the 11-week study was noted, but there were no significant differences in measured hemodynamic parameters (e.g., heart rate, systolic blood pressure, and diastolic blood pressure) over the course of the phase II trial.

- For the phase III trials, lisdexamfetamine had a similar safety and tolerability profile. At 12 weeks, there were increases in hemodynamic measures with a 4.41–6.31 bpm increase in heart rate, 0.2–1.45 mm Hg for systolic blood pressure, 1.06–1.83 mm Hg for diastolic pressure in subjects receiving lisdexamfetamine. There were also no differences in ACSA (Amphetamine Cessation Symptom Assessment) scores in lisdexamfetamine and placebo groups at any time point, which indicates lisdexamfetamine (50 or 70 mg/day) over a 12- week time period does not result in amphetamine withdrawal symptoms.

- In the open-label 12-month extension trial of the phase II and phase III studies, the greatest mean change in heart rate demonstrated on the ECG was 7.26 ± 10.21 bpm (SD) at 36 weeks. A reduction in body weight from baseline was observed at week 44 (−8.21%), which was maintained until study completion.

- Based on the conversion of lisdexamfetamine to amphetamine and potential for abuse and dependence, the Drug Enforcement Agency (DEA) has classified lisdexamfetamine dimesylate as a Schedule II controlled medication. The abuse potential and safety of lisdexamfetamine was compared with amphetamine and amphetamine derivative in a double-blind cross-over study (n = 36). For the study, subjects were given single doses of placebo, lisdexamfetamine (50 mg, 100 mg, and 150 mg), d-amphetamine (40 mg) and diethylpropion (200 mg), a Schedule IV amphetamine derivative. Abuse potential was assessed by clinically respected questionnaires.

- For the DRQS (Drug Rating Quesionnaire-Subject), there was an approximate 2- fold change in scoring of lisdexamfetamine 50 mg and 100 mg compared with placebo, but these changes were not significant. Liking scoring of lisdexamfetmine was only significantly different from placebo at 150 mg dose (p < 0.01).
- In contrast, amphetamine and diethylproprion (Tenuate) showed > 4-fold change in liking scoring from placebo (p < 0.01) and both medications had significantly higher scores from the 50 mg and 100 mg lisdexamfetamine (p < 0.05 for both). Results were similar for the DRQO assessment, in that amphetamine, diethlypropion, and lisdexamfetamine (150 mg) were rated significantly higher than placebo (p<0.05). One difference from the DRQS was that 100 mg lisdexamfetamine was rated significantly higher than placebo (p < 0.05).
- For the ARCI (Addiction Research Center Inventory) lisdexamfetamine (100 mg and 150 mg) were significantly higher than placebo (p < 0.05), but the 50 mg dose was significantly lower than amphetamine (p < 0.05).
- Taken together, **the data suggest that at the 50 mg dose, lisdexamfetamine has low abuse potential.**

Conclusion

- Both FDA-approved medications, fluoxetine and lisdexamfetamine, are overall safe medications with few adverse effects. The most common adverse effect with fluoxetine appears to be insomnia and not abuse potential Lisdexamfetamine has side effects of dry mouth, headache, and insomnia. There are also increases in heart rate and blood pressure that are positively associated with longer length of treatment. Lisdexamfetamine does have an abuse potential and is a schedule II classification by the DEA.

The popularity of competitive speed eating, the overuse of the term "binge" by advertisers, and the focus on body image by social media contributes to an environment of endorsing disordered eating behavior (Bello & Yeomans, 2018).

Use of Lisdexamfetamine to Treat Obesity in an Adolescent with Severe Obesity and Binge Eating.

Obesity: A Clinical Review

- Approximately two-thirds of US children and adolescents have either obesity or overweight status, with almost 24% of adolescents (ages 12‒19 years) afflicted with severe obesity.

- A 9-year-old girl was referred with a BMI of 32.5 kg/m^2 (1.4 × the 95th BMI percentile for age/gender). The patient underwent neuropsychiatric evaluation at the age of 6 years for developmental delay and autism spectrum diagnoses. By the age of 16 years, the patient's weight had approached 273.8 pounds with a BMI of 48.68.

- Laboratory evaluation revealed total cholesterol of 375 mg/dL, fasting blood glucose of 90 mg/dL, TSH 2.83 mIU/L. A polysomnogram showed mild sleep apnea.

- Evaluation of binge eating disorder (BED) and Attention Deficit Disorder (ADD) revealed positive results. A pharmacotherapy trial of lisdexamfetamine to address both BED, ADD and severe adolescent obesity was initiated. at 20 mg once daily.

- After one year of treatment the patient lost a total of 39.4 lbs, with a reduction of BMI from 48.49 to 40.91 on 50 mg/day.

- The association between obesity and Attention Deficit Hyperactivity Disorder (ADHD) and BED is well-known.

- Unfortunately, there are currently only two available FDA-approved anti-obesity medications with pediatric indications

- (1) Orlistat approved for age ≥12 years and (2) phentermine for age >16 years—Neither of these medications are approved for binge eating disorder in children. Interestingly, lisdexamfetamine is approved for the long-term treatment of ADHD in children and adolescents ages 6–17 years.

- It is FDA-approved for ADHD in children/adolescents and BED in adults. Suppression of growth without rebound may occur in pediatric patients (average height decline of ~2 cm less over 12 months and 2.7 kg less growth in weight over 2 years). The most common adverse reactions in children and adolescents were similar in adults with binge eating disorder prescribed lisdexamfetamine.

- Compared to the other obesity pharmacotherapeutic options utilized in adults, lisdexamfetamine has a long, safe history of use in children (Srivastava, O'Hara, & Browne, 2019).

Definition and diagnostic criteria for orthorexia nervosa: a narrative review of the literature.

- In some cases, detrimental consequences on health are generated by self-imposed dietary rules intended to promote health. The pursuit of an "extreme dietary purity" due to an exaggerated focus on food may lead to a disordered eating behavior called "orthorexia nervosa" (ON).

- There is no universally shared definition of orthorexia nervosa (ON), the diagnostic criteria are under debate. This narrative review of the literature aims at assessing orthorexia nervosa.

- Methods: Literature search into Pubmed/Medline, Scopus, Embase and Google Scholar (last access on 07 August 2018).
  Results:

- All these studies indicated as primary diagnostic criteria: (a) obsessional or pathological preoccupation with healthy nutrition; (b) emotional consequences (e.g. distress, anxieties) of non-adherence to self-imposed nutritional rules; (c) psychosocial impairments in relevant areas of life as well as malnutrition and weight loss. The ORTO-15 and the Orthorexia Self-Test developed by Bratman were the most used psychometric tools (Cena, et al., 2019).

Chapter 45: Orthopedics

"Operating rooms can be a gated community for BMI's less than 40".

The outcomes of total knee arthroplasty in morbidly obese patients: a systematic review of the literature.

- This systematic review aims to compare the long-term revision rates, functional outcomes and complication rates of TKAs in morbidly obese versus non-obese patients.
- A search of PubMed, EMBASE and PubMed Central was conducted to identify studies that reported revision rates in a cohort of morbidly obese patients (BMI $\geq$ 40 kg/m^2) that underwent primary TKA, compared to non-obese patients (BMI $\leq$ 30 kg/m^2).
- Nine studies were included in this review. There were 624 TKAs in morbidly obese patients and 9,449 TKAs in non-obese patients, average BMI values were 45.0 kg/m^2 and 26.5 kg/m^{2}respectively.
- The average follow-up time was 4.8 years and 5.2 years respectively, with a revision rate of 7% and 2% ($p < 0.001$) respectively.
- All functional scores improved after TKA ($p < 0.001$).
- Overall complication rates, including infection, were higher in morbidly obese patients.
- This review suggests an increased mid to long-term revision rate following primary TKA in morbidly obese patients, however, these patients have a functional recovery which is comparable to non-obese individuals.

- There is also an increased risk of perioperative complications, such as superficial wound infection. Morbidly obese patients should be fully informed of these issues prior to undergoing primary TKA (Boyce, et al., 2019).

Complications and Obesity in Arthroplasty-A Hip is Not a Knee.

- The purpose of this study was to compare the effects of obesity and body mass index (BMI) to determine whether the magnitude of the effect was similar for total hip and knee arthroplasties (THA and TKA)
- We queried the American College of Surgeons National Surgical Quality Improvement Program database.
- We identified 64,648 patients who underwent THA and 97,137 patients who underwent TKA.

Obese THA patients had significantly higher rates of

- wound complications (1.53% vs 0.96%)
- deep infection (0.31% vs 0.17%),
- reoperation rate (2.11% vs 1.02%),
- total complications (5.22% vs 4.63%) compared with obese TKA patients.

Morbidly obese THA patients had significantly higher rates of

- wound complications (3.25% vs 1.52%)
- deep infection (0.84% vs 0.23%)
- reoperation rate (3.65% vs 1.60%)
- total complications (7.36% vs 5.57%)

This study demonstrates that the impact of obesity on postoperative complications is higher for THA than TKA (DeMik, et al., 2018).

Does bariatric surgery prior to total hip or knee arthroplasty reduce post-operative complications and improve clinical outcomes for obese patients? Systematic review and meta-analysis.

- 657 patients who had bariatric surgery were compared with 23,348 who did not.

- There was no statistically significant difference in outcomes such as superficial wound infection , deep wound infection , PE , revision surgery, or mortality between the two groups. The answer to the question was surprisingly no. Bariatric surgery prior to THA or TKA does not significantly reduce the complication rates or improve the clinical outcome.
- (Smith, Aboelmagd, Hing, & MacGregor, 2016).

Obesity Increases the Risk of Postoperative Complications and Revision Rates Following Primary Total Hip Arthroplasty: An Analysis of 131,576 Total Hip Arthroplasty Cases.

- Evaluate the association of body mass index (BMI) and the risk of postoperative complications, mortality, and revision rates following primary total hip arthroplasty.
- Using nationwide billing data for inpatient hospital treatment of the biggest German healthcare insurance, 131,576 total hip arthroplasties in 124,368 patients between January 2012 and December 2014 were included.

BMI had a significant effect on overall complications (compared to BMI less than 30)

- BMI 30-34: OR 1.1 (Risk-adjusted odds ratios)
- BMI 35-39: OR 1.5
- BMI ≥40: OR 2.1

The Odds Ratios for 1-year revision procedures

- BMI 30-34: OR 1.2
- BMI 35-39: OR 1.6
- BMI ≥40: OR 2.4

- **90-day surgical complications increased with every BMI category. For mortality and periprosthetic fractures there was a higher risk only for patients with BMI ≥40.**
- **BMI increases the risk of revision rates in a liner trend. Therefore, the authors believe that patients with a BMI >40 kg/m^2 should be sent to obesity medicine physicians in order to decrease the body weight prior elective surgery** (Jeschke, et al., 2018).

Weighing in on Body Mass Index and Infection After Total Joint Arthroplasty: Is There Evidence for a Body Mass Index Threshold?

Is there a BMI cutoff threshold that is associated with increased risk for periprosthetic joint infection (PJI)?

Is the risk of PJI increased in higher obesity classes?

Methods:

- A retrospective study was conducted of all primary THAs and TKAs performed at one institution between 2006 and 2015.
- 18,173 patients (8757 TKAs and 9416 THAs). PJI was defined within 90 days of the index surgery.

Results:

- Among the BMI classes, patients with class III obesity ($\geq$ 40 kg/m) were the only ones showing a higher risk for PJI within 90 days (odds ratio 3.09)
- **patients with a BMI > 40 kg/m carried a threefold higher risk for PJI and for these patients, the risks of surgery must be carefully weighed against its benefits** (Shohat, Fleischman, Tarabichi, Tan, & Parvizi, 2018).

Surgical Risks and Costs of Care are Greater in Patients Who Are Super Obese and Undergoing THA.

We sought to quantify (1) the surgical risk, and (2) the costs associated with complications after THA in patients who were morbidly obesity (BMI $\geq$ 40 kg/m^2) or super obese (BMI $\geq$ 50 kg/m^2).

This is a retrospective study of patients who underwent THA with morbid obesity and super obesity from October 1, 2010 through December 31, 2014. Patients without any BMI-related diagnosis codes were used as the control group. Twelve complications occurring during the 90 days after THA were analyzed. In addition, hospital charges and payments were compared from primary surgery through the subsequent 90 days.

Patients with morbid obesity had increased postoperative complications

- prosthetic joint infection (hazard ratio [HR], 3.71)
- revision (HR, 1.91)

- wound dehiscence (HR, 3.91)
- risk of deep vein thrombosis (HR, 1.43)
- pulmonary embolism (HR, 1.57)
- implant failure (HR, 1.48)
- acute renal failure (HR, 1.68)
- all-cause readmission (HR, 1.48).
- death (HR, 0.94)
- acute myocardial infarction (HR, 0.94)
- dislocation (HR 1.07) were not different between patients in the control and morbidly obese groups.

Super obese patients

- risk of infection (HR, 6.48)
- wound dehiscence (HR, 9.81)
- readmission (HR, 2.16) compared with patients with normal BMI.
- Each THA had mean total hospital charges of USD 88,419 among patients who were super obese compared with USD 73,827 for the control group, a difference of USD 14,591.
- Medicare payment for the patients who were super obese also was higher, but only by USD 3631.

Conclusion:

Patients who are super obese (BMI ≥ 50 kg/m².) are at increased risk for serious complications compared with patients with morbid obesity (BMI ≥ 40 kg/m²), whose risks are elevated relative to patients whose BMI is less than 40 kg/m². Costs of care for patients who were super obese, likewise, were increased (Meller, et al., 2016).

WHO Class of Obesity Influences Functional Recovery Post-TKA.

- No study in the literature has compared early functional recovery following total knee arthroplasty (TKA) in the obese with the nonobese using World Health Organization (WHO) classes of obesity.
- Records of 885 consecutive primary TKA patients (919 knees) operated by a single surgeon were reviewed. The first 35 knees in each class I (BMI 30-34.9), class II (BMI

35-39.9) and class III (BMI 40+) obesity group were matched with a similar number of knees in nonobese TKA patients. Functional scores recorded pre- and postoperatively at 3 months and 1 year using Western Ontario and McMaster Osteoarthritis Index (WOMAC), Short-Form Health Survey (SF-12) score, and Knee Society Score (KSS).

• .

Conclusion:

- The class I obese group can expect good early and late functional recovery as the nonobese group. The class II obese group can expect comparable early functional recovery as the nonobese group but their late function may be lesser. The class III obese group would have poorer functional scores and lesser knee flexion postoperatively compared to the nonobese group. However, compared to their own preoperative status, there is definite improvement in function and knee flexion (Maniar, Maniar, Singhi, & Gangaraju, 2018)

Does BMI influence hospital stay and morbidity after fast-track hip and knee arthroplasty?

This was a prospective observational study involving 13,730 procedures (7,194 THA and 6,536 TKA operations) performed in a standardized fast-track setting. Complete 90-day follow-up was achieved.

Results:

- Median length of stay (LOS) was 2 days in all BMI groups.
- 30-day re-admission rates were around 6% for both THA (6.1%) and TKA (5.9%), without any statistically significant differences between BMI groups.
- 90-day re-admission rates were 8.6% for THA and 8.3% for TKA, which was similar among BMI groups.
- High BMI (BMI 35+) in THA patients was associated with a LOS of >4 days (p = 0.001), but not with re-admission. No such relationship existed for TKA.

- A fast-track setting resulted in similar length of hospital stay and re-admission rates regardless of BMI, except for very obese and morbidly obese THA patients (BMI 35+) (Husted, Jorgensen, & Kehlet, 2016).

Outcome of lumbar spinal fusion surgery in obese patients: a systematic review and meta-analysis.

- A systematic literature review and meta-analysis was made of those studies that compared the outcome of lumbar spinal fusion for LBP in obese and non-obese patients. A total of 17 studies were included in the meta-analysis.

- There was no difference in the pain and functional outcomes.

- Lumbar spinal fusion in the obese patient resulted in a statistically significantly greater intra-operative blood loss, more complications, and longer duration of surgery.

- Based on these results, obesity is not a contraindication to lumbar spinal fusion (Lingutla, et al., 2015).

The Impact of Obesity on the Outcome of Decompression Surgery in Degenerative Lumbar Spinal Canal Stenosis: Analysis of the Lumbar Spinal Outcome Study (LSOS): A Swiss Prospective Multicenter Cohort Study.

Prospective, multicenter cohort study including 8 medical centers of the Swiss states Zurich, Lucerne, and Thurgau, Switzerland.

- The aim of the study was to assess whether obese patients benefit after decompression surgery for degenerative lumbar spinal stenosis (DLSS).

Methods:
- Baseline patient characteristics and outcomes were analyzed at 6 and 12-month follow-up with multiple field proven questionnaires. Minimal clinically important differences (MCIDs) in SSM (spinal stenosis measure-scale of

symptoms) for different BMI categories were considered as main outcome.

Results:

- 166 patients met the inclusion criteria. Fifty had a BMI less than 25, 72 had a BMI between 25-30, and 44 patients had a BMI at least 30.
- 36% Obese patients reached MCID at 6 months, and 48% at 12 months. In the additional outcomes, field questionnaires showed statistically significant mean improvements in the 6 and 12-month follow-up.

Conclusion:

- Obese patients can expect clinical improvement after lumbar decompression for DLSS, but the percentage of patients with a meaningful improvement is lower than in the non-obese group of patients at 6 and 12 months (Burgstaller, et al., 2016).

The effect of high obesity on outcomes of treatment for lumbar spinal conditions: subgroup analysis of the spine patient outcomes research trial.

- To evaluate the effect of obesity on management of lumbar spinal stenosis, degenerative spondylolisthesis (DS), and intervertebral disc herniation (IDH).
- This study compares nonobese patients with those with class I obesity (body mass index=30-35 kg/m) and class II/III high obesity (body mass index≥35 kg/m).

Methods:

- For spinal stenosis, 250 of 634 nonobese patients, 104 of 167 obese patients, and 59 of 94 highly obese patients underwent surgery.
- For DS, 233 of 376 nonobese patients, 90 of 129 obese patients, and 66 of 96 highly obese patients underwent surgery.

- For IDH, 542 of 854 nonobese patients, 151 of 207 obese patients, and 94 of 129 highly obese patients underwent surgery.

- Outcomes included multiple industry questionnaires, operative events, complications, and reoperations.

Results:

- Highly obese patients (BMI 35+) had increased comorbidities. Baseline Short Form-36 physical function scores were lowest for highly obese patients.

- For spinal stenosis, groups were not significantly different.

- For DS, greatest treatment effect for the highly obese group was found in most primary outcome measures, and is attributable to the significantly poorer nonoperative outcomes.

- For IDH, highly obese patients experienced less improvement postoperatively compared with obese and nonobese patients. However, nonoperative treatment for highly obese patients was even worse, resulting in greater treatment effect in almost all measures. Blood loss and length of stay was greater for both obese cohorts.

Conclusion:

- Highly obese patients with DS experienced longer operative times and increased infection. Operative time was greatest for highly obese patients with IDH. DS and IDH saw greater surgical treatment effect for highly obese patients due to poor outcomes of nonsurgical management.

- This article emphasizes to me the best treatment for these types of patients is weight loss, weight loss and weight loss (McGuire, et al., 2014).

Patient Body Mass Index is an Independent Predictor of 30-Day Hospital Readmission After Elective Spine Surgery.

- Hospital readmission within 30 days of surgery is receiving increased scrutiny as an indicator of poor quality of care. Reducing readmissions achieves the dual benefit of improving quality and reducing costs. The aim of this study was to determine if obesity is an independent risk factor for unplanned 30-day readmissions after elective spine surgery.

Methods:
- The medical records of 500 patients (nonobese, n = 281; obese, n = 219) undergoing elective spine surgery at a major academic medical center were reviewed.

Results:
- 8.6% of patients were readmitted within 30 days of discharge; obese patients experienced a 2-fold increase in 30-day readmission rates (obese 12.33% vs. nonobese 5.69%, P = 0.01).

Conclusion:
- Preoperative obesity is an independent statistically significant risk factor for readmission within 30 days of discharge after elective spine surgery (P=0.001) (Elsamadicy, et al., 2016).

Impact of obesity on complications and outcomes: a comparison of fusion and nonfusion lumbar spine surgery.
- Prior studies have shown obesity to be associated with higher complication rates but equivalent clinical outcomes following lumbar spine surgery. These findings have been reproducible across lumbar spine surgery in general and for lumbar fusion specifically. Nevertheless, surgeons seem inclined to limit the extent of surgery, perhaps opting for decompression alone rather than decompression plus fusion, in obese patients.

- The purpose of this study was to ascertain any difference in clinical improvement or complication rates between obese and nonobese patients.

Results:
- In the nonobese cohort, 947 patients underwent decompression alone and 319 underwent decompression plus fusion.
- In the obese cohort, 844 patients had decompression alone and 337 had decompression plus fusion.
- There were no significant differences in the Oswestry Disability Index score or in leg pain improvement at 12 months.
- Absolute improvement in back pain was less in the obese group when decompression alone had been performed.
- Blood loss and operative time were lowest in the nonobese decompression only cohort and were higher in obese patients with or without fusion.
- Obese patients had a longer hospital stay (4.1 days) than the nonobese patients (3.3 days) when fusion had been performed.
- In-hospital stay was similar in both obese and nonobese decompression only cohorts. No significant differences were seen in 30-day readmission rates among the 4 cohorts.

Conclusions:
- Consistent with the prior literature, equivalent clinical outcomes were found among obese and non-obese patients treated for LSS. While obesity may influence the decision for or against surgery, the data suggest that obesity should not necessarily alter the appropriate procedure for well-selected surgical candidates (Onyekwelu, et al., 2017).

Chapter 46: Obstetrics

"A good life starts with good prenatal care"

The Risks Associated with Obesity in Pregnancy.

Approximately one-third of all women of childbearing age are overweight or obese. For these women, pregnancy is associated with increased risks for both mother and child.

Methods:

This review is based on PubMed search with special attention to current population-based cohort studies, systematic reviews, meta-analyses, and controlled trials.

Results:

- Obesity in pregnancy is associated with unfavorable clinical outcomes for both mother and child.

- Many of the risks have been found to depend linearly on the body-mass index (BMI). The probability of conception declines linearly, starting from a BMI of 29 kg/m2, by 4% for each additional 1 kg/m2 of BMI.

- A 10% increase of pre-gravid BMI increases the relative risk of gestational diabetes and that of preeclampsia by approximately 10% each.

- An estimated 11% of all neonatal deaths can be attributed to the consequences of maternal overweight and obesity.

Conclusion:

Preventive measures aimed at normalizing body weight before a woman becomes pregnant are, therefore, all the more important (Stubert, Reister, Hartmann, & Janni, 2018).

Maternal super obesity and risk for intensive care unit admission in the MFMU Cesarean Registry.

- Estimate the association between maternal obesity and ICU admission among women who delivered via cesarean section or vaginal birth after cesarean section (VBAC).
- This is a retrospective cohort analysis of women who delivered via VBAC or cesarean section in the Maternal-Fetal Medicine Unit (MFMU) Cesarean Registry.
- The primary outcome was ICU admission. Mediation analysis was used to estimate the proportion of ICU admission risk attributable specifically to obesity.
- We included 68 455 women; 40% non-obese, 46% class I or II obese, 12% morbidly obese, and 2% super obese (body mass index 50 kg/m^2 or greater)
- Super obese women were at higher risk for ICU admission compared with non-obese women (adjusted RR 1.61), after adjusting for confounders.
- Among super obese women, medical comorbidities mediated 58% of ICU admission risk, suggesting that a significant proportion of ICU admission is driven by maternal obesity.
- Super obese women who deliver by cesarean section or VBAC are at increased risk of peripartum ICU admission (Smid, et al., 2017).

Body Mass Index 50 kg/m2 and Beyond: Perioperative Care of Pregnant Women with Superobesity Undergoing Cesarean Delivery.

- Super-obesity, defined as body mass index 50 kg/m^2 or greater, is the fastest-growing obesity group in the United States. Currently, 2% of pregnant women in the United States are superobese, and 50% will deliver via cesarean delivery.
- Superobese women have a 30% to 50% risk of wound complications, a 20% risk of neonatal intensive care unit admission, and a 1% to 2% risk of maternal intensive care unit admission. Preoperative cefazolin with a 3-g dose, chlorhexidine skin preparation, and availability of adequate personnel for patient transfers are important evidence-

directed approaches to reducing maternal and personnel morbidity (Smid M. , Dotters-Katz, Silver, & Kuller, 2017).

Maternal obesity and major intraoperative complications during cesarean delivery.

- To estimate the association between maternal obesity at delivery and major intraoperative complications during cesarean delivery (CD).

Methods:

- This is a secondary analysis of the deidentified Maternal-Fetal Medicine Unit Cesarean Registry of women with singleton pregnancies.
- The primary outcome, any intraoperative complication, was defined as having at least 1 major intraoperative complication, including perioperative blood transfusion, intraoperative injury (bowel, bladder, ureteral injury; broad ligament hematoma), atony requiring surgical intervention, repeat laparotomy, and hysterectomy.

Results:

- A total of 51,218 women underwent CD; 38% had BMI 18.5 to 29.9, 47% BMI 30 to 39.9, 12% BMI 40 to 49.9 and 3% BMI ≥ 50.
- Having at least 1 intraoperative complication was uncommon at 3.4%:
- 3.8% for BMI 18.5 to 29.9
- 3.2% BMI 30 to 39.9
- 2.6% BMI 40 to 49.9
- 4.3% BMI ≥ 50 (P < .001).
- In contrast to the risk for post-cesarean complications, the risk of intraoperative complication does not appear to be increased in obese women, even among those with super obesity (Smid, et al., 2017).

The risk of perinatal mortality with each week of expectant management in obese pregnancies.

- Retrospective cohort study of singleton births between 2006 and 2011. For each BMI class, we calculated the rate of neonatal death and stillbirth at each week of gestation from 34 to 41 weeks.

Results:

- 2,149,771 births remained for analysis.
- Comparing normal weight to obese to morbidly obese, the stillbirth risk increased from 0.8 to 1.8 to 8.8 at 34 weeks to 5.7 to 10.5 to 83.7 at 42 weeks per 10,000 births.
- Comparing neonatal death risk of normal weight to obese to morbidly obese the risk decreased from 76.5 to 67.7 to 63.6 at 34 weeks to 30.4 to 26.2 to 15.5 at 42 weeks.
- It looks like the obesity paradox applies to neonatal death risk. If the baby can survive the stress of the pregnancy, then it usually survives the neonatal period.

Conclusion:

- The findings reported here suggest that delivery by 38 weeks in gestation minimizes perinatal mortality in pregnancies complicated by maternal morbid obesity (Yao, Schuh, & Caughey, 2019).

Prophylactic incisional negative pressure wound therapy reduces the risk of surgical site infection after caesarean section in obese women: a pragmatic randomised clinical trial.

- Multicentre randomised controlled trial involving 5 hospitals in Denmark
- Obese women (pre-pregnancy body mass index (BMI) ≥ 30 kg/m^2) undergoing elective or emergency caesarean section.

Methods:

- The primary outcome was surgical site infection requiring antibiotic treatment within the first 30 days after surgery.
- Incisional negative pressure wound therapy was applied to 432 women and 444 women had a standard dressing.
- Surgical site infection occurred in 20 (4.6%) women treated with incisional negative pressure wound therapy and in 41 (9.2%) women treated with a standard dressing (relative risk 0.50). Incisional negative pressure wound therapy significantly reduced wound exudate whereas no difference

was found for dehiscence and quality of life between the two groups.

Conclusion:

- Prophylactic use of incisional negative pressure wound therapy reduced the risk of surgical site infection in obese women giving birth by caesarean section (Hyldig, et al., 2019)

Risk assessment of morbidly obese parturient in cesarean section delivery: A prospective, cohort, single-center study.

- Up to 40% of women gain excessive weight during pregnancy. This study aimed to assess the safety and risk of obese women undergoing CS delivery with various perioperative anesthetic methods.

- Seven hundred ninety (790) parturient women underwent CS under general anesthesia (GA), intraspinal anesthesia including epidural anesthesia (EA) and combined spinal-epidural anesthesia (CSEA).

- They were divided into morbid (BMI 40+, n=255), severe obesity (BMI 30-40, n=274), and non-obesity (n=261) groups.

Results:

Between 2013 and 2016, 790 pregnant women were assessed. Compared with the non-obesity group, there were significantly more fetal distress, preeclampsia, multiparous, amniotic fluid abnormality, and high bleeding amounts in the morbid obesity group compared with the non-obesity group. Despite this GA, EA, and CSEA are safe and effective in severely or morbidly obese patients (An, et al., 2017).

Chapter 47: Cardiac Surgery

"Always protect the quarterback (heart)"

Influence of Body Mass Index on Outcomes of Patients Undergoing Surgery for Acute Aortic Dissection: A Propensity-Matched Analysis.

- To determine whether body mass index ≥30 kg/m² affects morbidity and mortality rates in patients undergoing surgery for type A acute aortic dissection, we conducted a retrospective study of 201 patients with type A dissection.
- Patients were divided into 2 groups according to body mass index (BMI): nonobese (BMI, <30; 158 patients) and obese (BMI, ≥30; 43 patients).
- The overall mortality rate was 19% (38/201 patients).
- The overall 5-year survival rates were 52.5% in the obese group and 70.3% in the nonobese group.
- Patients with obesity (BMI, ≥30 kg/m²) who underwent surgery for type A acute aortic dissection had higher operative mortality rates and an increased risk of low cardiac output syndrome, pulmonary complications, and other postoperative morbidities than did patients without obesity (Lio, et al., 2019).

Obesity Increases Risk-Adjusted Morbidity, Mortality, and Cost Following Cardiac Surgery.

- We hypothesized that increasing body mass index (BMI) is associated with worse risk-adjusted outcomes and higher cost.

- Medical records for 13 637 consecutive patients who underwent coronary artery bypass grafting (9702), aortic (1535) or mitral (837) valve surgery, and combined valve-coronary artery bypass grafting (1663) procedures.
- Patients were stratified by BMI: normal to overweight (BMI 18.5-30), obese (BMI 30-40), and morbidly obese (BMI >40).
- Morbidly obese patients incurred nearly 60% greater observed mortality than normal weight patients.
- morbidly obese patients had greater than 2-fold increase in renal failure and 6.5-fold increase in deep sternal wound infection.
- The risk-adjusted odds ratio for mortality for morbidly obese patients was 1.57 compared to normal patients.
- risk-adjusted total hospital cost increased with BMI, with 17.2% higher costs in morbidly obese patients (Ghanta, et al., 2017).

Chapter 48: Sumo Wrestling

Sumo wrestling is Japan's traditional national sport for over 300 years. Great prestige is given to Sumo champions.

- All Sumo wrestlers are obese and life as a wrestler is highly regimented, with rules regulated by the Japan Sumo Association. Most sumo wrestlers are required to live in communal sumo training stables, where all aspects of their daily lives—from meals to their manner of dress—are dictated by strict tradition. The word "sumo" means "to mutually rush at".
- The average weight of top division wrestlers has continued to increase:
  1. 125 kilograms (276 lb) in 1969
  2. 150 + kilograms (330 lb) by 1991
  3. 166 kilograms (366 lb) January 2019. "SUMO/ Heavier wrestlers blamed for increase in serious injuries". Asahi Shimbun. February 19, 2019.
- NFL lineman have had similar patterns.
  1. 1920s 6 foot, 211 lbs.
  2. 1940s 6 foot 1 ich, 221 lbs.
  3. 1970s 6 foot 3 inches, 255 lbs.
  4. 1990s 6 foot 4 inches, 300 lbs.
  5. 2000 6 foot 4 inches, 313 lbs.
  6. 2015 6 foot 5 inches, 312 lbs.
- Sumo wrestlers share many similarities to NFL lineman, they are massive people with great strength, dedication, discipline and athleticism. Unfortunately, their large size hurts them mechanically and metabolically with time. They put their career over health. The average lifespan for an

NFL lineman is about 55 years. Chronic disease such as hypertension, type 2 diabetes, obstructive sleep apnea and joint replacements are very common. Sumo wrestlers are a great example of the general principle that there are no healthy excess weight situations.

Higher Body Mass Index is a Predictor of Death Among Professional Sumo Wrestlers

- In previous studies on the life expectancies of professional Sumo wrestlers, the result suggested higher body weight led to shorter life expectancies compared to general population.
- The aim of the present study is to clarify if higher body mass index is a predictor of death among professional Sumo wrestlers.
- Data for all Sumo wrestlers who were promoted to the top division, generally called Nyuumaku, between the years of 1926 and 1989 were compiled using The Professional Sumo Wrestler Directory.
- Of the 430 wrestlers listed between 1926 to 1989, 73 were deceased. This study was a case-control study consisting of 73 deceased wrestlers born and 73 surviving wrestlers with matching birth years as controls.

Conclusion:

- Deceased wrestlers had higher body mass indexes with statistical significance as well as higher winning percentages, won more performance prizes in their careers, and more were ranked higher. BMI was a statistically significant death determinant among Sumo wrestlers.
- The present study suggests a higher BMI has strong effects on death and has statistical significance among Sumo wrestlers by case-control study, though we could not find an optimal BMI cutoff point for the prediction of death (Kanda, et al., 2009).

High REE in Sumo wrestlers attributed to large organ-tissue mass.

- It is unknown whether high resting energy expenditure (REE) in athletes is attributable to changes in organ-tissue mass and/or metabolic rate.
- The purpose of this study was to examine the contribution of organ-tissue mass of fat-free mass (FFM) components to REE for Sumo wrestlers who have large FFM and REE.

Methods:

- Ten Sumo wrestlers and 11 male untrained college students (controls) were recruited. FFM was estimated by two-component densitometry. Contiguous magnetic resonance imaging (MRI) images were used to measure tissue masses. The measured REE was determined by indirect calorimetry. The calculated REE was estimated as the sum of individual organ-tissue masses (seven body compartments) multiplied by their metabolic rate constants.

Results:

- The measured REE for Sumo wrestlers (2286 kcal) was higher (P<0.01) than for controls (1545 kcal). Sumo wrestlers had a greater amount of FFM and FFM components (e.g., SM, liver, and kidney), except for brain.

Conclusions:

- **The high REE for Sumo wrestlers can be attributed not to an elevation of the organ-tissue metabolic rate, but to a larger absolute amount of low and high metabolically active tissue including skeletal muscle, liver, and kidney.**
- **This article provides support that muscle mass essentially determines metabolic rate emphasizing the importance of maintaining muscle mass through exercise as we age** (Midorikawa, Kondo, Beekley, Koizumi, & Abe, 2007).

[Risk factors for mortality and mortality rate of sumo wrestlers].

- We compared the mortality rate of sumo wrestlers with that of the contemporaneous Japanese male population.
- The standardized mortality ratios (SMR) for sumo wrestlers were very high in each period, and also high for ages from 35 to 74.

- In the survival curves, the lower BMI group had good life expectancy compared with the higher BMI group.
- In sumo wrestlers, this study provides evidence that the higher overweight groups have substantially higher risks for mortality (Hoshiu & Inaba, 1995).

Some factors related to obesity in the Japanese sumo wrestler.

- Sumo is an ancient sport in Japan and there are at present over 800 professional sumo wrestlers (rikishis).
- After entrance into the wrestler society a wrestler takes strenuous daily training together with a very high calorie diet (more than 5,000 kcal). Frequency of food intake is twice a day.
- The average diet of Japanese people contains 2,279 calories and the meal frequency is generally three times a day.
- In 96 wrestlers, the average actual body weight was 100.4 kg.
- Mean serum levels of triglyceride, phospholipid, uric acid, and total protein were significantly higher than those obtained in 89 age-matched healthy males.
- The incidence of diabetes mellitus, gout, and hypertension in wrestlers were considerably higher than in controls.
- Weight correlated significantly with skinfold thickness, diastolic blood pressure, total cholesterol, and uric acid in each group. Obesity, hyperlipidemia, and hyperuricemia in wrestlers were presumed to be caused chiefly by the high calorie diet (Nishizawa, Akaoka, Nishida, Kawaguchi, & Hayashi, 1976).

Grand Sumo Tournaments and Out-of-Hospital Cardiac Arrests in Tokyo.

- We aimed to evaluate the association between sumo wrestling tournaments and the rate of out-of-hospital cardiac arrests.

Methods and Results:

- We counted the daily number of patients aged 18 to 110 years who had an out-of-hospital cardiac arrest of presumed-cardiac origin in the Tokyo metropolis between 2005 and 2014. Exposure days were the days on which a sumo tournament was held and broadcast, whereas control days were all other days. Risk ratios for out-of-hospital cardiac arrests on Grand Sumo tournaments days compared with control days were estimated.

- In total, 71 882 out-of-hospital cardiac arrests met the inclusion criteria.

- We recorded a 9% increase in the occurrence of out-of-hospital cardiac arrests on the day of a sumo tournament compared with control days.

- In patients aged 75 to 110 years, we found a 13% increase in the occurrence of out-of-hospital cardiac arrests on the day of a sumo tournament compared with control days.

Conclusions:

- We found a significant increase in the occurrence of out-of-hospital cardiac arrests on the days of sumo tournaments compared with control days in the Tokyo metropolis between 2005 and 2014. Further studies are needed to verify these initial findings on sumo tournaments and cardiovascular events (Hagihara, Onozuka, Hasegawa, Miyazaki, & Nagata, 2018).

Comparison of Normalized Maximum Aerobic Capacity and Body Composition Of Sumo Wrestlers To Athletes In Combat And Other Sports

- To win in sumo wrestling, one must push one's opponent out of the ring, or cause the opponent to touch the ground with any part of the body except the soles of the feet.

- The purpose of this study is to compare the maximum aerobic capacity and body composition of sumo wrestlers with untrained controls, and other combative, aerobic, and power sports. Untrained controls were used as a reference level.

- Eight untrained college undergraduates (22.2 yrs) and eight highly trained, championship-level (21.1 yrs). members of Japan's number one collegiate team that included a champion of the Japan Amateur Open were evaluated.

- Maximal oxygen uptake (VO_2max) was assessed by graded work on a cycle ergometer. The participants started to exercise at 30 Watts for 2 min, and the load was increased by 15 Watts every minute until exhaustion. The exercise was terminated when the participants failed to maintain the prescribed pedaling frequency of 60 rpm
- Fat-free mass (FFM) was estimated from body density using ultrasound. FFM was derived by subtracting fat mass from total body mass.

Results & Discussion:

- Heart rate at maximum was not different between sumo wrestlers and controls.
- In order to make better comparisons of VO_2max, we divided VO_2max by the amount of predicted skeletal muscle mass. The calculation of VO_2max /SMM should provide an indication of the "aerobic muscle quality" of the athlete's skeletal muscle. We use the term "aerobic muscle quality to refer to the amount of oxygen consumed per skeletal muscle mass. The higher this value, the higher the aerobic muscle quality.
- Relative VO_2max to body mass, however, was significantly lower in sumo wrestlers compared to untrained controls.
- Mean VO_2max/SMM (ml/kg SMM per min)
  1. aerobic athletes 164.8
  2. combat athletes 131.4
  3. Untrained college 22 years old 128.6
  4. power athletes 96.5
  5. sumo wrestlers 71.4
- **We found that sumo wrestlers have a low "aerobic muscle quality" (low VO_2max /SMM), compared to untrained controls and other combat sports, and aerobic and power sports**.
- The training and competition style of sumo is very brief and anaerobic - most competitions are over in < 1 minute. Thus, the aerobic energetic system probably receives little stress during sumo training and competition.
- Sumo wrestlers have a higher fat-free mass (FFM), fat mass, and predicted skeletal muscle mass (SMM) compared to other combative sports. Indeed, sumo wrestlers have some

of the largest absolute FFM (and thus, SMM) measured in humans.

- It is well known that energy cost per distance increases with increases in body mass in humans. VO_2max /SMM is negatively related to percent body fat, indicating that excess fat is detrimental to work because it increases the carried load, which increases oxygen costs (Beekley, Abe, Kondo, Midorikawa, & Yamauchi, 2006).

Conclusion

To summarize, obesity is a complicated heterogenous disease with no easy solutions. EAT LESS, MOVE MORE oversimplifies the disease and its treatment. A less judgmental attitude along with stressing the great benefits of healthier living and exercise may increase success at dealing with unhealthy BMIs. Less fear using obesity medicines along with the appreciation of how our body starts to fail at 35 years old and the importance of taking care of ourselves is the message I am trying to convey. A 2004 study revealed that greater than one third of obese patients are willing to risk death to lose 10% of body weight (Wee, Hamel, Davis, & Phillips, 2004). Suffering from obesity is painful both mentally and physically as outlined in my actual patient examples. Knowledge can be powerful and motivational.

I am going to repeat a paragraph from my preface since the idea has "sticking power" **"Mrs. And Mr. American waste valuable dollars and invaluable time in the pursuit of slimness through get-thin-quick drugs and dreams. The physician has to doff the robes of medicine and don the flannels of Madison Avenue. He has to be a counter-salesman, battling all the sources of misleading misinformation with convincing, correct, information. He has to prove to his patient that "reducing" foods do not reduce, that there are no "fattening" foods or "slimming" foods, just too much food."** (Alexander & Stare, 1967). **Knowledge can be powerful and motivational. As the great wordsmith Yogi Berra said "I'm not going to buy my kids an encyclopedia. Let them walk to school like I did"**

References

Abbate, V., Kicman, A., Evans-Brown, M., McVeigh, J., Cowan, D., Wilson, C., . . . Walker, C. (2015, Jul). Anabolic steroids detected in bodybuilding dietary supplements - a significant risk to public health. *Drug testing and analysis, 7*(7), 609-618. doi:10.1002/dta.1728

Abdelbasset, W., Tantawy, S., Kamel, D., Alqahtani, B., & Soliman, G. (2019). A randomized controlled trial on the effectiveness of 8-week high-intensity interval exercise on intrahepatic triglycerides, visceral lipids, and health-related quality of life in diabetic obese patients with nonalcoholic fatty liver disease. *Medicine (Baltimore), 98*(12), e14918. doi:10.1097/MD.0000000000014918

Abdullah, S., Barkley, K., Bhella, P., Hastings, J., Matulevicius, S., Fujimoto, N., . . . Levine, B. (2016). Lifelong Physical Activity Regardless of Dose Is Not Associated with Myocardial Fibrosis. *Circulation: Cardiovascular Imaging, 9.* doi:https://doi.org/10.1161/CIRCIMAGING.116.005511

Achar, S., Rostamian, A., & Narayan, S. (2015, Sep 15). Cardiac and metabolic effects of anabolic-androgenic steroid abuse on lipids, blood pressure, left ventricular dimensions, and rhythm. *American Journal of Cardiology, 106*(6), 893-901. doi:10.1016/j.amjcard.2010.05.013

Afilalo, J., Lauck, S., Kim, D., Lefèvre, T., Piazza, N., Lachapelle, K., . . . Perrault, L. P. (2017, Aug 8). Frailty in Older Adults Undergoing Aortic Valve Replacement: The FRAILTY-AVR Study. *Journal of the American College of Cardiology, 70*(6), 689-700. doi:10.1016/j.jacc.2017.06.024

Ahlskog, J., Geda, Y., Graff-Radford, N., & Petersen, R. (2011, Sept). Physical exercise as a preventive or disease-modifying treatment of dementia and brain aging. *Mayo Clinic*

Proceedings, 86(9), 876-84.
doi:https://doi.org/10.4065/mcp.2011.0252

Ahmed, A. (2002, Apr). History of diabetes mellitus. *Saudi medical journal, 23*(4), 373-8.

Albertson, T., Chenoweth, J., Colby, D., & Sutter, M. (2016). The Changing Drug Culture: Use and Misuse of Appearance- and Performance-Enhancing Drugs. *FP Essentials, 441*, 30-43.

Alexander, M., & Stare, F. (1967, Jun). Overweight, Obesity and Weight Control. *California medicine, 106*(6), 437-443.

Allan, C., Strauss, B., Forbes, E., Paul, E., & McLachlan, R. (2011). Variability in total testosterone levels in ageing men with symptoms of androgen deficiency. *International Journal of Andrology, 34*(3), 212-216.
doi:https://doi.org/10.1111/j.1365-2605.2010.01071.x

Almukhtar, S., Abbas, A., Muhealdeen, D., & Hughson, M. (2015, Aug). Acute kidney injury associated with androgenic steroids and nutritional supplements in bodybuilders†. *Clinical Kidney Journal, 8*(4), 415-419. doi:10.1093/ckj/sfv032

Amiri, M., Ghiasvand, R., Kaviani, M., Forbes, S., & Salehi-Abargouei, A. (2018, Jun 19). Chocolate milk for recovery from exercise: a systematic review and meta-analysis of controlled clinical trials. *European journal of clinical nutrition*.
doi:10.1038/s41430-018-0187-x

Amory, J., Chansky, H., Chansky, K., Camuso, M., Hoey, C., Anawalt, B., . . . Bremner, W. (2002). Preoperative Supra-physiological Testosterone in Older Men Undergoing Knee Replacement Surgery. *Journal of the American Geriatrics Society, 50*(10), 1698-1701. doi:10.1046/j.1532-5415.2002.50462.x

An, X., Zhao, Y., Zhang, Y., Yang, Q., Wang, Y., Cheng, W., & Yang, Z. (2017, Oct). Risk assessment of morbidly obese parturient in cesarean section delivery: A prospective, cohort, single-center study. *Medicine, 96*(42), e8265.
doi:10.1097/MD.0000000000008265

Andreassen, M., Raymond, I., Kistorp, C., Hildebrandt, P., Faber, J., & Kristensen, L. (2009). IGF1 as predictor of all-cause mortality and cardiovascular disease in an elderly population. *European Journal of Endocrinology, 160*(1), 25-31.
doi:https://doi.org/10.1530/EJE-08-0452

References

Anton, S., Moehl, K., Donahoo, W., Marosi, K., Lee, S., Mainous III, A., & Leeuwenburgh, C. (2018). Flipping the Metabolic Switch: Understanding and Applying Health Benefits of Fasting. *Obesity, 26*(2), 254-268. doi:10.1002/oby.22065

Anyanwagu, U., Mamza, J., Donnelly, R., & Idris, I. (2018). Association between insulin-induced weight change and CVD mortality: Evidence from a historic cohort study of 18,814 patients in UK primary care. *Diabetes/metabolism research and reviews., 34*(1). doi:10.1002/dmrr.2945.

Apovian, C., Aronne, L., Bessesen, D., McDonnell, M., Murad, M., Pagotto, U., . . . Still, C. (2015, Feb 1). Pharmacological Management of Obesity: An Endocrine Society Clinical Practice Guideline. *Journal of Clinical Endocrinology and Metabolism, 100*(2), 342-362. doi:10.1210/jc.2014-3415

Appelman, Y., Rijn, v., BB, Ten Haaf, M., Boersma, E., & Peters, S. (2015). Sex differences in cardiovascular risk factors and disease prevention. *Atherosclerosis, 241*(1), 211-8. doi:https://doi.org/10.1016/j.atherosclerosis.2015.01.027

Arapis, K., Macrina, N., Kadouch, D., Ribeiro-Parenti, L., Marmuse, J., & Hansel, B. (2019). Outcomes of Roux-en-Y gastric bypass versus sleeve gastrectomy in super-super-obese patients (BMI ≥60 kg/m2): 6-year follow-up at a single university. *Surgery for obesity and related disease, 15*(1), 23-33. doi:10.1016/j.soard.2018.09.487

Araujo, A., Dixon, J., Suarez, E., Murad, M., Guey, L., & Wittert, G. (2011). Clinical review: Endogenous testosterone and mortality in men: a systematic review and meta-analysis. *The Journal of Clinical Endocrinology and Metabolism, 96*(10), 3007-3019. doi:https://doi.org/10.1210/jc.2011-1137

Arnett, S., Laity, J., Agrawal, S., & Cress, M. (2008). Aerobic reserve and physical functional performance in older adults. *Age and Ageing, 37*(4), 384-9. doi:https://doi.org/10.1093/ageing/afn022

Arnold, M., Schlosser, K., Otero, J., Prasad, T., Lincourt, A., Gersin, K., . . . Colavita, P. (2019, Mar 1). Laparoscopic Weight Loss Surgery in the Elderly: An ACS NSQIP Study on the Effect of Age on Outcomes. *The American surgeon, 85*(3), 273-279.

Asbun, J., & Villareal, F. (2006, Feb 21). The pathogenesis of myocardial fibrosis in the setting of diabetic cardiomyopathy. *Journal of the American College of Cardiology, 47*(4), 693-700. doi:10.1016/j.jacc.2005.09.050

Ashrafian, H., Monnich, M., Braby, T., Smellie, J., Bonanomi, G., & Efthimiou, E. (2018, Nov). Intragastric balloon outcomes in super-obesity: a 16-year city center hospital series. *Surgery for Obesity and Related Disease, 14*(11), 1691-1699. doi:10.1016/j.soard.2018.07.010

Atkinson, R., Srinivas-Shankar, U., Roberts, S., Connolly, M., Adams, J., Oldham, J., . . . Narici, M. (2010). Effects of Testosterone on Skeletal Muscle Architecture in Intermediate-Frail and Frail Elderly Men. *J Gerontol A Biol Sci Med Sci, 65a*(11), 1215-1219. doi:https://doi.org/10.1093/gerona/glq118

Baas, W., & Köhler, T. (2016). Testosterone replacement therapy and voiding dysfunction. *Translational Andrology and Urology, 5*(6), 890-897. doi:https://dx.doi.org/10.21037%2Ftau.2016.08.11

Baillargeon, J., Deer, R., Kuo, Y., Zhang, D., Goodwin, J., & Volpi, E. (2016). Androgen Therapy and Re-hospitalization in Older Men With Testosterone Deficiency. *Mayo Clinic Proceedings, 91*(5), 587-95. doi:https://doi.org/10.1016/j.mayocp.2016.03.016

Baillargeon, J., Urban, R., Kuo, Y., Ottenbacher, K., Raji, M., Du, F., . . . Goodwin, J. (2014). Risk of Myocardial Infarction in Older Men Receiving Testosterone Therapy. *Annals of Pharmacotherapy, 48*(9), 1138-1144. doi:https://doi.org/10.1177/1060028014539918

Bann, D., Hire, D., Manini, T., Cooper, R., Botoseneanu, A., McDermott, M., . . . Group, L. S. (2013, Feb 3). Light Intensity physical activity and sedentary behavior in relation to body mass index and grip strength in older adults: cross-sectional findings from the Lifestyle Interventions and Independence for Elders (LIFE) study. *Plos one, 10*(2). doi:https://doi.org/10.1371/journal.pone.0116058

Basaria, S., Coviello, A., Travison, T., Storer, T., Farwell, W., Jette, A., . . . Aggarwal, S. (2010). Adverse events associated with testosterone administration. *New England Journal of Medicine, 363*(2), 109-22. doi:https://doi.org/10.1056/NEJMoa1000485

References

Bauman, W., La Fountaine, M., Cirnigliaro, C., Kirshblum, S., & Spungen, A. (2015). Lean tissue mass and energy expenditure are retained in hypogonadal men with spinal cord injury after discontinuation of testosterone replacement therapy. *The Journal of Spinal Cord Medicine, 38*(1), 38-47. doi:https://doi.org/10.1179/2045772314Y.0000000206

Bays, H., Perdomo, C., Nikonova, E., Knoth, R., & Malhotra, M. (2018). Lorcaserin and metabolic disease: weight-loss dependent and independent effects. *Obesity Science and Practice, 4*(6), 499-505. doi:10.1002/osp4.296

Beekley, M., Abe, T., Kondo, M., Midorikawa, T., & Yamauchi, T. (2006, Jul). Comparison of Normalized Maximum Aerobic Capacity and Body Composition Of Sumo Wrestlers To Athletes In Combat And Other Sports. *Journal of sports science & medicine, 5*, 13-20.

Bello, N., & Yeomans, B. (2018, Jan). Safety of pharmacotherapy options for bulimia nervosa and binge eating disorder. *Expert Opinion on Drug Safety, 17*(1), 17-23. doi:10.1080/14740338.2018.1395854

Bermon, S. (2017, Jun). Androgens and athletic performance of elite female athletes. *Current Opinion in Endocrinology, Diabetes, and Obesity, 24*(3), 246-251. doi:10.1097/MED.0000000000000335.

Bhasin, S., Brito, J., Cunningham, G., Hayes, F., Hodis, H., Matsumoto, A., . . . Yialamas, M. (2018, May 1). Testosterone Therapy in Men With Hypogonadism: An Endocrine Society Clinical Practice Guideline. *Journal of Clinical Endocrinology and Metabolism, 103*(5), 1715-1744. doi:10.1210/jc.2018-00229

Bhasin, S., Woodhouse, L., Casaburi, R., Singh, A., Bhasin, D., Berman, N., . . . Storer, T. (2001). Testosterone dose-response relationships in healthy young men. *The American Journal of Physiology, Endocrinology, and Metabolism, 281*(6). Retrieved from http://ajpendo.physiology.org/content/281/6/E1172.long

Bhasin, S., Woodhouse, L., Casaburi, R., Singh, A., Mac, R., Lee, M., . . . Storer, T. (2005). Older Men Are as Responsive as Young Men to the Anabolic Effects of Graded Doses of Testosterone on the Skeletal Muscle. *Journal of Clinical*

Endocrinology and Metabolism, 90(2), 678-688.
doi:https://doi.org/10.1210/jc.2004-1184

Bischoff-Ferrari, H., Orav, E., & Dawson-Hughes, B. (2008).
Additive benefit of higher testosterone levels and vitamin
D plus calcium supplementation in regard to fall risk
reduction among older men and women. *Osteoporosis
International, 19*(9), 1307-14.
doi:https://doi.org/10.1007/s00198-008-0573-7

Blackman, M., Sorkin, J., Münzer, T., Bellantoni, M., Busby-
Whitehead, J., Stevens, T., . . . Harman, S. (2002). Growth
Hormone and Sex Steroid Administration in Healthy Aged
Women and Men. A Randomized Controlled Trial. *JAMA,
288*(18), 2282-92. doi:10.1001/jama.288.18.2282

Blagrove, R., Howatson, G., & Hayes, P. (2018, May). Effects of
Strength Training on the Physiological Determinants of
Middle- and Long-Distance Running Performance: A
Systematic Review. *Sports Medicine, 48*(5), 1117-1149.
doi:1007/s40279-017-0835-7

Blind, E., Janssen, H., Dunder, K., & de Graeff, P. (2018). The
European Medicines Agency's approval of new medicines
for type 2 diabetes. *Diabetes, obesity, and metabolism, 20*(9),
2059-2063. doi:10.1111/dom.13349.

Boolell, M., Allen, M., Ballard, S., Gepi-Attee, S., Muirhead, G.,
Naylor, A., . . . Gingell, C. (1996). Sildenafil: an orally active
type 5 cyclic GMP-specific phosphodiesterase inhibitor for
the treatment of penile erectile dysfunction. *International
Journal of Impotence Research, 8*(2), 47-52.

Boolell, M., Gepi-Attee, S., Gingell, J., & Allen, M. (1996).
Sildenafil, a novel effective oral therapy for male erectile
dysfunction. *British Journal of Urology, 78*(2), 257-61.

Borst, S., & Yarrow, J. (2015). Injection of testosterone may be
safer and more effective than transdermal administration
for combating loss of muscle and bone in older men. *The
American Journal of Physiology. Endocrinology and Metabolism,
308*(12), e1035-1042.
doi:https://doi.org/10.1152/ajpendo.00111.2015

Borz, C., Bara, T., Bara, T., Suciu, A., Denes, M., Borz, B., . . .
Jimborean, G. (2017). Laparoscopic gastric plication for the
treatment of morbid obesity by using real-time imaging of
the stomach pouch. *Annali Italiani de chiurgia, 6*, 392-398.

References

Bowditch, M., & Villar, R. (1999). Do obese patients bleed more? A prospective study of blood loss at total hip replacement. *Annals of the Royal College of Surgeons of England, 81*(3), 198-200. Retrieved from https://www.researchgate.net/publication/12933968_Do_obese_patients_bleed_more_A_prospective_study_of_blood_loss_at_total_hip_replacement

Boyce, L., Prasad, A., Barrett, M., Dawson-Bowling, S., Millington, S., Hanna, S., & Achan, P. (2019, Apr). The outcomes of total knee arthroplasty in morbidly obese patients: a systematic review of the literature. *Archives of orthopaedic and trauma surgery, 139*(4), 553-560. doi:10.1007/s00402-019-03127-5

Brambilla, D., Matsumoto, A., Araujo, A., & McKinlay, J. (2009). The Effect of Diurnal Variation on Clinical measurement of Serum Testosterone and Other Sex Hormone Levels in Men. *Journal of Clinical Endocrinology and Metabolism, 94*(3), 907-913. doi:https://doi.org/10.1210/jc.2008-1902

Bray, G., Frühbeck, G., Ryan, D., & Wilding, J. (2016, May 7). Management of obesity. *Lancet, 387*(10031), 1947-56. doi:10.1016/S0140-6736(16)00271-3

Brennan, B., Kanayama, G., & Pope Jr., H. (2013, March). Performance-Enhancing Drugs on the Web: A Growing Public-Health Issue. *The American Journal of Addictions, 22*(2), 158-161. doi:10.1111/j.1521-0391.2013.00311.x

Brook, M., Wilkinson, D., Mitchell, W., Lund, J., Phillips, B., Szewczyk, N., . . . Atherton, P. (2016). Synchronous deficits in cumulative muscle protein synthesis and ribosomal biogenesis underlie age-related anabolic resistance to exercise in humans. *Journal of Physiology, 594*(24), 7399-7417. doi:https://dx.doi.org/10.1113%2FJP272857

Brooke, J., Walter, D., Kapoor, D., Marsh, H., Muraleedharan, V., & Jones, T. (2014). Testosterone deficiency and severity of erectile dysfunction are independently associated with reduced quality of life in men with type 2 diabetes. *Andrology, 2*(2), 205-211. doi:https://doi.org/10.1111/j.2047-2927.2013.00177.x

Brown, A. (2017, Sep). An overview of herb and dietary supplement efficacy, safety and government regulations in the United States with suggested improvements. *Food and*

Chemical Toxicology, 107(A), 449-471.
doi:10.1016/j.fct.2016.11.001

Brown, J., Harhay, M., & Harhay, M. (2014, Sep). Walking cadence and mortality among community-dwelling older adults. *Journal of general internal medicine, 29*(9), 1263-1269. doi:10.1007/s11606-014-2926-6

Budnitz, D. L., & Richards, C. (2011, Nov 24). Emergency Hospitalizations for Adverse Drug Events in Older Americans. *New England Journal of Medicine, 365*, 2002-2012. doi:10.1056/NEJMsa1103053

Burgstaller, J., Held, U., Brunner, F., Porchet, F., Farshad, M., Steurer, J., & Ulrich, N. (2016, Jan). The Impact of Obesity on the Outcome of Decompression Surgery in Degenerative Lumbar Spinal Canal Stenosis: Analysis of the Lumbar Spinal Outcome Study (LSOS): A Swiss Prospective Multicenter Cohort Study. *Spine, 41*(1), 82-9. doi:10.1097/BRS.0000000000001128

Butler, S., & Cole, L. (2016, November). Evidence for, and Associated Risks with, the Human Chorionic Gonadotropin Supplemented Diet. *13*(6), 694-9. doi:10.3109/19390211.2016.1156208

Buvat, J., Maggi, M., Guay, A., & Torres, L. (2013). Testosterone Deficiency in Men: Systematic Review and Standard Operating Procedures for Diagnosis and Treatment. *Journal of Sexual Medicine, 10*(1), 245-284. doi:https://doi.org/10.1111/j.1743-6109.2012.02783.x

Campbell, J., Bellman, S., Stephenson, M., & Lisy, K. (2017). Metformin reduces all-cause mortality and diseases of ageing independent of its effect on diabetes control: A systematic review and meta-analysis. *Ageing research reviews, 40*, 31-44. doi:10.1016/j.arr.2017.08.003

Campoverde Reyes, K., Misra, M., Lee, H., & Stanford, F. (2019). Weight Loss Surgery Utilization in Patients Aged 14-25 With Severe Obesity Among Several Healthcare Institutions in the United States. *Frontiers in pediatrics, 6*(251). doi:10.3389/fped.2018.00251

Candow, D., Vogt, E., Johannsmeyer, S., Forbes, S., & Farthing, J. (2015). Strategic creatine supplementation and resistance training in healthy older adults. *Applied Physiology, Nutrition,*

References

and Metabolism, 40(7), 689-94.
doi:https://doi.org/10.1139/apnm-2014-0498

Cannel, H. (1992, Aug). Enforced Intermaxillary Fixation (IMF) as a Treatment of Obesity. *Obesity Surgery, 2*(3), 225-230.

Carbajo, M., Gonzalez-Ramirez, G., Jimenez, J., Luque-de-Leon, E., Ortiz-de-Solorzano, J., Castro, M., & Ruiz-Trovar, J. (2019, May 1). A 5-Year Follow-up in Children and Adolescents Undergoing One-Anastomosis Gastric Bypass (OAGB) at a European IFSO Excellence Center (EAC-BS). *Obesity Surgery.* doi:10.1007/s11695-019-03908-2

Carling, M., Jeppsson, A., Eriksson, B., & Brisby, H. (2015). Transfusions and blood loss in total hip and knee arthroplasty: a prospective observational study. *Journal of Orthopaedic Surgery and Research, 10*(48). Retrieved from https://josr-online.biomedcentral.com/articles/10.1186/s13018-015-0188-6

Castleberry, T., Irvine, C., Deemer, S., Brisebois, M., Gordon, R., Oldham, M., . . . Ben-Ezra, V. (2019, July). Consecutive days of exercise decrease insulin response more than a single exercise session in healthy, inactive men. *European journal of applied physiology., 119*(7), 1591-1598. doi:10.1007/s00421-019-04148-z

Castro, A., Gomez-Arbelaez, D., Crujeiras, A., Granero, R., Aguera, Z., Jimenez-Murcia, S., . . . Gasanueva, F. (2018). Effect of A Very Low-Calorie Ketogenic Diet on Food and Alcohol Cravings, Physical and Sexual Activity, Sleep Disturbances, and Quality of Life in Obese Patients. *Nutrients, 10*(10), E1348. doi:10.3390/nu10101348

Catenacci, V., Pan, Z., Thomas, J., Ogden, L., Roberts, S., Wyatt, H., . . . Hill, J. (2014, Oct). Low/No calorie sweetened beverage consumption in the National Weight Control Registry. *Obesity (Silver Spring), 22*(10), 2244-51. doi:10.1002/oby.20834

Cena, H., Barthels, F., Cuzzolaro, M., Bratman, S., Brytek-Matera, A., Dunn, T., . . . Donini, L. (2019). Definition and diagnostic criteria for orthorexia nervosa: a narrative review of the literature. *Eating and weight disorders, 24*(2), 209-246. doi:10.1007/s40519-018-0606-y

Chapma, A. (1951, Jun 8). Weight Control: A Simplified Concept. *Public Health Reports (1896-1970), 66*(23), 725-731.

Cheetham, T., An, J., Jacobson, S., Niu, F., Sidney, S., Quesenbury, C., & VanDenEeden, S. (2017, Apr 1). Association of Testosterone Replacement With Cardiovascular Outcomes Among Men With Androgen Deficiency. *Jama Internal Medicine, 177*(4), 491-499. doi:10.1001/jamainternmed.2016.9546

Cheung, A., Tinson, A., Milevski, S., Hoermann, R., Zajac, J., & Grossmann, M. (2018, Jul). Persisting adverse body composition changes 2 years after cessation of androgen deprivation therapy for localized prostate cancer. *European Journal of Endocrinology, 179*(1), 21-29. doi:10.1530/EJE-18-0117

Christou, G., Christou, K., Nikas, D., & Goudevenos, J. (2016). Acute myocardial infarction in a young bodybuilder taking anabolic androgenic steroids: A case report and critical review of the literature. *European Journal of Preventative Cardiology, 23*(16), 1785-1796. doi:https://doi.org/10.1177/2047487316651341

Christou, M., Christou, P., Markozannes, G., Tsatsoulis, A., Mastorakos, G., & Tigas, S. (2017). Effects of Anabolic Androgenic Steroids on the Reproductive System of Athletes and Recreational Users: A Systematic Review and Meta-Analysis. *Sports Medicine.* doi:https://doi.org/10.1007/s40279-017-0709-z

Chu, L., Howell, B., Steinberg, A., Bar-Dayan, A., Toulany, A., Langer, J., & Hamilton, J. (2019, Mar 6). Early weight loss in adolescents following bariatric surgery predicts weight loss at 12 and 24 months. *Pediatric Obesity*, e12519. doi:10.1111/ijpo.12519

Cohen, P., Goday, A., & Swann, J. (2012). The Return of Rainbow Diet Pills. *American journal of public health, 102*(9), 1676-1686. doi:10.2105/AJPH.2012.300655.

Colman, E., Golden, J., Roberts, M., Egan, A., Weaver, J., & Rosebraugh, C. (2012, Oct 25). The FDA's Assessment of Two Drugs for Chronic Weight Management. *New England Journal of Medicine, 367*, 1577-79. doi:10.1056/NEJMp1211277

References

Connolly HM, C. J. (1997, August 28). Valvular heart disease associated with fenfluramine-phentermine. *New England Journal of Medicine, 337*(9), 581-8. doi: 10.1056/NEJM199708283370901

Corona, G., & Rastrelli, G. (2017, Dec). Meta-analysis of Results of Testosterone Therapy on Sexual Function Based on International Index of Erectile Function Scores. *European Urology 2017, 72*(6), 1000-1011. doi:10.1016/j.eururo.2017.03.032

Corona, G., Dicuio, M., Rastrelli, G., Maseroli, E., Lotti, F., Sforza, A., & Maggi, M. (2017, Aug). Testosterone treatment and cardiovascular and venous thromboembolism risk: what is 'new'? *Journal of Investigative Medicine, 65*(6), 964-973. doi:10.1136/jim-2017-000411.

Corona, G., Maseroli, E., & Maggi, M. (2014). Injectable testosterone undecanoate for the treatment of hypogonadism. *Expert Oninion on Pharmacotherapy*, 1903-26.

Corona, G., Maseroli, E., Rastrelli, G., Isidori, A., Sforza, A., Mannucci, E., & Maggi, M. (2014). Cardiovascular risk associated with testosterone-boosting medications: a systematic review and meta-analysis. *Expert Opinions on Drug Safety, 13*(10), 1327-1351. doi:https://doi.org/10.1517/14740338.2014.950653

Corona, G., Monami, M., Rastrelli, G., Aversa, A., Sforza, A., Lenzi, A., . . . Maggi, M. (2010). Type 2 diabetes mellitus and testosterone: a meta-analysis study. *International Journal of Andrology, 34*(6), 528-40. doi:https://doi.org/10.1111/j.1365-2605.2010.01117.x

Corona, G., Rastrelli, G., Monami, M., Saad, F., Luconi, M., Lucchese, M., . . . Maggi, M. (2003, May). Body weight loss reverts obesity-associated hypogonadotropic hypogonadism: a systematic review and meta-analysis. *European journal of Endocrinology, 168*(6), 829-43. doi:https://doi.org/10.1530/EJE-12-0955

Costa, R., Reichert, T., Coconcelli, L., Simmer, N., Bagatini, N., Buttelli, A., . . . Kruel, L. (2017). Short-term water-based aerobic training promotes improvements in aerobic conditioning parameters of mature women. *Complementary therapies in clinical practice, 28*, 131-135. doi:10.1016/j.ctcp.2017.06.001

Coto-Montes, A., Boga, J., Tan, D., & Reiter, R. (2016). Melatonin
as a Potential Agent in the Treatment of Sarcopenia.
International Journal of Molecular Sciences, 17(10), 1771.
doi:https://doi.org/10.3390/ijms17101771

Courcoulas, A., King, W., Belle, S., Berk, P., Flum, D., Garcia, L., .
. . Yanovski, S. (2018, May 1). Seven-Year Weight
Trajectories and Health Outcomes in the Longitudinal
Assessment of Bariatric Surgery (LABS) Study. *JAMA
Surgery, 153*(5), 427-434. doi:10.1001/jamasurg.2017.5025

Crewther, B., Cook, C., Cardinale, M., Weatherby, R., & Lowe, T.
(n.d.). Two Emerging Concepts for Elite Athletes. The
Short-Term Effects of Testosterone and Cortisol on the
Neuromuscular System and the Dose-Response Training
Role of these Endogenous Hormones. *Sports Medicine, 41*(2),
103-123. doi:https://doi.org/10.2165/11539170-
000000000-00000

Crewther, B., Cronin, J., Keogh, J., & Cook, C. (2008). The Salivary
Testosterone and Cortisol Response to Three Loading
Schemes. *Journal of Strength and Conditioning Research, 22*(1),
250-255.
doi:https://doi.org/10.1519/JSC.0b013e31815f5f91

Cui, T., Kovell, R., Brooks, D., & Terlecki, R. (2015, Nov 3). A
Urologist's Guide to Ingredients Found in Top-Selling
Nutraceuticals for Men's Sexual Health. *The Journal of Sexual
Medicine, 12*(11), 2105-2117. doi:10.1111/jsm.13013

Cummings, D., Purnell, J., Frayo, R., Schmidova, K., Wisse, B., &
Weigle, D. (2001, August). A preprandial rise in plasma
ghrelin levels suggests a role in meal initiation in humans.
Diabetes, 50(8), 1714-9.
doi:https://doi.org/10.2337/diabetes.50.8.1714

Cunningham, G., & Toma, S. (2011). Clinical review: Why is
androgen replacement in males controversial? *The Journal of
Clinical Endocrinology and Metabolism, 96*(1), 38-52.
doi:https://doi.org/10.1210/jc.2010-0266

Daka, B., Langer, R., Larsson, C., Rosén, T., Jansson, P., Råstam,
L., & Lindblad, U. (2015). Low concentrations of serum
testosterone predict acute myocardial infarction in men
with type 2 diabetes mellitus. *BMC Endocr Disord, 15*(35).
doi:https://doi.org/10.1186/s12902-015-0034-1

References

Dang, J., Switzer, N., Sun, W., Raghavi, F., Birch, D., & Karmali, S. (2018, Dec). Evaluating the safety of intragastric balloon: An analysis of the Metabolic and Bariatric Surgery Accreditation and Quality Improvement Program. *Surgery for Obesity and Related Diseases, 14*(9), 1340-1347. doi:10.1016/j.soard.2018.05.003

Dansinger, M., Tatsioni, A., Wong, J., Chung, M., & Balk, E. (2007, July 3). Meta-analysis: the effect of dietary counseling for weight loss. *Annals of Internal Medicine, 147*(1), 41-50.

Darke, S., Duflou, J., Kaye, S., Farrell, M., & Lappin, J. (2019). Body mass index and fatal stroke in young adults: A national study. *Journal of forensic and legal medicine, 63*, 1-6. doi:10.1016/j.jflm.2019.02.003

Davis, S., & Wahlin-Jacobsen, S. (2015). Testosterone in women- the clinical significance. *The Lancet. Diabetes and Endocrinology, 3*(12), 980-92. doi:https://doi.org/10.1016/S2213-8587(15)00284-3

De Spiegeleer, A., Beckwée, D., Bautmans, I., Petrovic, M., & (BSGG), S. G. (2018, Aug). Pharmacological Interventions to Improve Muscle Mass, Muscle Strength and Physical Performance in Older People: An Umbrella Review of Systematic Reviews and Meta-analyses. *Drugs and Aging, 35*(8), 719-734. doi:10.1007/s40266-018-0566-y

DeAntonio, J., Cockrell, H., Kang, H., Bean, M., Thompson, N., Brengman, M., . . . Wickham, E. 3. (2019, Jan 23). A pilot study of laparoscopic gastric plication in adolescent patients with severe obesity. *Journal of pediatric surgery*, S0022-3468(19)30011-9. doi:10.1016/j.jpedsurg.2019.01.004

DeFronzo, R. (2009, April). From the Triumvirate to the Ominous Octet: A New Paradigm for the Treatment of Type 2 Diabetes Mellitus. *Diabetes, 58*(4), 773-795. doi: 10.2337/db09-9028

DeMik, D., Bedard, N., Dowdle, S., Elkings, J., Brown, T., Gao, Y., & Callaghan, J. (2018, Oct). Complications and Obesity in Arthroplasty-A Hip is Not a Knee. *Journal of Athroplasty, 33*(10), 3281-3287. doi:10.1016/j.arth.2018.02.073

Dev, R., Bruera, E., & Del Fabbro, E. (2014). When and when not to use testosterone for palliation in cancer care. *Current Oncology Reports, 16*(4), 378. doi:https://doi.org/10.1007/s11912-014-0378-0

Dev, R., Hui, D., Fabbro, D., E, Delgado-Guay, MO, . . . Bruera, E. (2014). The Association Among Hypogonadism, Symptom Burden, and Survival in Male Patients with Advanced Cancer. . *Cancer, 120*(10), 1586-1593. doi:https://dx.doi.org/10.1002%2Fcncr.28619

Devrim, A., Bilfic, P., & Hongu, N. (2018, Sep). Is There Any Relationship Between Body Image Perception, Eating Disorders, and Muscle Dysmorphic Disorders in Male Bodybuilders? *American Journal of Mens Health, 12*(5), 1746-1758. doi:10.1177/1557988318786868

Dhindsa, S., Ghanim, H., Batra, M., Kuhadiya, N., Abuaysheh, S., Green, K., . . . Dandona, P. (2016). Effect of testosterone on hepcidin, ferroportin, ferritin, and iron binding capacity in patients with hypogonadotropic hypogonadism and type 2 diabetes. *Clinical Endocrinology, 85*(5), 772-780. doi:https://doi.org/10.1111/cen.13130

Dhindsa, S., Ghanim, H., Batra, M., Kuhadiya, N., Abuaysheh, S., Sandhu, S., . . . Dandona, P. (2016). Insulin Resistance and Inflammation in Hypogonadotropic Hypogonadism and Their Reduction After Testosterone Replacement in Men With Type 2 Diabetes. *Diabetes Care, 39*(1), 82-91. doi:https://doi.org/10.2337/dc15-1518

Dhindsa, S., Irwig, M., & Wyne, K. (2018, Apr). GONADOPENIA AND AGING IN MEN. *Endocrine Practice, 24*(4), 375-385. doi:doi: 10.4158/EP-2017-0131.

Dhindsa, S., Miller, M., McWhirter, C., Mager, D., Ghanim, H., Chaudhuri, A., & Dandona, P. (2010). Testosterone concentrations in diabetic and nondiabetic obese men. *Diabetes care, 33*(6), 1186-92. doi:https://doi.org/10.2337/dc09-1649

Dimitrakakis, C., & Bondy, C. (2009). Androgens and the breast. *Breast Cancer Research, 11*(5), 212. doi:https://dx.doi.org/10.1186%2Fbcr2413

Ding, E., Song, Y., Malik, V., & Liu, S. (2006). Sex differences of endogenous sex hormones and risk of type 2 diabetes: a systematic review and meta-analysis. *JAMA, 295*(11), 1288-99. doi:https://doi.org/10.1001/jama.295.11.1288

Discrepancy between self-reported and actual caloric inake and exerise in obese subjects. (1992, Dec 31). *New England Journal of medicine, 327*(27), 1893-1898.

References

Douthwaite, A. (1934, Apr 21). On the control of obesity. *The british medical journal, 1*(3824), 699-702.

Duan, C., & Xu, L. (2018, Mar 9). Testosterone and androstanediol glucuronide among men in NHANES III. *BMC Public Health, 18*(1), 339. doi:10.1186/s12889-018-5255-6

Dunstan, D., Daly, R., Owen, N., Jolley, D., Vulikh, E., Shaw, J., & Zimmet, P. (2005, Jan). Home-based resistance training is not sufficient to maintain improved glycemic control following supervised training in older individuals with type 2 diabetes. *Diabetes Care, 28*(1), 3-9. doi:https://doi.org/10.2337/diacare.28.1.3

Dwyer, T., Pezic, A., Sun, C., Cochrane, J., Venn, A., Srikanth, V., . . . Ponsonby, A. (2015, Nov 4). Objectively Measured Daily Steps and Subsequent Long Term All-Cause Mortality: The Tasped Prospective Cohort Study. *PLoS one, 10*(11), e0141274. doi:10.1371/journal.pone.0141274

Ekelund, U., Steene-Johannessen, J., Brown, W., Fagerland, M., Owen, N., Powell, K., . . . Group., L. S. (2016, Sep 24). Does physical activity attenuate, or even eliminate, the detrimental association of sitting time with mortality? A harmonised meta-analysis of data from more than 1 million men and women. *Lancet, 388*(10051), 1302-1310. doi:10.1016/S0140-6736(16)30370-1

Elraiyah, T., Sonbol, M., Wang, Z., Khairalseed, T., Asi, N., Undavalli, C., . . . MH, M. (2014). Clinical review: The benefits and harms of systemic testosterone therapy in postmenopausal women with normal adrenal function: a systematic review and meta-analysis. *Journal of Clinical Endocrinology and Metabolism, 99*(10), 3543-50. doi:https://doi.org/10.1210/jc.2014-2262

Elsamadicy, A., Adogwa, O., Vuong, V., Mehta, A., Vasquez, R., Cheng, J., & Karikari, I. B. (2016, Dec). Patient Body Mass Index is an Independent Predictor of 30-Day Hospital Readmission After Elective Spine Surgery. *World neurosurgery, 96*, 148-151. doi:10.1016/j.wneu.2016.08.097

Engel, F., Holmberg, H., & Sperlich, B. (2016, Dec). Is There Evidence that Runners can Benefit from Wearing Compression Clothing? *Sports Medicine, 46*(12), 1939-1952. doi:10.1007/s40279-016-0546-5

Engel, M., Kern, H., Brenna, J., & Mitmesser, S. (2018, Jan). Micronutrient Gaps in Three Commercial Weight-Loss Diet Plans. *Nutrients, 10*(1), 108. doi:10.3390/nu10010108

English, K., Steeds, R., Jones, T., Diver, M., & Channer, K. (2000). Low-dose transdermal testosterone therapy improves angina threshold in men with chronic stable angina: A randomized, double-blind, placebo-controlled study. *Circulations, 102*(16), 1906-11. doi:https://doi.org/10.1161/01.CIR.102.16.1906

English, W., DeMaria, E., Brethauer, S., Mattar, S., Rosenthal, R., & Morton, J. (2018, Mar). American Society for Metabolic and Bariatric Surgery estimation of metabolic and bariatric procedures performed in the United States in 2016. *Surgery for Obesity and Related Diseases, 14*(3), 259-263. doi:10.1016/j.soard.2017.12.013

Escobar-Morreale, H., Santacruz, E., Luque-Ramírez, M., & Botella Carretero, J. (2017). Prevalence of 'obesity-associated gonadal dysfunction' in severely obese men and women and its resolution after bariatric surgery: a systematic review and meta-analysis. *Human Reproduction Update, 9*, 1-19. doi:https://doi.org/10.1093/humupd/dmx012

Etminan, M., Skeldon, S., Goldenberg, S., Carleton, B., & Brophy, J. (2015). Testosterone therapy and risk of myocardial infarction: a pharmacoepidemiological study. *Pharmacotherapy, 35*(1), 72-78. doi:DOI: 10.1002/phar.1534

Evans, F. (1928). The Radical Cure of Simple Obesity by Dietary Measures Alone. *Transactions of the American Climatological and Clinical Association, 44*, 189-195.

Evans, M., Cogan, K., & Egan, B. (2017, May 1). Metabolism of ketone bodies during exercise and training: physiological basis for exogenous supplementation. *J Physiol, 595*(9), 2857-2871. doi:10.1113/JP273185

Fava, G., Benasi, G., Lucente, M., Offidani, E., Cosci, F., & Guidi, J. (2018). Withdrawal Symptoms after Serotonin-Noradrenaline Reuptake Inhibitor Discontinuation: Systematic Review. *Psychotherapy and psychosomatics, 87*(4), 195-203. doi:10.1159/000491524

Fayad, L., Adam, A., Dunlap, M., Badurdeen, D., Hill, C., Ajayi, T., . . . Kumbhari, V. (2019, Apr). Endoscopic sleeve gastroplasty versus laparoscopic sleeve gastrectomy: a case-

References

matched study. *Gastrointestinal Endoscopy, 89*(4), 782-788. doi:10.1016/j.gie.2018.08.030

Fennig, U., Snir, A., Halifa-Kurzman, I., Sela, A., Hadas, A., & Fennig, S. (2019, Apr). Pre-surgical Weight Loss Predicts Post-Surgical Weight Loss Trajectories in Adolescents Enrolled in a Bariatric Program. *Obesity Surgery, 29*(4), 1154-1163. doi:10.1007/s11695-018-03649-8.

Fiatarone, M., O'Neill, E., Ryan, N., Clements, K., Solares, G., Nelson, M., . . . Evans, W. (1994). Exercise Training and Nutritional Supplementation for Physical Frailty in Very Elderly People. *NEJM, 330*(25), 1769-1775. doi:https://doi.org/10.1056/NEJM199406233302501

Field, A., Camargo, C. J., & Ogino, S. (2013, Novembr 27). The merits of subtyping obesity: one size. *Jama, 310*(20), 2147-8. doi:10.1001/jama.2013.281501

Finer, N., Ryan, D., Renz, C., & Hewkin, A. (2005, March 23). Prediction of response to sibutramine therapy in obese non-diabetic and diabetic patients. *Diabetes, Obesity, and Metabolism, 8*(2), 206-213. doi:10.1111/j.1463-1326.2005.00481.x

Finkelstein, E., Trogdon, J., Cohen, J., & Dietz, W. (2009, September). Annual medical spending attributable to obesity: payer-and service-specific estimates. *Health Affaris, 28*(5), 822-31. doi:doi: 10.1377/hlthaff.28.5.w822

Finkle, W., Greenland, S., Ridgeway, G., Adams, J., Frasco, M., Cook, M., . . . Hoover, R. (2014). Increased risk of non-fatal myocardial infarction following testosterone therapy prescription in men. *PLoS one, 9*(1). doi:https://doi.org/10.1371/journal.pone.0085805

Fitts, R., Peters, J., Dillon, E., Durham, W., Sheffield-Moore, M., & Urban, R. (2015). Weekly Versus Monthly Testosterone Administration on Fast and Slow Skeletal Muscle Fibers in Older Adult Males. *Journal of Clinical Endocinology and Metabolism, 100*(2), D223-31. doi:https://doi.org/10.1210/jc.2014-2759

Fitts, R., Romatowski, J., Peters, J., Paddon-Jones, D., Wolfe, R., & Ferrando, A. (2007). The deleterious effects of bed rest on human skeletal muscle fibers are exacerbated by hypercortisolemia and ameliorated by dietary supplementation. *American Psychological Society, 293*(1), c313-320. doi:https://doi.org/10.1152/ajpcell.00573.2006

Fleishman, S., Khan, H., Homel, P., Suhail, M., Strebel-Amrhein, R., Mohammad, F., . . . Suppiah, K. (2010). Testosterone levels and quality of life in diverse male patients with cancers unrelated to androgens. *Journal of Clinical Oncology, 28*(34), 5054-60. doi:https://doi.org/10.1200/JCO.2010.30.3818

Fletcher, P., & Kenny, P. (2018, Dec). Food addiction: a valid concept? *Neuropsychopharmacology, 43*(13), 2506-2513. doi:10.1038/s41386-018-0203-9

Fortes, C., Mastroeni, S., Sperati, A., Pacifici, R., Zuccaro, P., Francesco, F., . . . Ebrahim, S. (2013, Mar). Walking four times weekly for at least 15 min is associated with longevity in a cohort of very elderly people. *Maturitas, 74*(3), 246-251.

Francomano, D., Bruzziches, R., Barbaro, G., Lenzi, A., & Aversa, A. (2014, Apr). Effects of testosterone undecanoate replacement and withdrawal on cardio-metabolic, hormonal and body composition outcomes in severely obese hypogonadal men: a pilot study. *Journal of Endocrinological Investigation, 37*(4), 401-411. doi:10.1007/s40618-014-0066-9

Froylich, D., Sadeh, O., Mizrahi, H., Kafri, N., Pascal, G., Daigle, C., . . . Hazzan, D. (2018, OCT). Midterm outcomes of sleeve gastrectomy in the elderly. *Surgery for Obesity and Related Diseases, 14*(10), 1495-1500. doi:10.1016/j.soard.2018.07.020

Frustaci, A., Kaistura, J., Chimenti, C., Jakoniuk, I., Leri, A., Maseri, A., . . . Anversa, P. (2000). Myocardial cell death in human diabetes. *Circulation Research, 87*(12), 1123-32.

Gafoor, R., Booth, H., & Gulliford, M. (2018, Apr). Antidepressant utilisation and incidence of weight gain during 10 years' follow-up: population-based cohort study. *BMJ, 361*, k1951.

Gargallo-Vaamonde, J., Perdomo, C., de la Higuera, M., & Frubeck, G. (2019). Is pharmacotherapy enough for urgent weight loss in severely obese patients? *Expert Opinion of Pharmacotherapy, 20*(4), 367-371. doi:10.1080/14656566.2018.1559818

Garvey, W. T. (2013, Sept). NEW TOOLS FOR WEIGHT-LOSS THERAPY ENABLE A MORE ROBUST MEDICAL MODEL FOR OBESITY TREATMENT: RATIONALE

References

FOR A COMPLICATIONS-CENTRIC APPROACH. *Endocrine Practice : Official Journal of the American College of Endocrinology and the American Association of Clinical Endocrinologists, 19*(5), 864–874. doi:10.4158/EP13263.RA

Gebel, K., Ding, D., Chey, Stamatakis, E., Brown, W., & Bauman, A. (2015, June). Effect of Moderate to Vigorous Physical Activity on All-Cause Mortality in Middle-aged and Older Australians. *JAMA, 175*(6), 970-7. doi:https://doi.org/10.1001/jamainternmed.2015.0541

Gelesis. (2019, April 14). *Gelesis.* Retrieved from Gelesis Granted FDA Clearance to Market PLENITY for Weight Loss: https://www.gelesis.com/2019/04/14/gelesis-granted-fda-clearance-to-market-plenitytm-a-new-prescription-aid-to-weight-management/

Gentil, P., de Lira, C., Paoli, A., Dos Santos, J., da Silva, R., Junior, J., . . . Magosso, R. (2017). Nutrition, Pharmacological and Training Strategies Adopted by Six Bodybuilders: Case Report and Critical Review. *European Journal of Translational Myology, 27*(1), 2647. doi:https://dx.doi.org/10.4081%2Fejtm.2017.6247

Gera, R., Tayeh, S., Chehade, H., & Mokbel, K. (2018, Dec). Does Transdermal Testosterone Increase the Risk of Developing Breast Cancer? A Systematic Review. *Anticancer research, 38*(12), 6615-6620. doi:10.21873/anticanres.13028

Gerich, J. (2002, Feb). Is reduced first-phase insulin release the earliest detectable abnormality in individuals destined to develop type 2 diabetes. *Diabetes, 51*, s117-21. doi:https://doi.org/10.2337/diabetes.51.2007.S117

Ghanta, R., LaPar, D., Zhang, Q., Devarkonda, V., Isbell, J., Yarboro, L., . . . Ailawadi, G. (2017, Mar 8). Obesity Increases Risk-Adjusted Morbidity, Mortality, and Cost Following Cardiac Surgery. *Journal of the American Heart Association, 6*(3), 3831. doi:10.1161/JAHA.116.003831

Giannoulis, M., Martin, F., Nair, K., Umpleby, A., & Sonksen, P. (2012). Hormone replacement therapy and physical function in healthy older men. Time to talk hormones? *Endocrine Reviews, 33*(3), 314-77. doi:https://doi.org/10.1210/er.2012-1002

Gibney, J., Healy, M., & Sönksen, P. (2007). The Growth Hormone/Insulin-Like Growth Factor-1 Axis in Exercise

and Sport. *Endocrine Reviews, 28*(6), 603-624.
doi:https://doi.org/10.1210/er.2006-0052

Gibson, A., Seimon, R., Lee, C., Ayre, J., Franklin, J., Markovic, T., . . . Sainsbury, A. (2015, Jan). Do ketogenic diets really suppress appetite? A systematic review and meta-analysis. *Obesity Review, 16*(1), 64-76. doi:10.1111/obr.12230

Giel, K., Thiel, A., Teufel, M., Mayer, J., & Zipfel, S. (2010). Weight Bias in Work Settings – a Qualitative Review. *Obesity facts, 3*(1), 33-40.

Gill, H., Kang, S., Lee, Y., Rosenblat, J., Brietzke, E., Zuckerman, H., & McIntyre, R. (2019, March 1). The long-term effect of bariatric surgery on depression and anxiety. *Journal of affective disorders, 246*, 886-894. doi:10.1016/j.jad.2018.12.113

Giordano, R., Bonelli, L., Marinazzo, E., Ghigo, E., & Arvat, E. (2008). Growth hormone treatment in human ageing: benefits and risks. *Hormones, 7*(2), 133-139. Retrieved from http://www.hormones.gr/216/article/article.html

Giugliano, D., Maiorino, M., Bellastella, G., & Esposito, K. (2018, Sep). More sugar? No, thank you! The elusive nature of low carbohydrate diets. *Endocrine, 61*(3), 383-387. doi:10.1007/s12020-018-1580-x

Glaser, R., & Dimitrakakis, C. (2013). Reduced breast cancer incidence in women treated with subcutaneous testosterone, or testosterone with anastrozole: A prospective, observational study. *Maturitas, 76*(4), 342-9. doi:https://doi.org/10.1016/j.maturitas.2013.08.002

Godfrey, J., Rothstein, R., & Gonzalez-Campoy, M. (2019, May 3). *Emerging Non-Surgical Gastric Devices Gain Approval for Weight Management.* Retrieved from Endocrine Web: https://www.endocrineweb.com/professional/obesity/em erging-endoscopic-devices-gain-approval-weight-management

Goldstein, I., Stecher, V., & Carlsson, M. (2017). Treatment response to sildenafil in men with erectile dysfunction relative to concomitant comorbidities and age. *International Journal of Clinical Practice, 71*, 3-4. doi:https://doi.org/10.1111/ijcp.12939

Gomez, G., & Stanford, F. (2018, Mar). US health policy and prescription drug coverage of FDA-approved medications for the treatment of obesity. *International Journal of Obesity,* *42*(3), 495-500. doi:10.1038/ijo.2017.287

Gomez-Cabrera, M., Domenech, E., & Viña, J. (2008, Jan 15). Moderate exercise is an antioxidant: upregulation of antioxidant genes by training. *Free Radical biology and medicine,* *44*(2), 126-31. doi:https://doi.org/10.1016/j.freeradbiomed.2007.02.001

Goodman, N., Guay, A., Dandona, P., Dhindsa, S., Faiman, C., & Cunningham, G. (2015). AMERICAN ASSOCIATION OF CLINICAL ENDOCRINOLOGISTS AND AMERICAN COLLEGE OF ENDOCRINOLOGY POSITION STATEMENT ON THE ASSOCIATION OF TESTOSTERONE AND CARDIOVASCULAR RISK. *Endocrine Practice, 21,* 1066-1073. doi:https://doi.org/10.4158/EP14434.PS

Gorgey, A., Khalil, R., Gill, R., O'Brien, L., Lavis, T., Castillo, T., . . . Adler, R. (2017). Effects of Testosterone and Evoked Resistance Exercise after Spinal Cord Injury (TEREX-SCI): study protocol for a randomised controlled trial. *BMJ open,* *7*(4). doi:https://doi.org/10.1136/bmjopen-2016-014125

Gorin, A., Lenz, E., Cornelius, T., Huedo-Medina, T., Wojtanowski, A., & Foster, G. (2018, Mar). Randomized Controlled Trial Examining the Ripple Effect of a Nationally Available Weight Management Program on Untreated Spouses. *Obesity, 26*(3), 499-504. doi:10.1002/oby.22098

Goss, A. (1980). Treatment of massive obesity by prolonged jaw immobilization for edentulous patients. *International journal of oral surgery, 9*(4), 253-258.

Gouveia, M., Sanches, R., Andrade, S., Carmona, S., & Ferreira, C. (2018, Nov 30). The Role of Testosterone in The Improvement of Sexual Desire in Postmenopausal Women: An Evidence-Based Clinical Review. *Acta Medica Portuguesa, 31*(11), 680-690. doi:10.20344/amp.9277

Gravisse, N., Vibarel-rebot, N., Labsy, Z., Do, M., Gagey, O., Dubourg, C., . . . Collomp, K. (2018, Sep). Short-term Dehydroepiandrosterone Intake and Supramaximal Exercise in Young Recreationally-trained Women. *International Journal of Sports Medicine, 39*(9), 712-719. doi:10.1055/a-0631-3008

Greene, D., Varley, B., Hartwig, T., Chapman, P., & Rigney, M. (2018, Dec). A Low-Carbohydrate Ketogenic Diet Reduces Body Mass Without Compromising Performance in Powerlifting and Olympic Weightlifting Athletes. *Journal of Strength and Conditioning Research, 32*(12), 3373-3382. doi:10.1519/JSC.0000000000002904

Grossmann, M. (2018, Jul). Hypogonadism and male obesity: Focus on unresolved questions. *Clinical Endocrinology, 89*(1), 11-21. doi:10.1111/cen.13723

Guerrero Pérez, F., Sánchez-González, J., Sánchez, I., Jiménez-Murcia, S., Granero, R., Simó-Servat, A., . . . Monasterio, C. (2018, Nov). Food addiction and preoperative weight loss achievement in patients seeking bariatric surgery. *European Eating disorders review, 26*(6), 645-656. doi:10.1002/erv.2649

Guo, C., Gu, W., Liu, M., Peng, B., Yao, X., Yang, C., & Zheng, J. (2016, Mar). Efficacy and safety of testosterone replacement therapy in men with hypogonadism: A meta-analysis study of placebo-controlled trials. *Experimental and Theraputic Medicine, 11*(3), 853-863. doi:10.3892/etm.2015.2957

Hackett, G. (2016). Testosterone Replacement Therapy and Mortality in Older Men. *Drug Safety, 39*, 117-130. doi:https://doi.org/10.1007/s40264-015-0348-y

Hackett, G. I., Cole, N. S., Deshpande, A. A., Popple, M. D., Kennedy, D., & Wilkinson, P. (2009). Biochemical hypogonadism in men with type 2 diabetes in primary care practice. *The British Journal of Diabetes & Vascular Disease, 9*(5), 226-31. doi:http://dx.doi.org/10.1177%2F1474651409342635

Hackett, G., Jones, P., Strange, R., & Ramachandran, S. (2017, Mar 15). Statin, testosterone and phosphodiesterase 5-inhibitor treatments and age-related mortality in diabetes. *World Journal of Diabetes, 8*(3), 104-111. doi:10.4239/wjd.v8.i3.104

Hackney, A., & Aggon, E. (2018, Feb). Chronic Low Testosterone Levels in Endurance Trained Men: The Exercise-Hypogonadal Male Condition. *Journal of Biochemical Physiology, 1*(1), 103.

Hackney, A., Moore, A., & Brownlee, K. (2005). Testosterone and endurance exercise: development of the "exercise-hypogonadal male condition". *Acta Physiologica Hungarica, 92*(2), 121-137.

Hagihara, A., Onozuka, D., Hasegawa, M., Miyazaki, S., & Nagata, T. (2018, Jul 6). Grand Sumo Tournaments and Out-of-Hospital Cardiac Arrests in Tokyo. *Journal of the American Heart Association, 7*(14), e009163. doi:10.1161/JAHA.118.009163

Haiat, F., Leibovitz, E., & Shimonov, M. (2018, Aug). [BARIATRICS IN GERIATRICS - IS AGE AN OBSTACLE FOR BARIATRIC SURGERY?]. *Harefuah, 157*(8), 498-502.

Haider, A., Yassin, A., Haider, K., Doros, G., Saad, F., & Rosano, G. (2016). Men with testosterone deficiency and a history of cardiovascular diseases benefit from long-term testosterone therapy: observational, real-life data from a registry study. *Health Risk Management, 12*, 251-61. doi:https://doi.org/10.2147/VHRM.S108947

Hajimonfarednejad, M., Nimrouzi, M., Heydari, M., Zarshenas, M., Raee, M., & Jahromi, B. (2018). nsulin resistance improvement by cinnamon powder in polycystic ovary syndrome: A randomized double-blind placebo controlled clinical trial. *Phytotherapy research, 32*(2), 276-283. doi:10.1002/ptr.5970.

Hajna, S., Ross, N., & Dasgupta, K. (2018, Feb). Steps, moderate-to-vigorous physical activity, and cardiometabolic profiles. *Preventive medicine, 107*, 69-74. doi:10.1016/j.ypmed.2017

Hallam, K., Bilsborough, S., & de Courten, M. (2018, Jan 24). "Happy feet": evaluating the benefits of a 100-day 10,000 step challenge on mental health and wellbeing. *BMC Psychiatry, 18*(1), 19. doi:10.1186/s12888-018-1609-y

Halpern, B., & Halpern, A. (2015, Feb 14). Why are anti-obesity drugs stigmatized? *Expert Opinion on Drug Safety, 14*(2), 185-189. doi:10.1517/14740338.2015.995088

Halpern, B., & Mancini, M. (2017, Jan). Safety assessment of combination therapies in the treatment of obesity: focus on naltrexone/bupropion extended release and phentermine-topiramate extended release. (39, Ed.) *Expert Opinion on Drug Safety, 16*(1), 27. doi:http://dx.doi.org/10.1080/14740338.2017.1247807

hamidi Madani, A., Asadolahzade, A., Mokhtari, G., Shahrokhi Damavand, R., Farzan, A., & Esmaeili, S. (2013, April). • Assessment of the efficacy of combination therapy with folic acid and tadalafil for the management of erectile dysfunction in men with type 2 diabetes mellitus. *The Journal of Sexual Medicine, 10*(4), 1146-1150. doi:10.1111/jsm.12047

Hampp, C., Kang, E., & Borders-Hemphill, V. (2019, September 9). Use of Prescription Antiobesity Drugs in the United States. *Pharmacotherapy, 33*(12), 1299-1307. doi: 10.1002/phar.1342

Handley, R., Bentley, R., Brown, T., & Annan, A. (2018). Successful treatment of obesity and insulin resistance via ketogenic diet status post Roux-en-Y. *BMJ Case Report.* doi:10.1136/bcr-2018-225643

Hariri, K., Guevara, D., Dong, M., Kini, S., Herron, D., & Fernandez-Ranvier, G. (2018). Is bariatric surgery effective for co-morbidity resolution in the super-obese patients? *Surgery for obesity and related disease, 14*(9), 1261-68. doi:10.1016/j.soard.2018.05.015

Hasnain, M., Vieweg, W., & Fredrickson, S. (2010, March). Metformin for atypical antipsychotic-induced weight gain and glucose metabolism dysregulation: review of the literature and clinical suggestions. *CNS Drugs, 24*(3), 193-206. doi:10.2165/11530130-000000000-00000

Haynes, A., Kersbergen, I., Sutin, A., Daly, M., & Robinson, E. (2018, Mar). A systematic review of the relationship between weight status perceptions and weight loss attempts, strategies, behaviours and outcomes. *Obesity Reviews, 19*(3), 347-363. doi:10.1111/obr.12634

Hazell, T., Islam, H., Townsend, L., Schmale, M., & Copeland, J. (2016, Mar 1). Effects of exercise intensity on plasma concentrations of appetite-regulating hormones: Potential mechanisms. *Appetite, 98*, 80-8. doi:https://doi.org/10.1016/j.appet.2015.12.016

Healthcare Cost and Utilization Project (HCUP). (2014). *HCUP National Inpatient Sample (NIS).* Rockville, MD: Agency for Healthcare Research and Quality. Retrieved from https://www.hcup-us.ahrq.gov/db/nation/nis/tools/stats/NIS_2014_Masked Stats_Core_Weighted.PDF

References

Hell, E., & Miller, K. (2002). [Bariatric surgery -- stereotypes and paradigms]. *Zentralblatt fur Chirurgie, 127*(12), 1032-4. doi:10.1055/s-2002-36374

Hellman, B., Gylfe, E., Grapengiesser, E., Dansk, H., & Salehi, A. (2007). [Insulin oscillations--clinically important rhythm. Antidiabetics should increase the pulsative component of the insulin release]. *Lakartidningen, 104*(32-33), 2236-9. Retrieved from https://www.ncbi.nlm.nih.gov/pubmed/17822201

Hendricks, E., & Greenway, F. (2011, July). A Study of Abrupt Phentermine Cessation in Patients in a Weight Management Program. *American Journal of Theraputics, 18*(4), 292-299. doi:10.1097/MJT.0b013e3181d070d7

Hendricks, E., Rothman, R., & Greenway, F. (2009, Sept). How physician obesity specialists use. *Obesity, 17*(9), 1730-5. doi:10.1038/oby.2009.69

Himmelstein, M., Puhl, R., & Quinn, D. (2018, Jun). Weight Stigma in Men: What, When, and by Whom? *Obesity, 26*(6), 968-976. doi:10.1002/oby.22162

Hirsh, S., Pons, M., Joval, S., & Swick, A. (2019). Avoiding holiday seasonal weight gain with nutrient-supported intermittent energy restriction: a pilot study. *Journal of Nutritional Science, 8*, e11. doi:10.1017/jns.2019

Hodish, I. (2018). Insulin therapy, weight gain and prognosis. *Diabetes, Obesity, and metabolism, 20*(9), 2085-2092. doi:10.1111/dom.13367

Högström, G., Nordström, A., & Nordström, P. (2016, Aug). Aerobic fitness in late adolescence and the risk of early death: a prospective cohort study of 1.3 million Swedish men. *International Journal of Epidemeiology, 45*(4), 1159-1168. doi:https://doi.org/10.1093/ije/dyv321

Holmboe, S., Skakkebaek, N., Juul, A., Scheike, T., Jensen, T., Linneberg, A., . . . Andersson, A. (2018). Individual testosterone decline and future mortality risk in men. *European Journal of Endocinology, 178*, 11-128. doi:doi: 10.1530/EJE-17-0280

Homola, J., & Hieber, R. (2018, Mar 26). Combination of venlafaxine and phentermine/ topiramate induced psychosis: A case report. *The Mental Health Clinician, 8*(2), 95-99. doi:10.9740/mhc.2018.03.095

Hooper, D., & Tenford, A. H. (2018, Nov). Treating exercise associated low testosterone and its related symptoms. *The pysician and Sports medicine, 46*(4), 427-434. doi:10.1080/00913847.2018.1507234

Hooper, D., Kraemer, W., Saenz, C., Schill, K., Focht, B., Volek, J., & Maresh, C. (2017, Jul). The presence of symptoms of testosterone deficiency in the exercise-hypogonadal male condition and the role of nutrition. *European Journal of applied Physiology, 117*(7), 1349-1357. doi:10.1007/s00421-017-3623-z

Hooper, D., Kraemer, W., Stearns, R., Kupchak, B., Volk, B., DuPont, W., . . . Casa, D. (2019, Feb). Evidence of the Exercise Hypogonadal Male Condition at the 2011 Kona Ironman World Championships. *International journal of sports physiology and performance, 14*(2), 170-175. doi:0.1123/ijspp.2017-0476

Hope, S., Knight, B., Shields, B., Hill, A., Choudhary, P., Strain, W., . . . Jones, A. (2018). Random non-fasting C-peptide testing can identify patients with insulin-treated type 2 diabetes at high risk of hypoglycaemia. *Diabetelogia, 61*(1), 66-74. doi:10.1007/s00125-017-4449-2

Horstman, A., Dillon, E., Urban, R., & Sheffield-Moore, M. (2012). The Role of Androgens and Estrogens on Healthy Aging and Longevity. *The Journals of Gerentology. Series A, Biological Sciences and Medical Sciences, 67*(11), 1140-1152. doi:https://doi.org/10.1093/gerona/gls068

Hoshiu, A., & Inaba, Y. (1995, Aug). [Risk factors for mortality and mortality rate of sumo wrestlers]. *Japanese Journal of Hygeine, 50*(3), 730-6.

Houghton, D., Alsawas, M., Barrioneuvo, P., Tello, M., Farah, W., Beuschel, B., . . . Moll, S. (2018, Dec). Testosterone therapy and venous thromboembolism: A systematic review and meta-analysis. *Thrombosis Research, 172*, 94-103. doi:10.1016/j.thromres.2018.10.023.

Huang, G., Basaria, S., Travison, T., Ho, M., Davda, M., Mazer, N., . . . Bhasin, S. (2014, Jun). Testosterone dose-response relationships in hysterectomized women with or without oophorectomy: effects on sexual function, body composition, muscle performance and physical function in a randomized trial. *menopause, 21*(6), 612-623. doi:10.1097/GME.0000000000000093

Hulmi, J., Volek, J., Selänne, H., & Mero, A. (2005). Protein Ingestion Prior to Strength Exercise Affects Blood Hormones and Metabolism. *Medicine and Science in Sports and Exercise, 37*(11), 1990-7. Retrieved from https://www.ncbi.nlm.nih.gov/pubmed/16286871

Huo, S., Scialli, A., McGarvey, S., Hill, E., Tügertimur, B., Hogenmiller, A., . . . Fugh-Berman, A. (2016). Treatment of Men for "Low Testosterone": A Systematic Review. *PLoS one, 11*(9). doi:https://doi.org/10.1371/journal.pone.0162480

Husted, H., Jorgensen, C. G., & Kehlet, H. (2016, Oct). Does BMI influence hospital stay and morbidity after fast-track hip and knee arthroplasty? *Acta Orthopaedica, 87*(5), 466-72. doi:10.1080/17453674.2016.1203477

Hyde, Z., Flicker, L., Almeida, O., Hankey, G., McCaul, K., Chubb, S., & Yeap, B. (2010). Low free testosterone predicts frailty in older men: the health in men study. *The Journal of Clinical Endocrinology and Metabolism, 95*(7), 3165-72. doi:https://doi.org/10.1210/jc.2009-2754

Hyldig, N., Vinter, C., Kruse, M., Mogensen, O., Bille, C., Sorensen, J., . . . Joergensen, J. (2019, Apr). Prophylactic incisional negative pressure wound therapy reduces the risk of surgical site infection after caesarean section in obese women: a pragmatic randomised clinical trial. *BJOG, 126*(5), 628-635. doi:10.1111/1471-0528.15413

Ingargiola, M., Motakef, S., Chung, M., Vasconez, H., & Sasaki, G. (2015, June). Cryolipolysis for Fat Reduction and Body Contouring: Safety and Efficacy of Current Treatment Paradigms. *Plastic and Reconstructive Surgery, 135*(6), 1581-1590. doi:10.1097/PRS.0000000000001236

Institute of Medicine (US) Committee on Assessing the Need for Clinical Trials. (2004). Testosterone and Aging: Clinical Research Directions. *National Academic Press.*

International Osteoporosis Foundation. (2017). *Facts and Statistics.* Retrieved from International Osteoporosis Foundation: https://www.iofbonehealth.org/facts-statistics

Ip, E., Trinh, K., Tenerowicz, M., Pal, J., Lindfelt, T., & Perry, P. (2015, Oct). Characteristics and Behaviors of Older Male

Anabolic Steroid Users. *Journal of pharmacy practice, 28*(5), 450-456. doi:10.1177/0897190014527319

Islam, R., Bell, R., Green, S., & Davis, S. (2019, Jan 11). Effects of testosterone therapy for women: a systematic review and meta-analysis protocol. *Systematic reviews, 8*(1), 19. doi:10.1186/s13643-019-0941-8

Ito, K., Colley, T., & Mercado, N. (2012). Geroprotectors as a novel therapeutic strategy for COPD, an accelerating aging disease. *International journal of chronic obstructive pulmonary disorder, 7*, 641-652. doi:10.2147/COPD.S28250

Ivesaj, V., Wiedermann, A., Lawson, J., & Grilo, C. (2019). Food Addiction in Sleeve Gastrectomy Patients with Loss-of-Control Eating. *Obesity Surgery, 29*(7), 2071-2077. doi:10.1007/s11695-019-03805-8

Ivezaj, V., Fu, E., Lydecker, J., Duffy, A., & Grilo, C. (2019, May). Racial Comparisons of Postoperative Weight Loss and Eating-Disorder Psychopathology Among Patients Following Sleeve Gastrectomy Surgery. *Obesity (Silver Spring), 27*(5), 740-745. doi:10.1002/oby.22446

Jäger, R., Kerksick, C., Campbell, B., Cribb, P., Wells, S., Skwiat, T., ... Antonio, J. (2017, Jun 20). International Society of Sports Nutrition Position Stand: protein and exercise. *journal of the international society of sports medicine, 14*(20). doi:10.1186/s12970-017-0177-8

Jannah, N., Hild, J., Gallagher, C., & Dietz, W. (2018, Dec). Coverage for Obesity Prevention and Treatment Services: Analysis of Medicaid and State Employee Health Insurance Programs. *Obesity, 26*(12), 1834-1840. doi:10.1002/oby.22307

Janssen, H., Samson, M., & Verhaar, H. (2002). Vitamin D deficiency, muscle function, and falls in elderly people. *The American Journal of Clinical Nutrition, 75*(4), 611-5. Retrieved from http://ajcn.nutrition.org/content/75/4/611.long

Jayasena, C., Alkaabi, F., Liebers, C., Handley, T., Franks, S., & Dhillo, W. (2018, Nov 29). A systematic review of randomized controlled trials investigating the efficacy and safety of testosterone therapy for female sexual dysfunction in postmenopausal women. *Clinical Endocrinology, 90*(3), 391-414. doi:10.1111/cen.13906

References

Jeschke, E., Citak, M., Gunster, C., Halder, A., Heller, K., Malzahn, J., . . . Gehrke, T. (2018, Jul). Obesity Increases the Risk of Postoperative Complications and Revision Rates Following Primary Total Hip Arthroplasty: An Analysis of 131,576 Total Hip Arthroplasty Cases. *Journal of Arthroplasty, 33*(7), 2287-2292. doi:10.1016/j.arth.2018.02.036

Jha, M., Wakhlu, S., Dronamraju, N., Minhajuddin, A., Greer, T., & Trivedi, M. (2018, Jul). Validating pre-treatment body mass index as moderator of antidepressant treatment outcomes: Findings from CO-MED trial. *Journal of Effective Disorders, 234*, 34-37. doi:10.1016/j.jad.2018.02.089

Johnston, C., Moreno, J., Hernandez, D., Link, B., Chen, T., Wojtanowski, A., . . . Foreyt, J. (2019, Jan). Levels of adherence needed to achieve significant weight loss. *International Journal of Obesity, 43*(1), 125-131. doi:10.1038/s41366-018-0226-7

Jones, T. (2010). Testosterone deficiency: a risk factor for cardiovascular disease? *Trends in Endocrinology and Metabolism, 21*(8), 496-503. doi:https://doi.org/10.1016/j.tem.2010.03.002

Kanayama, G., Hudson, J., DeLuca, J., Isaacs, S., Baggish, A., Weiner, R., . . . Pope, H. J. (2015). Prolonged Hypogonadism in Males Following Withdrawal from Anabolic-Androgenic Steroids: an Underrecognized Problem. *Addictions, 110*(5), 823-831. doi:https://dx.doi.org/10.1111%2Fadd.12850

Kanda, H., Hayakawa, T., Tsuboi, S., Mori, Y., Takahashi, T., & Fukushima, T. (2009, Dec). Higher Body Mass Index is a Predictor of Death Among Professional Sumo Wrestlers. *Journal of sports science & medicine, 8*(4), 711-712.

Karakas, M., Schäfer, S., Appelbaum, S., Ojeda, F., Kuulasmaa, K., Brückmann, B., . . . Zeller, T. (2018, Aug 20). Testosterone Levels and Type 2 Diabetes-No Correlation with Age, Differential Predictive Value in Men and Women. *Biomolecules, 8*(3). doi:10.3390/biom8030076

Khaw, K., Dowsett, M., Folkerd, E., Bingham, S., Wareham, N., Luben, R., . . . Day, N. (2007). Endogenous Testosterone and Mortality Due to All Causes, Cardiovascular Disease, and Cancer in Men. *Circulation, 116*, 2694-2701.

doi:https://doi.org/10.1161/CIRCULATIONAHA.107.71 9005

Kim, J., Oh, S., Shin, J., Hwang, S., Hyun, S., Yang, H., & Lee, G. (2013). Testosterone related good neurologic outcome on the patients with return of spontaneous circulation after cardiac arrest: a prospective cohort study. *Resuscitation, 84*(5), 645-50. doi:https://doi.org/10.1016/j.resuscitation.2012.10.022

Kim, M., Han, K., Koh, E., Kim, E., Lee, M., Nam, G., & Kwon, H. (2019, Mar). Weight change and mortality and cardiovascular outcomes in patients with new-onset diabetes mellitus: a nationwide cohort study. *Cardiovascular diabetology, 18*(1), 36. doi:10.1186/s12933-019-0838-9.

Kim, S. (2014). Testosterone Replacement Therapy and Bone Mineral Density in Men with Hypogonadism. *Endocrinology and Metabolism, 29*(1), 30-32. doi:https://dx.doi.org/10.3803%2FEnM.2014.29.1.30

King, G., & Thamrin, C. (2019). Obesity and the lungs: Not just a crush. *Respirology, 24*(6), 502-503. doi:10.1111/resp.13532

King, W., Chen, J., Belle, S., Courcoulas, A., Dakin, G., Elder, K., . . . Yanovski, S. (2016). Change in Pain and Physical Function Following Bariatric Surgery for Severe Obesity. *JAMA, 315*(13), 1362-1371. doi:10.1001/jama.2016.3010

Klein, S., Fontana, L., Young, V., Coggan, A., Kilo, C., Patterson, B., & Mohammed, B. (2004, June 17). Absence of an effect of liposuction on insulin action and risk factors for coronary heart disease. *New England Journal of Medicine, 350*(25), 2549-2557. doi:10.1056/NEJMoa033179

Klotzbuecher, C., Ross, P., Landsman, P., Abbott, T. 3., & Berger, M. (2000). Patients with prior fractures have an increased risk of future fractures: a summary of the literature and statistical synthesis. *J Bone Miner Res, 15*(4), 721-39. doi:https://doi.org/10.1359/jbmr.2000.15.4.721

Knechtle, B. (2014, Jun). Relationship of Antropometric and Training Characteristics with Race Performance in Endurance and Ultra-Endurance Athletes. *Asian Journal of Sports Medicine, 5*(2), 73-90.

Knechtle, B., Rust, C., Knechtle, P., & Rosemann, T. (2012, Dec). Does Muscle Mass Affect Running Times in Male Long-distance Master Runners? *Sports Medicine, 3*(4), 247-256.

References

Koeslag, J., Saunders, P. T., & Terblanche, E. (2003, Apr 25). reappraisal of the blood glucose homeostat which comprehensively explains the type 2 diabetes mellitus–syndrome X complex. *The Journal of Physiology*, 333-346. doi: 10.1113/jphysiol.2002.037895

Koh, C., Inaba, C., Sujatha-Bhaskar, S., & Nguyen, N. (2018, Oct). Outcomes of Laparoscopic Bariatric Surgery in the Elderly Population. *The American surgeon, 84*(10), 1600-1603.

Koltyn, K., Brellenthin, A., Cook, D., Sehgal, N., & Hillard, C. (2014, Dec). Mechanisms of Exercise-Induced Hypoalgesia. *Journal of Pain, 15*(12), 1294-1304.

Kovac, J., Rajanahally, S., Smith, R., Coward, R., Lamb, D., & Lipshultz, L. (2014). Patient satisfaction with testosterone replacement therapies: the reasons behind the choices. *Journal of Sexual Medicine, 11*(2), 553-62. doi:https://doi.org/10.1111/jsm.12369

Kraemer, W., & Ratamess, N. (2005). Hormonal Responses and Adaptations to Resistance Exercise and Training. *Sports Medicine, 35*(4), 339-61.

Kraemer, W., Häkkinen, K., Newton, R., Nindl, B., Volek, J., McCormick, M., . . . Evans, W. (1999). Effects of heavy-resistance training on hormonal response patterns in younger vs. older men. *Journal of Applied Physiology, 87*(3), 982-992. Retrieved from http://jap.physiology.org/content/87/3/982.long

Krasnoff, J., Basaria, S., Pencina, M., Jasuja, G., Vasan, R., Ulloor, J., . . . Murabito, J. (2010). Free testosterone levels are associated with mobility limitation and physical performance in community-dwelling men: the Framingham Offspring Study. *The Journal of Clinical Endocrinology and Metabolism, 95*(6), 2790-9. doi:https://doi.org/10.1210/jc.2009-2680

Kreider, R., Kalman, D., Antonio, J., Zeigenfuss, T., Wildman, R., Collins, R., . . . Lopez, H. (2017, Jun). International Society of Sports Nutrition position stand: safety and efficacy of creatine supplementation in exercise, sport, and medicine. *Journal of the International Society of Sports Nutrition, 14*, eCollection. doi:10.1186/s12970-017-0173-z

Kreider, R., Kalman, D., Antonio, J., Zeigenfuss, T., Wildman, R., Collins, R., . . . Lopez, H. (2017). International Society of

Sports Nutrition position stand: safety and efficacy of creatine supplementation in exercise, sport, and medicine. *Journal of the International Society for Sports Nutrition, 14*, 18. doi:10.1186/s12970-017-0173-z

Kuller, L. (2009, August 24). Weight Loss and Reduction of Blood Pressure and Hypertension. *Hypertension, 54*(4), 700-01. doi:10.1161/HYPERTENSIONAHA.109.138891

Kumar, N. (2017). Gastric Plication. *Gastrointestinal endoscopy clinics of North America, 27*(2), 257-265. doi:10.1016/j.giec.2016.12.003.

Kunnumakkara, A., Bordoloi, D., Padmavathi, G., Monisha, J., Roy, N., Prasad, S., & Aggarwal, B. (2017). Curcumin, the golden nutraceutical: multitargeting for multiple chronic diseases. *British Journal of Pharmacology, 174*(11), 1325-1348. doi:10.1111/bph.13621

Kvorning, T., Andersen, M., Brixen, K., & Madsen, K. (2006). Suppression of endogenous testosterone production attenuates the response to strength training: a randomized, placebo-controlled, and blinded intervention study. *American Journal of Physiology. Endocrinology and Metabolism, 291*(6), e1325-1332. doi:https://doi.org/10.1152/ajpendo.00143.2006

Laaksonen, D., Niskanen, L., Punnonen, K., Nyyssönen, K., Tuomainen, T., Valkonen, V., . . . Salonen, J. (2004). Testosterone and sex hormone-binding globulin predict the metabolic syndrome and diabetes in middle-aged men. *Diabetes Care, 27*(5), 1036-41. doi:https://doi.org/10.2337/diacare.27.5.1036

Lane, A., & Hackney, A. (2014). Reproductive Dysfunction from the Stress of Exercise Training is not Gender Specific: The "Exercise-Hypogonadal Male Condition". *Journal of Endocrinology and Diabetes, 1*(2), 4. doi:10.15226/2374-6890/1/2/00108

Laughlin, G., Barrett-Connor, E., & Bergstrom, J. (2008). Low serum testosterone and mortality in older men. *The Journal of Clinical Endocrinology and Metabolism, 93*(1), 68-75. doi:https://doi.org/10.1210/jc.2007-1792

Laughlin, G., Goodell, V., & Barrett-Connor, E. (2010). Extremes of Endogenous Testosterone Are Associated with Increased Risk of Incident Coronary Events in Older

References

Women. *Journal of Clinical Endocrinology and Metabolism, 95*(2), 740-7. doi:https://doi.org/10.1210/jc.2009-1693

LeBlanc, E., Nielson, C., Marshall, L., Lapidus, J., Barrett-Connor, E., Ensrud, K., . . . Orwoll, E. (2009). The effects of serum testosterone, estradiol, and sex hormone binding globulin levels on fracture risk in older men. *Journal of Clinical Endocrinology and Metabolism, 94*(9), 3337-46. doi:https://doi.org/10.1210/jc.2009-0206

Leblanc, E., O'Connor, E., Whitlock, E., Patnode, C., & Kapka, T. (2011, Oct 4). Effectiveness of primary care-relevant treatments for obesity in adults: a systematic evidence review for the U.S. Preventive Services Task Force. *Annals of Internal Medicine, 155*(7), 434-37. doi:10.7326/0003-4819-155-7-201110040-00006

Leder, B., Rohrer, J., Rubin, S., Gallo, J., & Longcope, C. (2004). Effects of Aromatase Inhibition in Elderly Men with Low or Borderline-Low Serum Testosterone Levels. *Journal of Clinical Endocrinology and Metabolism, 89*(3), 1174-1180. doi:https://doi.org/10.1210/jc.2003-031467

Leighton, E., Sainsbury, C., & Jones, G. (2017, Jun). A Practical Review of C-Peptide Testing in Diabetes. *Diabetes therapy, 8*(3), 475-487. doi:10.1007/s13300-017-0265-4

Levin, P., Wei, W., Zhou, S., Xie, L., & Baser, O. (2014). Outcomes and treatment patterns of adding a third agent to 2 OADs in patients with type 2 diabetes. *Journal of managed care and specialty pharmacy, 20*(5), 501-12. doi:10.18553/jmcp.2014.20.5.501

Lewis, K., Fischer, H., Ard, J., Barton, L., Bessesen, D., Daley, M., . . . Arterburn, D. (2019, Apr). Safety and Effectiveness of Longer-Term Phentermine Use: Clinical Outcomes from an Electronic Health Record Cohort. *Obesity, 27*(4), 591-602. doi:10.1002/oby.22430

Li, H., Guo, Y., Yang, Z., Roy, M., & Guo, Q. (2016). The efficacy and safety of oxandrolone treatment for patients with severe burns: A systematic review and meta-analysis. *Burns, 42*(4), 717-27. doi:https://doi.org/10.1016/j.burns.2015.08.023

Li, J., O'Connor, L., Zhou, J., & Campbell, W. (2014, Jul). Exercise patterns, ingestive behaviors, and energy balance. *Physiology and behavior, 134*, 70-75. doi:10.1016/j.physbeh.2014.04.023.

Li, J., Pursey, K., Duncan, M., & Burrows, T. (2018). Addictive Eating and Its Relation to Physical Activity and Sleep Behavior. *Nutrients, 10*(10), e1428. doi:10.3390/nu10101428

Li, L., Yu, H., Liang, J., Guo, Y., Peng, S., Luo, Y., & Wang, J. (2019, Mar). Meta-analysis of the effectiveness of laparoscopic adjustable gastric banding versus laparoscopic sleeve gastrectomy for obesity. *Medicine, 98*(9), e14735. doi:10.1097/MD.0000000000014735

Li, T., Sun, X., & Chen, L. (2019, Jan 18). Free testosterone value before radical prostatectomy is related to oncologic outcomes and post-operative erectile function. *BMC Cancer, 19*(1), 87. doi:10.1186/s12885-018-5148-1.

Liakopoulos, V., Franzén, S., Svensson, A., Miftaraj, M., Ottosson, J., Näslund, I., . . . Eliasson, B. (2019). Pros and cons of gastric bypass surgery in individuals with obesity and type 2 diabetes: nationwide, matched, observational cohort study. *BMJ Open, 9*(1), e023882. doi:10.1136/bmjopen-2018-023882

Lim, S., Rogers, L., Tessler, O., Mundinger, G., Rogers, C., & Lau, F. (2018, Oct). Phentermine: A Systematic Review for Plastic and Reconstructive Surgeons. *Annals of Plastic Surgery, 81*(4), 503-507. doi:10.1097/SAP.0000000000001478

Lingutla, K., Pollock, R., Benomran, E., Purushothaman, B., Kasis, A., Bhatia, C., . . . Friesem, T. (2015, Oct). Outcome of lumbar spinal fusion surgery in obese patients: a systematic review and meta-analysis. *Bone & joint journal, 97-B*(10), 1395-1404. doi:10.1302/0301-620X.97B10.35724

Lio, A., Bovio, E., Nicolo, F., Saitto, G., Scafuri, A., Bassano, C., . . . Ruvolo, G. (2019, Feb 1). Influence of Body Mass Index on Outcomes of Patients Undergoing Surgery for Acute Aortic Dissection: A Propensity-Matched Analysis. *Texas Heart Institute journal., 46*(1), 7-13. doi:10.14503/THIJ-17-6365

Liu, H., Bravata, D., Olkin, I., Nayak, S., Roberts, B., Garber, A., & Hoffman, A. (2007). Systematic Review: The Safety and Efficacy of Growth Hormone in the Healthy Elderly. *Annals of Internal Medicine, 146*(2), 104-115. doi:10.7326/0003-4819-146-2-200701160-00005

Longo, V., Antebi, A., Bartke, A., Barzilai, N., Brown-Borg, H. M., Caruso, C., . . . Fontana, L. (2015). Interventions to Slow

Aging in Humans: Are We Ready? *Aging cell, 14*(4), 497-510. doi:https://doi.org/10.1111/acel.12338

Lundeen, E., Park, S., Pan, L., & Blanck, H. (2018, Dec). Daily Intake of Sugar-Sweetened Beverages Among US Adults in 9 States, by State and Sociodemographic and Behavioral Characteristics, 2016. *Preventing Chronic Disease, 15*, e154. doi:10.5888/pcd15.180335

Maggio, M., Lauretani, F., Ceda, G., Bandinelli, S., Ling, S., Metter, E., . . . Ferrucci, L. (2007). Relationship Between Low Levels of Anabolic Hormones and 6-Year Mortality in Older MenThe Aging in the Chianti Area (InCHIANTI) Study. *Arch Intern Med, 167*(20), 2249-2254. doi:10.1001/archinte.167.20.2249

Maggio, M., Lauretani, F., De Vita, F., Basaria, S., Lippi, G., Butto, V., . . . Ceda, G. (2014). Multiple hormonal dysregulation as determinant of low physical performance and mobility in older persons. *Current Pharmeceutical Design*, 3119-48.

Maggio, M., Nicolini, F., Cattabiani, C., Beghi, C., Gherli, T., Schwartz, R., . . . Ceda, G. (2012). Effects of testosterone supplementation on clinical and rehabilitative outcomes in older men undergoing on-pump CABG. *Contemporary Clinical Trials, 33*(4), 730-8. doi:https://doi.org/10.1016/j.cct.2012.02.019

Magnussen, L., Hvid, L., Hermann, A., Hougaard, D., Gram, B., Caserotti, P., & Andersen, M. (2017, Sep). Testosterone therapy preserves muscle strength and power in aging men with type 2 diabetes-a randomized controlled trial. *Andrology, 5*(5), 946-953. doi:10.1111/andr.12396

Magon, N., Chopra, S., & Kumar, P. (2012). Geroprotection: A promising future. *Journal of mid-life health, 3*(2), 56-8. doi:10.4103/0976-7800.104449

Major, P., Wysocki, M., Dworak, J., Pedziwiatr, M., Pisarska, M., Wierdak, M., . . . Budzynski, A. (2018, Jun). Analysis of Laparoscopic Sleeve Gastrectomy Learning Curve and Its Influence on Procedure Safety and Perioperative Complications. *Obesity Surgery, 28*(6), 1672-1680. doi:10.1007/s11695-017-3075-x

Major, P., Wysocki, M., Torbicz, G., Gajewska, N., Dudek, A., Malczak, P., . . . Budzynski, A. (2018). Risk Factors for Prolonged Length of Hospital Stay and Readmissions After

Laparoscopic Sleeve Gastrectomy and Laparoscopic Roux-en-Y Gastric Bypass. *Obesity Surgery, 28*(2), 323-332. doi:10.1007/s11695-017-2844-x

Malkin, C., Pugh, P., Morris, P., Asif, S., Jones, T., & Channer, K. (2010). Low serum testosterone and increased mortality in men with coronary heart disease. *Heart, 96*(22), 1821-5. doi:https://doi.org/10.1136/hrt.2010.195412

Malkin, C., Pugh, P., Morris, P., Kerry, K., Jones, R., Jones, T., & Channer, K. (2004). Testosterone replacement in hypogonadal men with angina improves ischemic threshold and quality of life. *Heart, 90*(8), 871-6. doi:https://doi.org/10.1136/hrt.2003.021121

Malmberg, K., Yusuf, S., Gerstein, H., Brown, J., Zhao, F., Hunt, D., . . . Budaj, A. (2000). Impact of Diabetes on Long-Term Prognosis in Patients With Unstable Angina and Non-Q-Wave Myocardial Infarction : Results of the OASIS (Organization to Assess Strategies for Ischemic Syndromes) Registry. *Circulation, 102*, 1014-1019. doi:10.1161/01.CIR.102.9.1014

Mancini, A., Borel, A., Coumes, S., Wion, N., Arvieux, C., & Reche, F. (2018, Jul 20). Bariatric surgery improves the employment rate in people with obesity: 2-year analysis. *Obesity and Related Diseases, 14*(11), 1700-1704. doi:10.1016/j.soard.2018.06.026

Mangolim, A., Brito, L., & Nunes-Nogueira, V. (2018, Apr). Effectiveness of testosterone therapy in obese men with low testosterone levels, for losing weight, controlling obesity complications, and preventing cardiovascular events: Protocol of a systematic review of randomized controlled trials. *Medicine, 97*(17), e0842. doi:doi: 10.1097/MD.0000000000010482.

Maniar, R., Maniar, P., Singhi, T., & Gangaraju, B. (2018, Mar). WHO Class of Obesity Influences Functional Recovery Post-TKA. *Clinics in orthopedic surgery, 10*(1), 26-32. doi:10.4055/cios.2018.10.1.26

Maradit Kremers, H., Larson, D., Crowson, C., Kremers, W., Washington, R., Steiner, C., . . . Berry, D. (2015). Prevalence of Total Hip and Knee Replacement in the United States. *The Journal of Bone and Joint Surgery. American*

References

Volume., 97(17), 1386-1397.
doi:https://doi.org/10.2106/JBJS.N.01141

Marsh, C., Green, D., Naylor, L., & Guelfi, K. (2017, Sep 1). Consumption of dark chocolate attenuates subsequent food intake compared with milk and white chocolate in postmenopausal women. *Appetite, 116*, 544-551. doi:10.1016/j.appet.2017.05.050

Martinez, C., Suissa, S., Rietbrock, S., Katholing, A., Freedman, B., Cohen, A., & Handelsman, D. (2016). Testosterone treatment and risk of venous thromboembolism: population based case-control study. *BMJ*. doi:10.1136/bmj.i5968

Martone, A., Marzetti, E. C., Picca, A., Tosato, M., Santoro, L., Giorgio, D., . . . Landi, F. (2017, Mar 21). Exercise and Protein Intake: A Synergistic Approach against Sarcopenia. *Biomed Research International.* doi:10.1155/2017/2672435

Mazidi, M., Rezaie, P., Kengne, A., Mobarhan, M., & Ferns, G. (2016, April-June). Gut microbiome and metabolic syndrome. *Diabetes and Metabolic Syndrome: Clinical Research and Reviews, 10*(2 s1), s150-s157. doi:https://doi.org/10.1016/j.dsx.2016.01.024

McEvedy, S., Sullivan-Mort, G., McLean, S., Pascoe, M., & Paxton, S. (2017, Oct). Ineffectiveness of commercial weight-loss programs for achieving modest but meaningful weight loss: Systematic review and meta-analysis. *Journal of health psychology, 22*(12), 1614-1627. doi:10.1177/1359105317705983

McGuire, K., Khaleel, M., Rihn, J., Lurie, J., Zhao, W., & Weinstein, J. (2014, Nov 1). The effect of high obesity on outcomes of treatment for lumbar spinal conditions: subgroup analysis of the spine patient outcomes research trial. *Spine, 39*(23), 1975-1980. doi:10.1097/BRS.0000000000000577

McSwiney, F., Wardrop, B., Hyde, P., Lafountain, R., Volek, J., & Doyle, L. (2018, Apr). Keto-adaptation enhances exercise performance and body composition responses to training in endurance athletes. *Metabolism, 83*, 25-34. doi:10.1016/j.metabol.2017.11.016

Mechanick, J., Garber, A., Grunberger, G., Handelsman, Y., & Garvey, W. (2018, Nov). DYSGLYCEMIA-BASED

CHRONIC DISEASE: AN AMERICAN ASSOCIATION OF CLINICAL ENDOCRINOLOGISTS POSITION STATEMENT. *Endocrine Practice, 24*(11), 995-1011. doi:10.4158/PS-2018-0139

Mekala, K., & Tritos, N. (2009). Effects of Recombinant Human Growth Hormone Therapy in Obesity in Adults: A Meta-analysis. *Journal of Clinical Endocrinology and Metabolism, 94*(1), 130-137. doi:https://doi.org/10.1210/jc.2008-1357

Meller, M., Toossi, N., Gonzalez, M., Son, M., Lau, E., & Johanson, N. (2016, Nov). Surgical Risks and Costs of Care are Greater in Patients Who Are Super Obese and Undergoing THA. *Clinical orthopaedics and related research, 474*(11), 2472-2481.

Meltzer, H., & Roth, B. (2013, Dec 2). Lorcaserin and pimavanserin: emerging selectivity of serotonin receptor subtype–targeted drugs. *The Journal of Clinical Investigation, 123*(12), 4986-4991. doi: 10.1172/JCI70678

Menke, A., Guallar, E., Rohrmann, S., Nelson, W., Rifai, N., Kanarek, N., . . . Platz, E. (2010). Sex steroid hormone concentrations and risk of death in US men. *American Journal of Epidemiology, 17*(5), 583-92. doi:https://doi.org/10.1093/aje/kwp415

Midorikawa, T., Kondo, M., Beekley, M., Koizumi, K., & Abe, T. (2007, Apr). High REE in Sumo wrestlers attributed to large organ-tissue mass. *Medicine and science in sports and exercise., 39*(4), 688-93.

Miyake, H., Kanazawa, I., Tanaka, K., & Sugimoto, T. (2019, Apr 26). Low skeletal muscle mass is associated with the risk of all-cause mortality in patients with type 2 diabetes mellitus. *Theraputic advances in endocrinology and metabolism.* doi:10.1177/2042018819842971

Mo, J., Liu, L., Peng, W., Rao, J., Liu, Z., & Ciu, L. (2017, Jun 2). • The effectiveness of creatine treatment for Parkinson's disease: an updated meta-analysis of randomized controlled trials. *BMC Neurology, 17*(1), 105. doi:doi: 10.1186/s12883-017-0885-3

Molitch, M., Clemmons, D., Malozowski, S., Merriam, G., & Vance, M. (2011). Evaluation and Treatment of Adult Growth Hormone Deficiency: An Endocrine Society Clinical Practice Guideline. *Journal of Clinical Endocrinology*

and Metabolism, 96(6), 1587-1609.
doi:https://doi.org/10.1210/jc.2011-0179

Møller, N., & Jørgensen, J. (2009). Effects of Growth Hormone on Glucose, Lipid, and Protein Metabolism in Human Subjects. *Endocrine Reviews, 30*(2), 152-177. doi:https://doi.org/10.1210/er.2008-0027

Morano, S., Mandosi, E., Fallarino, M., Gatti, A., Tiberti, C., Sensi, M., . . . Lenzi, A. (2007, Dec). Antioxidant treatment associated with sildenafil reduces monocyte activation and markers of endothelial damage in patients with diabetic erectile dysfunction: a double-blind, placebo-controlled study. *European Urology, 52*(6), 1768-1774. doi:10.1016/j.eururo.2007.04.042

Morganteler, A. (2015). Testosterone deficiency and cardiovascular mortality. *Asian Journal of Andrology, 17*(1), 26-31. doi:https://dx.doi.org/10.4103%2F1008-682X.143248

Morgentaler, A., Zitzmann, M., Traish, A., Fox, A., Jones, T., Maggi, M., . . . Torres, L. (2016). Fundamental Concepts Regarding Testosterone Deficiency and Treatment: International Expert Consensus Resolutions. *Mayo Clinic Proceedings, 91*(7), 881-96. doi:http://dx.doi.org/10.1016/j.mayocp.2016.04.007

Moussa, O., Erridge, S., Chidambaram, S., Ziprin, P., Darzi, A., & Purkayastha, S. (2019, Jun). Mortality of the Severely Obese: A Population Study. *Annals of Surgery, 269*(6), 1087-1091. doi:10.1097/SLA.0000000000002730

Muniyappa, R., Sorkin, J., Veldhuis, J., Harman, S., Münzer, T., Bhasin, S., & Blackman, M. (2007). Long-term testosterone supplementation augments overnight growth hormone secretion in healthy older men. *American Journal of Physiology. Endocrinology and Metabolism, 293*(3), E769-E775. doi:https://doi.org/10.1152/ajpendo.00709.2006

Muraleedharan, V., Marsh, H., Kapoor, D., Channer, K., & Jones, T. (2013). Testosterone deficiency is associated with increased risk of mortality and testosterone replacement improves survival in men with type 2 diabetes. *European Journal of Endocrinology, 169*(6), 725-33. doi:https://doi.org/10.1530/EJE-13-0321

Myers, J., Kaykha, A., George, S., Abella, J., Zaheer, N., Lear, S., . . . Froelicher, V. (2004, Dec 15). Fitness versus physical activity patterns in predicting mortality in men. *American Journal of Medicine, 117*(12), 912-8. doi:https://doi.org/10.1016/j.amjmed.2004.06.047

Nakamura, K., & Ogata, T. (2016). Locomotive Syndrome: Definition and Management. *Clinical Reviews in Bone and Mineral Metabolism, 14*(2), 56-67. doi:0.1007/s12018-016-9208-2

Nareste, T., Nareste, M., Buckspan, R., & Ersek, R. (2012, Apr). Large-volume liposuction and prevention of type 2 diabetes: a preliminary report. *Aethetic Plastic Surgery, 36*(2), 438-442. doi:10.1007/s00266-011-9798-5

Nass, R., Park, J., & T. M. (2007). Growth hormone supplementation in the elderly. *Endocrinology and Metabolism clinics of North America, 36*(1), 233-45. doi:https://doi.org/10.1016/j.ecl.2006.08.004

Neto, W., Gama, E., Rocha, L., Ramos, C., Taets, W., Scapini, K., . . . Caperuto, É. (2015). Effects of testosterone on lean mass gain in elderly men: systematic review with meta-analysis of controlled and randomized studies. *Age, 37*(5), 9742. doi:https://doi.org/10.1007/s11357-014-9742-0

Ng Tang Fui, M., Hoermann, R., Zajac, J., & Grossmann, M. (2017, Oct). The effects of testosterone on body composition in obese men are not sustained after cessation of testosterone treatment. *Clinical Endocrinology, 87*(4), 336-343. doi:10.1111/cen.13385.

Ng Tang Fui, M., Prendergast, L. D., Raval, M., Strauss, B., Zajac, J., & Grossmann, M. (2016). Effects of testosterone treatment on body fat and lean mass in obese men on a hypocaloric diet: a rondomised controlled trial. *BMC Medicine, 14*, 153.

Nieschlag, E., & Vorona, E. (2015). MECHANISMS IN ENDOCRINOLOGY: Medical consequences of doping with anabolic androgenic steroids: effects on reproductive functions. *European Journal of Endocrinology, 173*(2), R47-58. doi:https://doi.org/10.1530/EJE-15-0080

Nijs, J., Kosek, E., Van Oosterwijck, J., & Meeus, M. (2012). Dysfunctional endogenous analgesia during exercise in patients with chronic pain: to exercise or not to exercise? *Pain Physician, 15*(3s), e205-213. Retrieved from http://www.painphysicianjournal.com/linkout?issn=1533-3159&vol=15&page=ES205

Ning, H., Le, J., Wang, Q., Young, C., Deng, B., Gao, P., . . . Qin, S. (2018). The effects of metformin on simple obesity: a meta-analysis. *Endocrine, 62*(3), 528-534. doi:10.1007/s12020-018-1717-y

Nishizawa, T., Akaoka, I., Nishida, Y., Kawaguchi, T., & Hayashi, E. (1976, Oct). Some factors related to obesity in the Japanese sumo wrestler. *American journal of clinical nutrition, 29*(10), 1167-74.

Norain, A., Arafat, M., & Burjonrappa, S. (2019, May 2). Trending Weight Loss Patterns in Obese and Super Obese Adolescents: Does Laparoscopic Sleeve Gastrectomy Provide Equivalent Outcomes in both Groups? *Obesity Surgery*, epub. doi:10.1007/s11695-019-03867-8

Norrback, M., Tynelius, P., Ahlstrom, G., & Rasmussen, F. (2019, Mar 28). The association of mobility disability and obesity with risk of unemployment in two cohorts from Sweden. *BMC Public Health, 19*(1), 347. doi:10.1186/s12889-019-6627-2

Oakland, K., Nadler, R., Cresswell, L., Jackson, D., & Coughlin, P. (2016). Systematic review and meta-analysis of the association between frailty and outcome in surgical patients. *Annals of the Royal College of Surgeons of England, 98*(2), 80-85. doi:https://doi.org/10.1308/rcsann.2016.0048

Obesity: Its Causes and Treatment. (1891, Oct 24). *Hospital (Lond 1886), 11*(265), 46.

Ofer, K., Ronit, L., Ophir, A., & Amir, K. (2019, Mar). Normal body mass index (BMI) can rule out metabolic syndrome: An Israeli cohort study. *Medicine, 98*(9), e14712. doi:10.1097/MD.0000000000014712

Ohlander, S., Lindgren, M., & Lipshultz, L. (2016). Testosterone and Male Infertility. *The Urologic Clinics of North America, 43*(2), 195-202. doi:https://doi.org/10.1016/j.ucl.2016.01.006

Ohlsson C, B.-C. E., Labrie, F., Karlsson, M., Ljunggren, O., Vandenput, L., Mellström, D., & Tivesten, A. (2011). High serum testosterone is associated with reduced risk of cardiovascular events in elderly men. The MrOS (Osteoporotic Fractures in Men) study in Sweden. *Journal of the American College of Cardiology, 58*(16), 1674-81. doi:https://doi.org/10.1016/j.jacc.2011.07.019

Oliver, T. (1880). Post-Mortem in a Case of Extreme Obesity. *Journal of anatomy and physiology, 14*(Pt 3), 345-347.

Onakpova, I., Heneghan, C., & Aronson, J. (2016). Post-marketing withdrawal of anti-obesity medicinal products because of adverse drug reactions: a systematic review. *BMC Med, 14*(1), 191. doi:https://doi.org/10.1186/s12916-016-0735-y

Onyekwelu, I., Glassman, S., Asher, A., Shaffrey, C., Mummaneni, P., & Carreon, L. (2017, Feb). Impact of obesity on complications and outcomes: a comparison of fusion and nonfusion lumbar spine surgery. *Journal of neurosurgery. Spine., 26*(2), 158-162. doi:10.3171/2016.7.SPINE16448

Painter, S., Ahmed, R., Hill, J., Kushner, R., Lindquist, R., Brunning, S., & Margulies, A. (2017, May). What Matters in Weight Loss? An In-Depth Analysis of Self-Monitoring. *Journal of Medical Internet Research, 19*(5), e160. doi:10.2196/jmir.7457

Pal, S., Cheng, C., & Ho, S. (2011, Mar 31). The effect of two different health messages on physical activity levels and health in sedentary overweight, middle-aged women. *BMC Public Health, 11*, 204. doi:10.1186/1471-2458-11-204

Pearl, R. A., & Wadden, T. (2017, Aug). Effects of medical trainees' weight-loss history on perceptions of patients with obesity. *Medical education, 51*(8), 802-811. doi:10.1111/medu.13275

Pederson, B. S. (2006, Feb 1). Evidence for prescribing exercise as therapy in chronic disease. *Scandinavian Journal of Medicine and Science in Sports, 16*(s1), 3–63. doi:10.1111/j.1600-0838.2006.00520.x

Perera, N., Steinbeck, K., & Shackel, N. (2013, Dec). 10.1210/jc.2013-2310. *Journal of clinical endocrinology and metabolism, 98*(12), 4613-4618. doi:10.1210/jc.2013-2310

Performance-Enhancing Drugs on the Web: A Growing Public-Health Issue. (n.d.).

Perreault, L. (2017, Jul). EMPA-REG OUTCOME: The Endocrinologist's Point of View. *American Journal of Cardiology, 120*(1S), S48-S52. doi:10.1016/j.amjmed.2017.04.005

Pham, N., Bena, J., Bhatt, D., Kennedy, L., Schauer, P., & Kashyap, S. (2018, Jan). Increased Free Testosterone Levels in Men with Uncontrolled Type 2 Diabetes Five Years After Randomization to Bariatric Surgery. *Obesity Surgery, 28*(1). doi:10.1007/s11695-017-2881-5

Pham, S., & Chilton, R. (2017, Jun). EMPA-REG OUTCOME: The Cardiologist's Point of View. *American Journal of Medicine, 130*(6S), S57-S62. doi:10.1016/j.amjmed.2017.04.006

Piacentino, D., Kotzalidis, G., del Casale, A., Aromatario, M., Pomara, C., Girardi, P., & Sani, G. (2015, Jan). Anabolic-androgenic Steroid use and Psychopathology in Athletes. A Systematic Review. *Current Neuropharmacology, 13*(1), 101-121. doi:10.2174/1570159X13666141210222725.

Picca, A., Fanelli, F., Calvani, R., Mulè, G., Pesce, V., Sisto, A., & Pantanelli, C. (2018, Jan 30). Gut Dysbiosis and Muscle Aging: Searching for. *Mediators of Inflammation.* doi:0.1155/2018/7026198

Picca, A., Pesce, V., & Lezza, A. (2017, Nov 8). Does eating less make you live longer and better? An update on calorie restriction. *Clinical interventions in aging, 12*, 1887-1902. doi:10.2147/CIA.S126458

Picca, A., Pesce, V., & Lezza, A. (2017, Nov). Does eating less make you live longer and better? An update on calorie restriction. *Clinical Interventions in Aging, 12*, 1887-1902. doi:10.2147/CIA.S126458

Pierpoint, T., McKeigue, P., Isaacs, A., Wild, S., & Jacobs, H. (1998). Mortality of women with polycystic ovary syndrome at long-term follow-up. *Journal of Clinical Epidemiology, 51*(7), 581-6. doi:http://dx.doi.org/10.1016/S0895-4356(98)00035-3

Pilone, V., Tramontano, S., Renzulli, M., Romano, M., Cobellis, L., Berselli, T., & Schiavo, L. (2018, Jul). Metabolic effects, safety, and acceptability of very low-calorie ketogenic dietetic scheme on candidates for bariatric surgery. *Surg Obes Relat Dis., 14*(7), 1013-1019. doi:10.1016/j.soard.2018.03.018

Pope, H. J., & Katz, D. (1994). Psychiatric and Medical effects of anaboli-androgenic steroid use. A controlled study of 160 athletes. *Archives of General Psychiatry, 51*(5), 375-82. doi:doi:10.1001/archpsyc.1994.03950050035004

Pope, H. J., Wood, R., Rogol, A., Nyberg, F., Bowers, L., & Bhasin, S. (2014, 2014). Adverse Health Consequences of Performance-Enhancing Drugs: An Endocrine Society Scientific Statement. *Endocrinology Review, 35*(3), 341-75. doi:https://doi.org/10.1210/er.2013-1058

Potter, J., & Fuller, B. (2015, DEC). The effectiveness of chocolate milk as a post-climbing recovery aid. *Journal of Sports medicine and physical fitness, 55*(12), 1438-1444.

Pouwels, S., Topal, B., Knook, M., Celik, A., Sundbom, M., Ribeiro, R., . . . Ugale, S. (2019, Mar). Interaction of obesity and atrial fibrillation: an overview of pathophysiology and clinical management. *Expert Rev Cardiovasc Ther, 17*(3), 209-223. doi:10.1080/14779072.2019.1581064

Puggaard, L. (2005). Age-Related Decline in Maximal Oxygen Capacity: Consequences for Performance of Everyday Activities. *Journal of the American Geriatrics Society, 53*(3), 546-7. doi:https://doi.org/10.1111/j.1532-5415.2005.53178_3.x

R, H., Donnelly, R., Bi, Y., Bashan, E., Minhas, R., & Hodish, I. (2016, Sep). Dynamics in insulin requirements and treatment safety. *Journal of Diabetes Complications, 30*(7), 1333-8. doi:10.1016/j.jdiacomp.2016.05.017

Rahnema, C., Crosnoe, L., & Kim, E. (2015). Designer steroids - over-the-counter supplements and their androgenic component: review of an increasing problem. *Andrology, 3*(2), 150-155. doi:https://doi.org/10.1111/andr.307

Ramsey-Stewart, G., & Martin, L. (1985, Apr). Jaw wiring in the treatment of morbid obesity. *Australian and New Zealand journal of surgery, 55*(2), 163-167.

Ranchordas, M., Rogerson, D., Soltani, H., & Costello, J. (2018). Antioxidants for preventing and reducing muscle soreness after exercise: a Cochrane systematic review. *British journal of sports medicine*, e. doi:10.1136/bjsports-2018-099599

Rand, C., & Macgregor, A. (1990, Dec). Morbidly obese patients' perceptions of social discrimination before and after surgery for obesity. *Southern medical journal, 83*(12), 1390-5.

Randeva, H., Tan, B., Weickert, M., Lois, K., Nestler, J., Sattar, N., & Lehnert, H. (2012). Cardiometabolic Aspects of the Polycystic Ovary Syndrome. *Endocrine Review, 33*(5), 812-841. doi:https://doi.org/10.1210/er.2012-1003

References

Rao, A., Steels, E., Inder, W., Abraham, S., & Vitetta, L. (2016, Jun). Testofen, a specialised Trigonella foenum-graecum seed extract reduces age-related symptoms of androgen decrease, increases testosterone levels and improves sexual function in healthy aging males in a double-blind randomised clinical study. *Aging Male, 19*(2), 134-142. doi:10.3109/13685538.2015.1135323

Rasmussen, J., Selmer, C., Østergren, P., Pedersen, K., Schou, M., Gustafsson, F., . . . Kistorp, C. (2016). Former Abusers of Anabolic Androgenic Steroids Exhibit Decreased Testosterone levels and Hypogonadal Symptoms Years after Cessation: A Case-Control Study. *PLoS One, 11*(8). doi:https://doi.org/10.1371/journal.pone.0161208

Rasmussen, R., Midttun, M., Kolenda, T., Ragle, A., Sørensen, T., Vinther, A., . . . Overgaard, K. (2018, Mar 2). Therapist-Assisted Progressive Resistance Training, Protein Supplements, and Testosterone Injections in Frail Older Men with Testosterone Deficiency: Protocol for a Randomized Placebo-Controlled Trial. *JMIR Research Protocols, 7*(3), e71. doi:10.2196/resprot.8854

Rastrelli, G., Corona, G., & Maggi, M. (2018, Jun). Testosterone and sexual function in men. *Maturitas, 112*, 46-52. doi:doi:10.1016/j.maturitas.2018.04.004.

Ravussin, E., & Ryan, D. (2018, Jan). Three New Perspectives on the Perfect Storm: What's Behind the Obesity Epidemic? *Obesity, 26*(1), 9-10. doi:10.1002/oby.22085

Regenbogen, S., Cain-Nielsen, A., Norton, E., Chen, L., Birkmeyer, J., & Skinner, J. (2017, March 22). Costs and Consequences of Early Hospital Discharge After Major Inpatient Surgery . *JAMA Surgery*. doi:10.1001/jamasurg.2017.0123

Regis, L., Celma, A., Planas, J., deTorres, I., Ferrer, R., & Morote, J. (2015). Determined Free Serum Testosterone is Better than Total Testosterone as a Predictor of Prostate Cancer Risk. *International Journal of Research Studies in Biosciences, 3*(9), 22-32. Retrieved from https://www.google.com/url?sa=t&rct=j&q=&esrc=s&source=web&cd=1&cad=rja&uact=8&ved=0ahUKEwiGw7a1zZXUAhWCPCYKHdo_ADwQFggtMAA&url=https%3A%2F%2Fwww.arcjournals.org%2Fpdfs%2Fijrsb%2Fv3-i9%2F4.pdf&usg=AFQjCNHkA-

NQf7uq42uokLL_340FycPeyA&sig2=Thr5berq4S3kOJAc
3v

Resnick, S., Matsumoto, A., Stephens-Shields, A., Ellenberg, S., Gill, T., Shumaker, S., . . . Snyder, P. J. (2017, Feb 17). Testosterone Treatment and Cognitive Function in Older Men With Low Testosterone and Age-Associated Memory Impairment. *JAMA, 317*(7), 717-727. doi:10.1001/jama.2016.21044

Rich, S., Rubin, L., Walker, A., Schneeweiss, S., & Abenhaim, L. (2000). Anorexigens and pulmonary hypertension in the United States: results from the surveillance of North American pulmonary hypertension. *Chest, 117*(3), 870-874. doi:https://doi.org/10.1378/chest.117.3.870

Rissenen, A., Lean, M., Rossner, S., Segal, K., & Sjostrom, L. (2003, Jan). Predictive value of early weight loss in obesity management with orlistat: an evidence-based assessment of prescribing guidelines. *Int J Obes Relat Metab Disord, 27*(1), 103-9. doi: 10.1038/sj.ijo.0802165

Robinson, B., & Coveleski, S. (2018, Feb). Don't Say That to ME: Opposition to Targeting in Weight-Centric Intervention Messages. *Health Communication, 33*(2), 139-147. doi:10.1080/10410236.2016.1250189

Rodgers, S., Burnet, R., Goss, A., Phillips, P., Goldney, R., Kimber, C., . . . Wise, P. (1977, Jun 11). Jaw wiring in treatment of obesity. *Lancet, 1*(8024), 1221-2. doi:https://doi.org/10.1016/S0140-6736(77)92434-5

Romero-Corral, A., Somers, V., Sierra-Johnson, J., Thomas, R., Bailey, K., Collazo-Clavell, M., . . . Lopez-Jiminez, F. (2008, Feb 19). Accuracy of Body Mass Index to Diagnose Obesity in the US Adult Population. *International Journal of Obesity, 32*(6), 959-966. doi:10.1038/ijo.2008.11

Rose, S., Poynter, P., Anderson, J., Noar, S., & Conigliaro, J. (2013, Jan). Physician weight loss advice and patient weight loss behavior change: a literature review and meta-analysis of survey data. *Int J Obes (Lond), 37*(1), 118-28. doi:10.1038/ijo.2012.24

Rosenbaum, D., Espel, H., Butryn, M., Zhang, F., & Lowe, M. (2017). Daily self-weighing and weight gain prevention: a longitudinal study of college-aged women. *Journal of*

References

Behavioral Medicine, 40(5), 846-853. doi:10.1007/s10865-017-9870-y

Ross, R., Hill, J., Latimer, A., & Day, A. (2016, Mar). Evaluating a small change approach to preventing long term weight gain in overweight and obese adults--Study rationale, design, and methods. *Contemporary Clinical Trials, 47*, 275-81. doi:https://doi.org/10.1016/j.cct.2016.02.001

Rossow, L., Fukuda, D., Fahs, C., Loenneke, J., & Stout, J. (2013). Natural bodybuilding competition preparation and recovery: a 12-month case study. *International Journal of Sports Physiology and Performance, 8*(5), 582-92. doi:10.1123/ijspp.8.5.582

Roth, B. (2007). Drugs and Valvular Heart Disease. *New England Journal of Medicine, 356*(1), 6-9. doi: 10.1056/NEJMp068265

Roy, C., Snyder, P., Stephens-Shields, A., Artz, A., Bhasin, S., Cohen, H., . . . Ellenberg, S. S. (2017). Association of Testosterone Levels With Anemia in Older Men: A Controlled Clinical Trial. *JAMA Internal Medicine, 177*(4), 480-490. doi:https://doi.org/10.1001/jamainternmed.2016.9540

Rudman, D., Feller, A., Nagraj, H., Gergans, G., Lalitha, P., Goldberg, A., . . . Mattson, D. (1990). Effects of Human Growth Hormone in Men Over 60 Years Old. *New England Journal of Medicine, 323*(1), 1-6. doi:https://doi.org/10.1056/NEJM199007053230101

Rynearson, E., & Sprague, A. (1940, Oct). Obesity. *California and western medicine., 53*(4), 158-44.

Saad F, Y. A. (2016). Effects of long-term treatment with testosterone on weight and waist size in 411 hypogonadal men with obesity classes I-III: observational data from two registry studies. *International Journal of Obesity, 40*(1), 162-70. doi:https://doi.org/10.1038/ijo.2015.139

Saad, F. (2017). Testosterone Therapy and Glucose Homeostasis in Men with Testosterone Deficiency (Hypogonadism). *Advances in Experimental Medicine and Biology, 1043*, 527-558. doi:10.1007/978-3-319-70178-3_23.

Saad, F., Yassin, A., Haider, A., Doros, G., & Gooren, L. (2015). Elderly men over 65 years of age with late-onset hypogonadism benefit as much from testosterone treatment as do younger men. *Korean Journal of Urology, 56,* 310-317. doi:https://doi.org/10.4111/kju.2015.56.4.310

Saitoh, M., Ebner, N., von Haehling, S., Anker, S., & Springer, J. (2018, Feb). Therapeutic considerations of sarcopenia in heart failure patients. *Expert Review of Cardiovascular Therapy, 16*(2), 133-142. doi:10.1080/14779072.2018.1424542

Salinero, J., Soriano, M., Ruiz-Vicente, D., Gonzalez-Millan, C., Areces, F., Gallo-Salazar, C., . . . Del Coso, J. (2016, Dec). Respiratory function is associated to marathon race time. *Journal of Sports Medicine and Physical Fitness, 56*(12), 1433-1438.

Samaras, N., Papadopoulou, M., Samaras, D., & Ongaro, F. (2014). Off-label use of hormones as an antiaging strategy: a review. *Clinical Interventions in Aging, 9,* 1175-1186. doi:https://dx.doi.org/10.2147%2FCIA.S48918

Samaras, N., Samaras, D., Lang, P., Forster, A., Pichard, C., Frangos, E., & Meyer, P. (2013). A view of geriatrics through hormones. What is the relation between andropause and well-known geriatric syndromes? *Maturitas, 74*(3), 213-9. doi:https://doi.org/10.1016/j.maturitas.2012.11.009

Sanchis-Gomar, F., Olaso-Gonzalez, G., Corella, D., Gomez-Cabrera, M., & Vina, J. (2011, Aug). Increased average longevity among the "Tour de France" cyclists. *International journal of sports medicine, 32*(8), 644-7. doi:https://doi.org/10.1055/s-0031-1271711

Santilli, F., Simeone, P., Guagnano, M., Leo, M., Maccarone, M., Di Castelnuovo, A., . . . Consoli, A. (2017, Nov). Effects of Liraglutide on Weight Loss, Fat Distribution, and β-Cell Function in Obese Subjects With Prediabetes or Early Type 2 Diabetes. *Diabetes Care, 40*(11), 1556-1564. doi:10.2337/dc17-0589

Santos, M., Sayegh, A., Groehs, R., Fonseca, G., Trombetta, I., Barretto, A., . . . Alves, M. (2015). Testosterone Deficiency Increases Hospital Readmission and Mortality Rates in Male Patients with Heart Failure. *Arquivos Brasileiros Cardiologia, 105*(3), 256–264. doi:https://dx.doi.org/10.5935%2Fabc.20150078

Sarwer, D., Spitzer, J., Wadden, T., Rosen, R., Mitchell, J., Lancaster, K., . . . Christian, N. (2015). Sexual functioning and sex hormones in men who underwent bariatric surgery. *Surgery for Obesity and Related Diseases, 11*(3), 643-51. doi:https://doi.org/10.1016/j.soard.2014.12.014

Sattler, F., Bhasin, S., He, J., Yarasheski, K., Binder, E., Schroeder, E., . . . Azen, S. (2011). Durability of the effects of testosterone and growth hormone supplementation in older community dwelling men: the HORMA trial. *Clinical Endocrinology, 75*(1), 103-111. doi:https://doi.org/10.1111/j.1365-2265.2011.04014.x

Schwartz, J., Bashian, C., Kushnir, L., Nituica, C., & Slotman, G. (2017, Sep 1). Variation in Clinical Characteristics of Women versus Men Preoperative for Laparoscopic Roux-en-Y Gastric Bypass: Analysis of 83,059 Patients. *The American surgeon, 83*(9), 947-951.

Scovell, J., Ramasamy, R., & Kovac, J. (2014). A critical analysis of testosterone supplementation therapy and cardiovascular risk in elderly men. *Canadian Urological Association Journal, 8*(5-6). doi:http://dx.doi.org/10.5489/cuaj.1962

Semenkovich, C. (2017, Jul). We Know More Than We Can Tell About Diabetes and Vascular Disease: The 2016 Edwin Bierman Award Lecture. *Diabetes, 66*(7), 1735-1741. doi:10.2337/db17-0093

Shea, B., Bovan, W. J., Botta, J., Ali, S., Fenig, Y., paulin, E., . . . Borao, F. (2017). Five Years, Two Surgeons, and over 500 Bariatric Procedures: What Have We Learned? *Obesity surgery, 27*(10), 2742-49. doi:10.1007/s11695-017-2873-

Sheehan, D., Gasior, M., McElroy, S., Radewonuk, J., Herman, B., & Hudson, J. (2018, Jun 1). Effects of Lisdexamfetamine Dimesylate on Functional Impairment Measured on the Sheehan Disability Scale in Adults With Moderate-to-severe Binge Eating Disorder. *Innovations in Clinical Neuroscience, 15*(5-6), 22-29.

Sheffield-Moore, M., Dillon, E., Casperson, S., Gilkison, C., Paddon-Jones, D., Durham, W., . . . Urban, R. (2011). A Randomized Pilot Study of Monthly Cycled Testosterone Replacement or Continuous Testosterone Replacement Versus Placebo in Older Men. *Journal of Clinical Endocrinology and Metabolism, 96*(11), E1831-1837. doi:https://doi.org/10.1210/jc.2011-1262

Shephard, R., & Futcher, R. (1997). Physical activity and cancer: how may protection be maximized. *Critical Reviews in Oncogenesis, 8*(2-3), 219-72. Retrieved from https://www.ncbi.nlm.nih.gov/pubmed/9570295

Sherman, M., Ungureanu, A., & Rey, J. (2016). Newly Approved Treatment Option for Chronic Weight Management in Obese Adults. *PT, 41*(3), 164-172.

Shin, Y., You, J., Cha, J., & Park, J. (2016). The relationship between serum total testosterone and free testosterone levels with serum hemoglobin and hematocrit levels: a study in 1221 men. *Aging Male, 19*(4), 209-214. doi:https://doi.org/10.1080/13685538.2016.1229764

Shohat, N., Fleischman, A., Tarabichi, M., Tan, T., & Parvizi, J. (2018, Oct). Weighing in on Body Mass Index and Infection After Total Joint Arthroplasty: Is There Evidence for a Body Mass Index Threshold? *Clinical orthopaedics and related research, 476*(10), 1964-69. doi:10.1007/s11999.0000000000000141

Shojaei, M., Alavinia, S., & Craven, B. (2017, Nov). Management of obesity after spinal cord injury: a systematic review. *The journal of spinal cord medicine, 40*(6), 783-794. doi:10.1080/10790268.2017.1370207

Shores, M., Arnold, A., Biggs, M., Longstreth, W. J., Smith, N., Kizer, J., . . . Matsumoto, A. (2014). Testosterone and Dihydrotestosterone and Incident Ischemic Stroke in Men in the Cardiovascular Health Study. *Clinical Endocrinology, 81*(5), 746-753. doi:https://doi.org/10.1111/cen.12452

Shores, M., Biggs, M., Arnold, A., Smith, N., Longstreth, W. J., Kizer, J., . . . Matsumoto, A. (2014). Testosterone, Dihydrotestosterone, and Incident Cardiovascular Disease and Mortality in the Cardiovascular Health Study. *Journal of Clinical Endocrinology and Metabolism, 99*(6), 2061-2068. doi:https://dx.doi.org/10.1210%2Fjc.2013-3576

Sievers, C., Klotsche, J., Pieper, L., Schneider, H., März, W., Wittchen, H., . . . Mantzoros, C. (2010). Low testosterone levels predict all-causes mortality and cardiovascular events in women: a prospective cohort study in German primary care patients. *European Journal of Endocrinology, 163*(4), 699-708. doi:https://doi.org/10.1530/EJE-10-0307

References

Smid, M., Dotters-Katz, S., Silver, R., & Kuller, J. (2017, Aug). Body Mass Index 50 kg/m2 and Beyond: Perioperative Care of Pregnant Women with Superobesity Undergoing Cesarean Delivery. *Obstetrics and gynecological survey, 72*(8), 500-510. doi:10.1097/OGX.0000000000000469

Smid, M., Dotters-Katz, S., Vaught, A., Vladutiu, C., Boggess, K., & Stamilio, D. (2017, Aug). Maternal super obesity and risk for intensive care unit admission in the MGMU Cesarean Registry. *Acta obstetrica et gynecologica Scandinavica, 96*(8), 976-983. doi:10.1111/aogs.13145

Smid, M., Vladutiu, C., Dotters-Katz, S., Boggess, K., Manuck, T., & Stamilio, D. (2017, Jun). Maternal obesity and major intraoperative complications during cesarean delivery. *American journal of obstetrics and gynecology, 216*(6), 614. doi:10.1016/j.ajog.2017.02.011

Smith, T., Aboelmagd, T., Hing, C., & MacGregor, A. (2016, Sep). Does bariatric surgery prior to total hip or knee arthroplasty reduce post-operative complications and improve clinical outcomes for obese patients? Systematic review and meta-analysis. *The Bone & Joint Journal, 98*(9), 1160-6. doi:https://doi.org/10.1302/0301-620X.98B9.38024

Snyder, G., & Shoskes, D. (2016). Hypogonadism and testosterone replacement therapy in end-stage renal disease (ESRD) and transplant patients. *Translational Andrology and Urology, 5*(6), 885-889. doi:https://dx.doi.org/10.21037%2Ftau.2016.08.01

Snyder, P. (2004). Hypogonadism in Elderly Men- What to Do Until the Evidence Comes. *New England Journal of Medicine, 350*(5), 440-2. doi:https://doi.org/10.1056/NEJMp038207

Sonksen, P., Holt, R., Bohning, W., Guha, N., Cowan, D., Bartlett, C., & Bohning, D. (2018, Feb 7). Why do endocrine profiles in elite athletes differ between sports? *Clinical Diabetes and Endocrinology, 4*(3). doi:10.1186/s40842-017-0050-3.

Speliotes, E. K., Willer, C. J., Berndt, S. I., Monda, K. L., Thorleifsson, G., Jackson, A. U., & ... Loos, R. J. (2010, October 10). (2010). Association analyses of 249,796 individuals reveal eighteen new loci associated with body

mass index. *Nature Genetics, 42*(11), 937–948.
doi:10.1038/ng.686

Spitzer, M., Huang, G., Basaria, S., Travison, T., & Bhasin, S.
(2013). Risk and benefits of testosterone therapy in older
men. *Nature Reviews. Endocrinology, 9*(7), 414-24.
doi:https://doi.org/10.1038/nrendo.2013.73

Srinivas-Shankar, U., Roberts, S., Connolly, M., O'Connell, M.,
Adams, J., Oldham, J., & Wu, F. (2010). Effects of
Testosterone on Muscle Strength, Physical Function, Body
Composition, and Quality of Life in Intermediate-Frail
Elderly Men: A Randomized, Double-Blind, Placebo-
Controlled Study. *Clinical Endocrinology and Metabolism, 95*(2),
639-650. doi:https://doi.org/10.1210/jc.2009-1251

Srivastava, G., O'Hara, V., & Browne, N. (2019, Feb 4). Use of
Lisdexamfetamine to Treat Obesity in an Adolescent with
Severe Obesity and Binge Eating. *Children (Basel), 6*(2), e22.
doi:10.3390/children6020022.

Stavrou, G., Tsaousi, G., & Kotzampassi, K. (2019). Life-
threatening visceral complications after intragastric balloon
insertion: Is the device, the patient or the doctor to blame?
Endoscopy International Open, 7(2), e122-e129. doi:10.1055/a-
0809-4994

Stephens, L., & Katz, S. (2005, Aug). Phentermine and anaesthesia.
Anaesthesia and Intensive Care, 33(4), 525-7. Retrieved from
http://www.aaic.net.au/document/?D=2005004

Stergiopoulos, K., Brennan, J., Mathews, R., Setaro, J., & Kort, S.
(2008). Anabolic steroids, acute myocardial infarction and
polycythemia: A case report and review of the literature.
Vascular Health Risk Management, 4(6), 1475-1480. Retrieved
from
https://www.ncbi.nlm.nih.gov/pmc/articles/PMC2663437
/?report=reader#__ffn_sectitle

Strohacker, K., McCaffery, J., MacLean, P., & Wing, R. (2014,
Mar). Adaptations of leptin, ghrelin or insulin during weight
loss as predictors of weight regain: a review of current
literature. *International Journal of Obesity, 38*(3), 388-396.
doi:10.1038/ijo.2013.118

Stubert, J., Reister, F., Hartmann, S., & Janni, W. (2018, Apre 20).
The Risks Associated with Obesity in Pregnancy. *Dtsch
Arztebl Int, 115*(16), 276-283. doi:10.3238/arztebl.2018.0276

References

Surve, A., Cottam, D., Zaveri, H., Cottam, A., Belnap, L., Richards, C., . . . D. (2018). Does the future of laparoscopic sleeve gastrectomy lie in the outpatient surgery center? A retrospective study of the safety of 3162 outpatient sleeve gastrectomies. *Surgery for Obesity and Related Disease, 14*(10), 1442-1447. doi:10.1016/j.soard.2018.05.027

Swiecicka, A., Eendebak, R., Lunt, M., O'Neill, T., Bartfai, G., Casanueva, F., . . . Gr, E. M. (2018, Feb 1). Reproductive Hormone Levels Predict Changes in Frailty Status in Community-Dwelling Older Men: European Male Ageing Study Prospective Data. *Journal of Clinical Endocrinology and Metabolism, 103*(2), 701-709. doi:10.1210/jc.2017-01172

Sylvetsky, A., & Rother, K. (2018, Apr). Nonnutritive Sweeteners in Weight Management and Chronic Disease: A Review. *Obesity, 26*(4), 635-640. doi:10.1002/oby.22139

Tang, W., & Hazen, S. (2014, Oct 1). The contributory role of gut microbiota in cardiovascular disease. *The Journal of Clinical Investigation, 124*(10), 4204–4211. doi:https://dx.doi.org/10.1172%2FJCI72331

Tappy, L. (2004). Metabolic consequences of overfeeding in humans. *Curr Opin Clin Nutr Metab Care, 7*(6), 623-8.

The GBD 2015 Obesity Collaborators. (2017, Jul 6). Health Effects of Overweight and Obesity in 195 Countries over 25 Years. *NEJM, 377*(1), 13-27. doi:10.1056/NEJMoa1614362

The Treatment of Obesity. (1890). *The Indian medical gazette, 21*(5), 21.

Thenappan, A., & Nadler, E. (2019). Bariatric Surgery in Children: Indications, Types, and Outcomes. *Current gastroenterology reports, 21*(6), 24. doi:10.1007/s11894-019-0691-8

Thomas, N., Lynam, A., Hill, A., Weedon, M., Shields, B., Oram, R., . . . Jones, A. (2018). Type 1 diabetes defined by severe insulin deficiency occurs after 30 years of age and is commonly treated as type 2 diabetes. *Diabetologia, 62*(7), 1167-1172. doi:10.1007/s00125-019-4863-8.

Thompson, P., Franklin, B., Balady, G., Blair, S., Corrado, D., Estes, N. 3., . . . Costa, F. (2007, May 1). Exercise and acute cardiovascular events placing the risks into perspective: a scientific statement from the American Heart Association Council on Nutrition, Physical Activity, and Metabolism and the Council on Clinical Cardiology. *Circulation, 115*(17),

2358-68.
doi:https://doi.org/10.1161/CIRCULATIONAHA.107.18
1485

Tiwari, N., Pasrija, S., & Jain, S. (2019, Jan 4). Randomised controlled trial to study the efficacy of exercise with and without metformin on women with polycystic ovary syndrome. *European Journal of Obstetrics, Gynecology, and Reproductive Biology, 234,* 149-154. doi:10.1016/j.ejogrb.2018.12.021

Tokarek, T., Dziewierz, A., Sorysz, D., Bagienski, M., Rzeszutko, Ł., Krawczyk-Ożóg, A., . . . Kleczyński, P. (2019). The obesity paradox in patients undergoing transcatheter aortic valve implantation: is there any effect of body mass index on survival? *Kardiolgia polska, 77*(2), 190-197. doi:10.5603/KP.a2018.0243

Tomova, A., Bukovsky, I., Rembert, E., Yonas, W., Alwarith, J., Barnard, N., & Kahleova, H. (2019, Apr). The Effects of Vegetarian and Vegan Diets on Gut Microbiota. *Frontiers in nutrition., 6*(47). doi:10.3389/fnut.2019.00047

Toth, A., Gomez, G., Shukla, A., Pratt, J., Cena, H., Biino, G., . . . Stanford, F. (2018, Aug 29). Weight Loss Medications in Young Adults after Bariatric Surgery for Weight Regain or Inadequate Weight Loss: A Multi-Center Study. *Children, 5*(9), e116. doi:10.3390/children5090116

Tracz, M., Sideras, K., Boloña, E., Haddad, R., Kennedy, C., Uraga, M., . . . Montori, V. (2006). Clinical Review: Testosterone Use in Men and Its Effects on Bone Health. A Systematic Review and Meta-analysis of Randomized Placebo-Controlled Trials. *The Journal of Clinical Endocrinology and Metabolism, 9*(16), 2011-2016. doi:https://doi.org/10.1210/jc.2006-0036

Travison, T., Basaria, S., Storer, T., Jette, A., Miciek, R., Farwell, W., . . . Brooks, B. (2011). Clinical Meaningfulness of the Changes in Muscle Performance and Physical and Function Associated with Testosterone Administration In Older Men With Mobility Limitation. *J Gerontol A Biol Sci Med Sci, 66*(10), 1090-99. doi:https://doi.org/10.1093/gerona/glr100

Travison, T., Morley, J., Araujo, A., O'Donnel, l. A., & McKinlay, J. (2006). The Relationship between Libido and Testosterone

Levels in Aging Men. *The Journal of Clinical Endocrinology and Metabolism, 91*(7), 2509-2513. doi:https://doi.org/10.1210/jc.2005-2508

Tricker, R., Casaburi, R., Storer, T., Clevenger, B., Berman, N., Shirazi, A., & Bhasin, S. (1996). The effects of supraphysiological doses of testosterone on angry behavior in healthy eugonadal men-a clinical research center study. *Journa of Clinical Endocrinology and Metabolism, 81*(10), 3754-8. doi:https://doi.org/10.1210/jcem.81.10.8855834

Tronieri, J., Wadden, T., Walsh, O., Berkowitz, R., Alamudden, N., Gruber, K., . . . Chao, A. (2019). Effects of liraglutide plus phentermine in adults with obesity following 1 year of treatment by liraglutide alone: A randomized placebo-controlled pilot trial. *Metabolism.* doi:10.1016/j.metabol.2019.03.005

Tsai AG, W. T. (2005). ystematic Review: An Evaluation of Major Commercial Weight Loss Programs in the United States. *Annals of Internal Medicine, 142*(1), 56-66. doi:10.7326/0003-4819-142-1-200501040-00012

Tsitsimpikou, C., Tsarouhas, K., Vasilaki, F., Papalexis, P., Dryllis, G., Choursalas, A., . . . Bacopoulou, F. (2018, Oct). Health risk behaviors among high school and university adolescent students. *Experimental and theraputic medicine, 16*(4), 3433-3438. doi:0.3892/etm.2018.6612

Tuccinardi, D., Farr, O., Upadhyay, J., Oussaada, S., Mathew, H., Paschou, S., . . . Mantzoros, C. (2019). Lorcaserin treatment decreases body weight and reduces cardiometabolic risk factors in obese adults: A six-month, randomized, placebo-controlled, double-blind clinical trial. *Diabetes, Obesity, and Metabolism, 21*(6), 1487-1492. doi:10.1111/dom.13655

Tudor-Lock, C., & Bassett, D. (2004). How many steps/day are enough? Preliminary pedometer indices for public health. *Sports Medicine, 34*(1), 1-8. doi:doi.org/10.2165/00007256-200434010-00001

van den Driessche, J., Plat, J., & Mensink, R. (2018, Apr 25). .Effects of superfoods on risk factors of metabolic syndrome: a systematic review of human intervention trials. *Food and function, 9*(4), 1944-1966. doi:10.1039/C7FO01792H.

Vandenput, L., Mellström, D., Laughlin, G., Cawthon, P., Cauley, J., Hoffman, A., . . . Ohlsson, C. (2017). Low Testosterone, but Not Estradiol, Is Associated With Incident Falls in Older Men: The International MrOS Study. *Journal of Bone and Mineral Research.* doi:https://doi.org/10.1002/jbmr.3088

Vermeulen, A., & Verdonck, G. (1992). Representativeness of a single point plasma testosterone level for the long term hormonal milieu in men. *Journal of Clinical Endocrinology and Metabolism, 74*(4), 939-42. doi:https://doi.org/10.1210/jcem.74.4.1548361

Vigen, R., O'Donnell, C., Barón, A., Grunwald, G., Maddox, T., Bradley, S., . . . Ho, P. (2013). Association of testosterone therapy with mortality, myocardial infarction, and stroke in men with low testosterone levels. *JAMA, 310*(17), 1829-36. doi:https://doi.org/10.1001/jama.2013.280386

Vilaca-Alves, J., Muller, F., Rosa, C., Payan-Carreira, R., Lund, R., Matos, F., . . . Machado Reis, V. (2018, Mar 1). Cardiorespiratory, enzymatic and hormonal responses during and after walking while fasting. *PLoS One, 13*(3). doi:10.1371/journal.pone.0193702

Vina, J., Sanchis-Gomar, F., Martinez-Bello, V., & Gomez-Cabrera, M. (2012, September). Exercise acts as a drug; the pharmacological benefits of exercise. *British Journal of Pharmacology, 167*(1), 1-12. doi:https://dx.doi.org/10.1111%2Fj.1476-5381.2012.01970.x

Vitale, G., Cesari, M., & Mari, D. (2016). Aging of the endocrine system and its potential impact on sarcopenia. *European Journal of Internal Medicine, 35*, 10-15. doi:https://doi.org/10.1016/j.ejim.2016.07.017

Volek, J., Freidenreich, D., Saenz, C., Kunces, L., Creighton, B., Bartley, J., . . . Phinney, S. (2016, Mar). Metabolic characteristics of keto-adapted ultra-endurance runners. *Metabolism, 65*(3), 100-10. doi:10.1016/j.metabol.2015.10.028

Wadden, T., & Stunkard, A. (1985, Dec). Social and psychological consequences of obesity. *Annals of internal medicine, 103*(Pt 2), 1062-1067.

Wang, F., Wu, Y., Zhu, Y., Ding, T., Batterham, R., Qu, F., & Hardimann, P. (2018). 5. Pharmacologic therapy to induce

References

weight loss in women who have obesity/overweight with polycystic ovary syndrome: a systematic review and network meta-analysis. *Obesity Review, 19*(10), 1424-1445. doi:10.1111/obr.12720

Wang, Y., Song, Y., Chen, J., Zhao, R., Xia, L., Cui, Y., . . . Wu, X. (2019). Roux-en-Y Gastric Bypass Versus Sleeve Gastrectomy for Super Super Obese and Super Obese: Systematic Review and Meta-analysis of Weight Results, Comorbidity Resolution. *Obesity Surgery, 29*(6), 1954-1964. doi:10.1007/s11695-019-03817-4

Wang, Y., Wan, H., Chen, Y., Xia, F., Zhang, W., Wang, C., . . . Lu, Y. (2019, Apr 23). Association of C-peptide with diabetic vascular complications in type 2 diabetes. *Diabetes and metabolism*, S1262-3636. doi:10.1016/j.diabet.2019.04.004

Wanner, C. (2017). EMPA-REG OUTCOME: The Nephrologist's Point of View. *American Journal of Medicine, 130*(6S), S63-S72. doi:10.1016/j.amjcard.2017.05.012

Warburton, D., Nicol, C., & Bredin, S. (2006, Mar 14). Health benefits of physical activity: the evidence. *Canadian Medical Association Journal, 174*(6), 801-809. doi:https://dx.doi.org/10.1503%2Fcmaj.051351

Ward, K., & Citrome, L. (2018, Feb). Lisdexamfetamine: chemistry, pharmacodynamics, pharmacokinetics, and clinical efficacy, safety, and tolerability in the treatment of binge eating disorder. *Epert Opinion on Drug Metabolism and Toxicology, 14*(2), 229-238. doi:10.1080/17425255.2018.1420163

Wardle, J., Carnell, S., Haworth, C., & Plomin, R. (2008, Feb). Evidence for a strong genetic influence on childhood adiposity despite the force of the obesogenic environment. *American Journal of Clinical Nutrition, 87*(2), 398-404. Retrieved from https://www.ncbi.nlm.nih.gov/pubmed/18258631

Weissberger, A., Anastasiadis, A., Sturgess, I., Martin, F., Smith, M., & Sönksen, P. (2003). Recombinant human growth hormone treatment in elderly patients undergoing elective total hip replacement. *Clinical Endocrinology, 58*(1), 99-107. doi:10.1046/j.1365-2265.2003.01700.x

Wen, C., Wai, J., Tsai, M., Yang, Y., Cheng, T., Lee, M., . . . Wu, X. (2011, Oct 1). Minimum amount of physical activity for reduced mortality and extended life expectancy: a prospective cohort study. *Lancet, 378*(9798), 1244-53. doi:http://dx.doi.org/10.1016/S0140-6736(11)60749-6

Westerman, M., Charchenko, C., Ziegelmann, M., Bailey, G., Nippoldt, T., & Trost, L. (2016). Heavy Testosterone Use Among Bodybuilders: An Uncommon Cohort of Illicit Substance Users. *Mayo Clinic Proceedings, 91*(2), 175-182. doi:https://doi.org/10.1016/j.mayocp.2015.10.027

WHO. (2016, June). *Obesity and Overweight*. Retrieved from World Health Organization: http://www.who.int/mediacentre/factsheets/fs311/en/

Wierman, M., Arlt, W., Basson, R., Davis, S., Miller, K., Murad, M., . . . Santoro, N. (2014). Androgen therapy in women: a reappraisal: an Endocrine Society clinical practice guideline. *Journal of Clinical Endocrinology and Metabolism, 99*(10), 3489-510. doi:https://doi.org/10.1210/jc.2014-2260

Wild, S., Pierpoint, T., McKeigue, P., & Jacobs, H. (2000). Cardiovascular disease in women with polycystic ovary syndrome at long-term follow-up: a retrospective cohort study. *Clinical Endocrinology, 52*(5), 595-600. doi:10.1046/j.1365-2265.2000.01000.x

Williams, P. (2011, Nov). Exercise attenuates the association of body weight with diet in 106,737 runners. *Medicine and Science in Sports and Exercise, 43*(11), 2120-2126. doi:10.1249/MSS.0b013e31821cd128

Williams, P., & Pate, R. (2005, Aug). Cross-sectional relationships of exercise and age to adiposity in 60,617 male runners. *Medicine and Science in Sports and Exercise, 37*(8), 1329-1337.

Williams, P., & Satariano, W. (2005, Aug). Relationships of age and weekly running distance to BMI and circumferences in 41,582 physically active women. *Obesity Research, 13*(8), 1370-1380.

Willoughby, D., Spillane, M., & Schwarz, N. (2014). Heavy Resistance Training and Supplementation with the Alleged Testosterone Booster NMDA Has No Effect on Body Composition, Muscle Performance, and Serum Hormones Associated with the Hypothalamus-Pituitary-Gonadal Axis in Resistance-Trained Males. *Journal of Sports Science and Medicine, 13*(1), 192-199. Retrieved from https://www.ncbi.nlm.nih.gov/pmc/articles/PMC3918557/

References

Woolston, C. (2011, September 12). The Healthy Skeptic: Products make testosterone claims. *Los Angeles Times*. Retrieved from http://articles.latimes.com/2011/sep/12/health/la-he-skeptic-testosterone-supplements-20110912

Xu, L., Freeman, G., Cowling, B., & Schooling, C. (2013). Testosterone therapy and cardiovascular events among men. A systematic review and meta-analysis of placebo-controlled randomized trials. *BMC Medicine, 11*(108). doi:https://doi.org/10.1186/1741-7015-11-108

Yamamoto, N., Miyazaki, H., Shimada, M., Nakagawa, N., Sawada, S., Nishimuta, M., . . . Yoshitake, Y. (2018, Apr 23). Daily step count and all-cause mortality in a sample of Japanese elderly people: a cohort study. *BMC Pulic Health, 18*(1), 540. doi:10.1186/s12889-018-5434-5

Yao, R., Schuh, B., & Caughey, A. (2019, Feb). The risk of perinatal mortality with each week of expectant management in obese pregnancies. *Journal of maternal-fetal and neonatal medicine, 32*(3), 434-441. doi:10.1080/14767058.2017.1381903.

Yassin DJ, Y. A. (2014). Combined testosterone and vardenafil treatment for restoring erectile function in hypogonadal patients who failed to respond to testosterone therapy alone. *Journal of Sexual Medicine, 11*(2), 543-52. doi:https://doi.org/10.1111/jsm.12378

Yeap, B., & Wu, F. (2019, Jan). Clinical practice update on testosterone therapy for male hypogonadism: Contrasting perspectives to optimize care. *Clinical Endocrinology, 90*(1), 56-65. doi:10.1111/cen.13888

Yeap, B., Alfonso, H., Chubb, S., Hankey, G., Handelsman, D., Golledge, J., . . . Norman, P. (2014). In older men, higher plasma testosterone or dihydrotestosterone are independent predictors for reduced incidence of stroke but not myocardial infarction. *Journal of Clinical Endocrinology and Metabolism, 99*(12), 4565-4573. doi:https://doi.org/10.1210/jc.2014-2664

Yeo, J., Cho, S., Park, S., Jo, S., Ha, J., Lee, J., . . . Park, M. (2018, May). Which Exercise Is Better for Increasing Serum Testosterone Levels in Patients with Erectile Dysfunction? *World Journal of Mens Heatlh, 36*(2), 147-152. doi:0.5534/wjmh.17030

Yheulon, C., Millard, A., Balla, F., Jonsson, A., Constantin, T., Singh, A., . . . Davis, S. J. (2019, Mar). Laparoscopic Sleeve Gastrectomy Outcomes in Patients with Polycystic Ovary Syndrome. *The American surgeon, 85*(3), 232-255.

Yoshihisa, A., Suzuki, S., Sato, Y., Kanno, Y., Abe, S., Miyata, M., . . . Oikawa, M. (2018, Jun 1). Relation of Testosterone Levels to Mortality in Men With Heart Failure. *American Journal of Cardiology, 121*(11), 1321-1327.

Zago, M., Capodaglio, P., Ferrario, C., Tarabini, M., & Galli, M. (2018). Whole-body vibration training in obese subjects: A systematic review. *PLoS One, 13*(9), e0202866. doi:10.1371/journal.pone.0202866

Zand, A., Ibrahim, K., & Patham, B. (2018). Prediabetes: Why Should We Care? *Methodist devakey Cardiovascular Journal, 14*(4), 289-297. doi:10.14797/mdcj-14-4-289

Zeller, M., Brown, J., Reiter-Purtill, J., Sarwer, D., Black, L., Jenkins, T., . . . Noll, J. (2019, Mar 20). Sexual behaviors, risks, and sexual health outcomes for adolescent females following bariatric surgery. *Surgery for Obesity and Related Disease*, S1550-7289. doi:10.1016/j.soard.2019.03.001.

Zeller, T., Schnabel, R., Appelbaum, S., Ojeda, F., Berisha, F., Schulte-Steinberg, B., . . . Karakas, M. (2018, Jul). Low testosterone levels are predictive for incident atrial fibrillation and ischemic stroke in men, but protective in women - results from the FINRISK study. *European Journal of Preventive Cardiology, 25*(11), 1133-1139. doi:10.1177/2047487318778346

Zhang, L., Shin, Y., Kim, J., & Park, J. (2016). Could Testosterone Replacement Therapy in Hypogonadal Men Ameliorate Anemia, a Cardiovascular Risk Factor? An Observational, 54-Week Cumulative Registry Study. *The Journal of Urology, 195*(4), 1057-64. doi:https://doi.org/10.1016/j.juro.2015.10.130

Zheng, Y., Shen, X., Zhou, Y., Ma, J., Shang, X., & Shi, y. (2015). Effect and safety of testosterone undecanoate in the treatment of late-onset hypogonadism: a meta-analysis. *PubMed Journals, 21*(3), 263-271. Retrieved from https://www.ncbi.nlm.nih.gov/labs/articles/25898560/

Made in the USA
Lexington, KY
02 September 2019